Fundamentals of
Children's Applied Pathophysiology

Fundamentals of Children's Applied Pathophysiology

An Essential Guide for Nursing and Healthcare Students

EDITED BY

LIZ GORMLEY-FLEMING
Associate Director
Academic Quality Assurance at University of Hertfordshire
Hatfield, UK

IAN PEATE OBE FRCN
Visiting Professor of Nursing
St George's University of London
Kingston University London, UK
Editor in Chief *British Journal of Nursing*
Head of School, School of Health Studies
University of Gibraltar

WILEY Blackwell

This edition first published 2019
© 2019 John Wiley & Sons Ltd

All rights reserved. No part of this publication may be reproduced, stored in a retrieval system, or transmitted, in any form or by any means, electronic, mechanical, photocopying, recording or otherwise, except as permitted by law. Advice on how to obtain permission to reuse material from this title is available at http://www.wiley.com/go/permissions.

The right of Elizabeth Gormley-Fleming and Ian Peate to be identified as the authors of the editorial material in this work has been asserted in accordance with law.

Registered Offices
John Wiley & Sons, Inc., 111 River Street, Hoboken, NJ 07030, USA
John Wiley & Sons Ltd, The Atrium, Southern Gate, Chichester, West Sussex, PO19 8SQ, UK

Editorial Office
9600 Garsington Road, Oxford, OX4 2DQ, UK

For details of our global editorial offices, customer services, and more information about Wiley products visit us at www.wiley.com.

Wiley also publishes its books in a variety of electronic formats and by print-on-demand. Some content that appears in standard print versions of this book may not be available in other formats.

Limit of Liability/Disclaimer of Warranty
The contents of this work are intended to further general scientific research, understanding, and discussion only and are not intended and should not be relied upon as recommending or promoting scientific method, diagnosis, or treatment by physicians for any particular patient. In view of ongoing research, equipment modifications, changes in governmental regulations, and the constant flow of information relating to the use of medicines, equipment, and devices, the reader is urged to review and evaluate the information provided in the package insert or instructions for each medicine, equipment, or device for, among other things, any changes in the instructions or indication of usage and for added warnings and precautions. While the publisher and authors have used their best efforts in preparing this work, they make no representations or warranties with respect to the accuracy or completeness of the contents of this work and specifically disclaim all warranties, including without limitation any implied warranties of merchantability or fitness for a particular purpose. No warranty may be created or extended by sales representatives, written sales materials or promotional statements for this work. The fact that an organization, website, or product is referred to in this work as a citation and/or potential source of further information does not mean that the publisher and authors endorse the information or services the organization, website, or product may provide or recommendations it may make. This work is sold with the understanding that the publisher is not engaged in rendering professional services. The advice and strategies contained herein may not be suitable for your situation. You should consult with a specialist where appropriate. Further, readers should be aware that websites listed in this work may have changed or disappeared between when this work was written and when it is read. Neither the publisher nor authors shall be liable for any loss of profit or any other commercial damages, including but not limited to special, incidental, consequential, or other damages.

A catalogue record for this book is available from the Library of Congress and the British Library.

ISBN 9781119232650

Cover image: © PIXOLOGICSTUDIO/SCIENCE PHOTO LIBRARY/Getty Images
Cover design by Wiley

Printed and bound by CPI Group (UK) Ltd, Croydon, CR0 4YY

C9781119232650_191023

Contents

List of contributors	vii
Preface	xiii
Acknowledgements	xv
About the companion website	xvii
How to use your textbook	xix

Chapter 1   **The cell and body tissue**   **1**
Peter S. Vickers

Chapter 2   **Genetics**   **27**
Peter S. Vickers

Chapter 3   **Cancer**   **51**
Tanya Urquhart-Kelly

Chapter 4   **Homeostasis**   **67**
Mary Brady

Chapter 5   **Inflammation, immune response and healing**   **83**
Alison Mosenthal

Chapter 6   **Shock**   **115**
Usha Chandran

Chapter 7   **Pain and pain management**   **133**
Helen Monks, Kate Heaton-Morley and Sarah McDonald

Chapter 8   **Disorders of the nervous system**   **159**
Petra Brown

Chapter 9   **Disorders of the cardiac system**   **179**
Sheila Roberts

Chapter 10   **Disorders of the respiratory system**   **213**
Elizabeth Mills, Rosemary Court and Susan Fidment

Chapter 11   **Disorders of the endocrine system**   **233**
Julia Petty

Contents

Chapter 12 Disorders of the digestive system   **257**
         Ann L. Bevan

Chapter 13 Disorders of the renal system   **279**
         Cathy Poole

Chapter 14 Disorders of the reproductive systems   **311**
         Michele O'Grady

Chapter 15 Disorders of the musculoskeletal system   **335**
         Liz Gormley-Fleming

Chapter 16 Disorders of the skin   **359**
         Liz Gormley-Fleming

Index   383

List of contributors

Ann L. Bevan RN, RSCN, PhD, MSc, FHEA, PGCED
Senior Lecturer, Children's and Young People's Nursing, Faculty of Health and Social Science, Bournemouth University, UK
Ann is senior lecturer in the Children's and Young People's nursing programme in the Faculty of Health and Social Science at Bournemouth University. She has been a registered nurse for nearly 40 years, has qualifications in adult nursing, midwifery and children's nursing, and is a qualified teacher. Ann has nursed in many areas in the UK and also in Hong Kong. She returned to the UK in January 2010 after nursing and teaching for 16 years in Canada. Research interests are children's nutrition and childhood obesity, and also all aspects of child health. Her primary research methodology is action research.

Mary Brady RN, RSCN, CHSM, BSc, PGCHE, MSc, SHEA
Senior Lecturer, Child Field Cohort Lead, Exams and Assessment Tutor, Kingston University, UK
Mary is a senior lecturer and field lead for children's nursing at Kingston University. She has a lengthy and extensive knowledge of the clinical care required for children in a variety of settings (neonatal units, paediatric intensive care and general paediatric wards). She has held posts as sister in neonatal/infant surgery, a neonatal unit and a general children's ward. Since 2004, she has been teaching pre- and post-registration nurses, midwives and paramedics. In 2016, she took on the role of Exams and Assessment Tutor for the School of Nursing. Mary is also an external examiner at Huddersfield University.

In January 2015, she joined the RCN Children and Young People's Professional Issues Forum and has contributed to RCN various publications.

Mary is interested in all aspects of children's nursing and more recently has researched the preparation of first-year student child nurses for their first clinical practice placements.

Petra Brown RGN, DP, SN, BSc (Hons), MA
Lecturer, Faculty of Health and Social Sciences, Bournemouth University, UK
Petra began her nursing a career in 1988 at Salisbury School of Nursing, becoming a staff nurse. She has worked in a variety of clinical areas including recovery, telephone triage, intensive and coronary care. On completion of her degree in critical care, Petra started her career in nurse education as a practice educator for critical care, A & E and orthopaedics. On completion of a Master's degree in health and social care practice education, she was appointed as a lecturer at Bournemouth University on the overseas and pre-registration nursing courses. Her key areas of interest are nursing practice, anatomy and physiology, nurse education, practice development, respiratory and critical care.

Usha Chandran RN (Mental Health, Adult, Child), PGCEA, MSc Critical Care Nursing (Adults), MSc Health and Disease
Lecturer/Practitioner Paediatric Intensive Care Unit (PICU), St George's Hospital, Tooting, UK
Senior Lecturer, Child Health, Kingston University, UK
Usha trained as a mental health, adult and children's nurse, specialising in postnatal mental health disorders and eating disorders in mental health and intensive and critical care nursing in adult and children's nursing.

Usha has extensive experience both as an expert clinical nurse, nurse manager and nurse lecturer. She managed a mother and baby mental health unit and functioned as a practice development nurse for a nurse-led eating disorder clinic (anorexia nervosa) at Springfield University Hospitals, Tooting, UK. Usha facilitated workshops at eating disorder nursing conferences delivered training as a nurse teacher for mental health nursing.

Usha is an expert intensive and critical care nurse with expertise in adult and children's critical care nursing and enjoys teaching this subject very much and helping new and novice nurses develop in this area of care. Her main specialities are in applied physiology and intensive care management and interventions. She worked in a combined cardiac and general adult intensive care unit in Melbourne, Australia for a period of eight months and presented a poster on sedation scales – the next generation at the British Association of Critical Care Nursing in York, UK. Usha is particularly interested in simulation training.

Usha is the lead nurse for children's critical care nurse training and development at St George's Hospital, Tooting, London, UK, the nursing PI for a multi-centre trial on sedation and weaning in children (SANDWICH) trial and the module leader for the PICU course modules at the joint faculty: Kingston University & St George's, University of London.

Rosemary Court RGN, RSCN, RNT, BSc (Hons), MSc, FHEA
Senior Lecturer in Children's Nursing, Sheffield Hallam University, Sheffield, UK
Rosemary began her nursing career in 1986 at Sheffield School of Nursing, becoming a registered general nurse and a registered sick children's nurse working in a neonatal intensive care unit. She completed a course in special and intensive care of newborns and worked as a neonatal sister for 13 years. Rosemary went on to work in the community, becoming a community specialist practitioner children's nurse and a nurse independent prescriber. She worked within a children's complex care team for 5 years before taking up a position in nurse education. In 2012, Rosemary joined Sheffield Hallam University as a senior lecturer in children's nursing, where she teaches on both pre- and post-registration nursing courses. Her key areas of interest are children's critical care nursing, children's respiratory nursing, public health, advancing practice, and nurse education.

Susan Fidment RGN, RSCN, RNT, BSc, MSc, FHEA
Senior Lecturer in Children's Nursing, Sheffield Hallam University, Sheffield, UK
Sue began her general nursing career in 1987 at Leeds General Infirmary. After she qualified as an RGN, she spent a brief period working in care of the elderly at Leicester General Hospital, before moving back to Leeds to commence a career in children's nursing. She has worked in children's orthopaedics and plastics at St James's Hospital, moved on to commence RSCN education and then worked at Killingbeck Hospital in children's cardiology. In 2012, after 16 years working within paediatric critical care both clinically and in education, she became a full-time lecturer. Sue has a specialist interest in critical care of the child and teaches on advanced paediatric life support programmes. She is particularly interested in using simulation as a teaching methodology.

Liz Gormley-Fleming RGN, RSCN, RNT, PGCert (Herts), PGDip HE (Herts), BSc (Hons), MA (Keele), SFHEA
Associate Director of Academic Quality Assurance, Centre for Academic Quality Assurance, University of Hertfordshire, UK
Liz commenced her nursing career in Ireland where she qualified as an RGN and RSCN. Initially working in paediatric oncology and bone marrow transplant, Liz moved to London and has held a variety of senior clinical nursing and leadership roles across a range of NHS Trusts both in the acute care setting and in the community. Liz has worked in education since 2001, initially as a clinical facilitator before moving into full-time higher education in 2003.

Liz has held a number of senior leadership positions in higher education: Head of Nursing (Children's, Learning Disability, Mental Health), Social Work Associate Dean of School, and Principal Lecturer in Learning and Teaching. Her areas of interest are care of the acutely ill child, healthcare law and ethics, the use of technology in higher education, curriculum development, and work-based learning.

Kate Heaton-Morley RNMH, RGN, RSCN, BSc (Hons), RNT, MSc, FHEA
Senior Lecturer Children's Nursing, Sheffield Hallam University, Sheffield, UK
Kate's career began in 1982 undertaking RNMH training (now RNLD) at Whittington Hall Hospital, Chesterfield. Subsequently training as a RGN and RSCN, Kate's practice since 1991 has been dedicated to children's nursing. She has worked and trained in the Sheffield Hospitals as a staff nurse, then sister, in acute and A & E settings. In 1998, Kate took up a senior sister post at Chesterfield Royal Hospital and, successively, positions of practice development advisor, matron, and senior matron. In 2007, to pursue her interest in nurse education, Kate joined Sheffield Hallam University as a senior lecturer in children's nursing. She maintains her clinical skills and passion for children's nursing through working as a staff nurse on the acute paediatric ward at Chesterfield Royal Hospital.

Sarah McDonald RSCN, BA (Hons), PGCert, RNT, FHEA
Senior Lecturer in Children's Nursing, Sheffield Hallam University, Sheffield, UK
Sarah completed her RSCN Honours degree at Sheffield Hallam University in 1995. She consolidated her degree as a staff nurse in acute medicine at Rotherham District General Hospital. This was followed by positions as staff nurse then senior staff nurse at Sheffield Children's Hospital in trauma, orthopaedics and plastics. Her other positions include sister in outpatient theatre at the Charles Clifford Dental Hospital and senior staff nurse in post-anaesthetic care. Sarah became a clinical nurse educator at Sheffield Children's Hospital in 2012. In 2014, she commenced a secondment as a lecturer in children's nursing and is now a full-time senior lecturer at Sheffield Hallam University. Sarah's teaching interests include pain, tissue viability, and practical nursing skills. She has published guidelines for clinical-skills.net.

Elizabeth Mills RGN, RSCN, RNT, BSc (Hons), PGCert, PGDip, MSc, FHEA
Senior Lecturer in Children's Nursing, Sheffield Hallam University, Sheffield, UK
Elizabeth began her nursing career in 1992 at West Yorkshire School of Nursing, Halifax, becoming a RGN and then a RSCN. After working in acute paediatric respiratory care, Elizabeth changed career direction and moved into neonatal intensive care, completing a course in the special and intensive care of newborns. Elizabeth worked in both district general and subregional neonatal intensive care units, and in 2005 she became a clinical educator within a large NHS Trust. In 2008, Elizabeth joined Sheffield Hallam University as a senior lecturer in children's nursing, where she teaches on both pre- and post-registration nursing courses. Her key areas of interest are children's critical care nursing, children's respiratory nursing, evidence-based practice, and nurse education.

Helen Monks RGN, RSCN, BSc (Hons), RNT, MSc, FHEA
Senior Lecturer in Children's Nursing, Sheffield Hallam University, Sheffield, UK
Helen started her career in 1986 and gained her RGN qualification at Bradford and a few years later her RSCN qualification at Manchester. She has experience in nursing children and families within the fields of general surgery, plastic surgery and general medicine. During her practice, Helen has sought to empower both families and nurses via education and partnership approaches. Her career progressed to sister and ward manager where she became more interested in education, took up project nurse roles within Bradford's

nursing development unit, and subsequently worked as a practice development nurse. She then commenced lecturing at the University of Bradford in 1997 where she was part of a team to set up the first children's nursing course there. Helen moved to Sheffield Hallam University in 2008 bringing her experience of course leadership and curriculum development. She has a research interest in the subjective nature of assessment of student nurses in the practice environment, and is currently undertaking a PhD in this subject.

Alison Mosenthal RGN, RSCN, Dip N (London), Dip Nursing Education, MSc
Senior Lecturer in Children's Nursing, School of Health and Social Work, University of Hertfordshire, UK
Alison began her nursing career at St Thomas' Hospital London before undertaking her RSCN training at Great Ormond Street in 1979. After qualifying, she worked in the respiratory intensive care unit and then moved into nurse education in the School of Nursing at Great Ormond Street in 1983.

After a career break raising her family Alison returned to clinical nursing working as a clinical nurse specialist in paediatric immunology nursing at St George's Healthcare NHS Trust in 1996. She remains in clinical practice part-time and in 2010 returned to teaching in higher education at the University of Hertfordshire, where she currently works part-time as a senior lecturer in paediatric nursing.

Michele O'Grady RGN, RSCN, MSc, PGCert
Senior Lecturer, University of Hertfordshire, UK
Michele trained in Dublin and worked as a qualified nurse until she went to Sudan with the voluntary agency GOAL, running a primary care programme. She moved to the UK in 1987 where she worked in several hospitals before moving to Oxford where she became the HIV liaison officer for 5 years. Michele returned to the NHS where she was a senior sister and an emergency nurse practitioner in the children's emergency department at Watford General Hospital. Michele joined the child nursing lecturing team at the University of Hertfordshire in 2015.

Michele has had an interest in sexual health and health promotion since her time in Sudan.

Julia Petty RGN, RSCN, MSc, PGCert, MA
Senior Lecturer in Children's Nursing, School of Health and Social Work, University of Hertfordshire, UK
Julia began her children's nursing career at Great Ormond Street Hospital. After a period in clinical practice and education, she moved into higher education and worked as a senior lecturer at City University, London for 12 years before commencing her current post in 2013. Her key interests are neonatal health, outcome of early care and most recently, the development of digital learning resources in neonatal/children's nursing care. Julia has a considerable publication portfolio and is on the editorial board of the *Journal of Neonatal Nursing*. She is a newborn life support instructor for the UK Resuscitation Council, executive member and chair of the Neonatal Nurses Association Special Interest Education and Research Group. Her recent research interest involves exploring the narratives and experiences of parents in neonatal care for the development and evaluation of a digital storytelling resource for children's nurses.

Cathy Poole RGN, RSCN, MSc, Public Sector Management PGDip Ed ENB 147
Training and Education Manager, Fresenius Medical Care, Birmingham, UK
Cathy started her career as a nursery nurse not knowing that her career would lead on to nursing and the private health education sector. With over 35 years' experience in a variety of health and education positions, Cathy has published several times and presented at

local, national and international conferences. Her main area of interest is renal nursing. Her current post allows her to combine her two passions of renal nursing and education. Not wanting to abandon her third passion of children's nursing, Cathy maintains her clinical practice as a bank staff nurse at Acorns Children's Hospice.

Sheila Roberts RGN, RSCN, RNT, BA (Hons), MA
Senior Lecturer in Children's Nursing, University of Hertfordshire, UK
Sheila began her nursing career in 1979 at the Queen Elizabeth School of Nursing in Birmingham, working primarily at Birmingham Children's Hospital. She moved to general paediatrics at Kidderminster, Ipswich and finally to Bedford Hospital where she became ward sister. Sheila moved into nurse education in 2006. Her areas of interest include nursing practice and teaching nursing skills to students, along with an interest in the cardiac and respiratory systems and child development. More recently, Sheila has been taking part in projects involving children as service users within the pre-registration nursing curriculum.

Tanya Urquhart-Kelly RGN, RSCN, MSc, NMP, Dip H Onc
Child Field Nursing Lecturer, Sheffield Hallam University, Sheffield, UK
Tanya graduated from Sheffield School of Nursing and Midwifery in March 1993 as an RGN/RSCN and has worked in a variety of roles within the field of paediatric oncology/haematology nursing since qualifying. Most recently she worked as a Macmillan clinical nurse specialist in paediatric and teenage and young adult late effects at Sheffield Children's NHS Foundation Trust. She has recently taken a substantive child field nursing lecturer post at Sheffield Hallam University. Her key areas of interest are teenagers and young adults with cancer, transition and survivorship; particularly the endocrine care for survivors of childhood cancer. She was awarded a distinction and the faculty prize for her contemporary Master's degree in the care of teenagers and young adults with cancer from Coventry University, and holds certificates in endocrine nursing and research studies. She is recognised in the international arena of late effects following cancer in childhood, and has presented at numerous international symposiums. She was the previous chair of the CAN UK Nurses group (Cancer Aftercare Nurses group) and an active member of the CCLG (Children's Cancer & Leukaemia Group) Late Effects group.

Peter S. Vickers Cert Ed, DipCD, RGN, RSCN, BA, PhD
Following several years as a schoolteacher, Peter began his nursing career in 1980 at York District Hospital, before specialising in paediatric nursing at The Hospital for Sick Children, Great Ormond Street. His nursing specialties were paediatric immunology and immunodeficiency, infectious diseases, and genetics. In 1999, he was awarded his PhD following his study of children with severe combined immunodeficiency who had survived bone marrow transplants in the UK and Germany (which was later published as a book). Following award of his PhD, Peter entered nurse education as a senior lecturer in paediatric nursing at the University of Hertfordshire, where he first began writing, and has gone on to publish widely in nursing textbooks and journals. He has also undertaken research into adult hospice care and written computer programmes on immunology for distance learning. He has also presented at conferences in many European countries, as well as North Africa. In 2012, Peter was elected President of INGID (the international organisation for immunology nurses), and in 2014, upon stepping down as INGID President, he was presented with a life-time achievement award in immunology nursing by INGID.

Preface

In order to provide safe and effective care to children and families, it is essential that those who are providing that care are able to understand the pathophysiology that underpins the child's condition.

The overall aim of this text is to help make the sometimes complex subject of pathophysiology accessible and exciting, and to enable the reader to apply their knowledge to various contexts of care. The body has an extraordinary ability to respond to disease in a variety of physiological and psychological ways. It is able to compensate for the changes that come about as a result of the disease process – the pathophysiological processes. The text can assist you in advancing your critical thinking; it fosters innovation and creativity in relation to the health and wellbeing of those to whom you have the privilege to offer care.

The text adopts a user-friendly approach – inviting you to delve deeper, discover new facts, and to engender curiosity. There are many illustrations, which are used in such a way as to explain and assist in understanding and appreciating the complex disease patterns that are being discussed. Applying a fundamental approach will provide you with a crucial understanding of applied pathophysiology, while emphasising that at all times the child and the family must be at the centre of all that is done.

A series of activities are provided, which are intended to help you learn in an engaged way and support you as you apply your learning in the various care settings, wherever these may be. This text offers an up-to-date overview of pathophysiology and the key issues associated with care provision.

The need to constantly consider the wider context of care provision, supplementing a nursing focus and recognising the broadening of the professional base, is emphasised. In providing care that is contemporary, safe and effective, an integrated, multidisciplinary approach is a key requirement. Healthcare students are important members of any multidisciplinary care team. It should also be acknowledged that contemporary care provision is delivered in ever-changing environments to a range of children, families, communities and circumstances.

Most chapters provide case studies that are related to chapter content. The chapters will stimulate reflection and further thought. In all case studies the names used are pseudonyms, in order to maintain confidentiality. Nurses owe a duty of confidentiality to all those who are receiving care (NMC, 2015). The majority of case studies have been extended further and include data concerning the patient's vital signs and blood analysis. This can help you to relate important concepts to care, offering you further insight into the patient's condition and therefore their needs. A selection of case studies include a Paediatric Early Warning Score (PEWS).

In England, nearly every hospital uses a different PEWS chart and calculates PEWS in varied ways. The PEWS charts included in this text are only there to demonstrate how they may be used. It must be remembered that infants (0–11 months), preschool children (1–4 years), school-age children (5–12 years), and teenagers (13–18 years) will all require a PEWS chart that is specific to their age. You should familiarise yourself with the PEWS chart used in the organisation where you work.

Where appropriate, significant information related to the chapter appears in boxed format to focus the reader, for example, red flags and medicines management. This can help you when you are offering care to children and families who may be vulnerable and scared.

A feature found in most chapters is the investigations box. One investigation has been chosen related to chapter content. This contains details about the test or investigation encouraging the reader to think about the pre-, peri- and post-procedural care that the child and family may require.

All chapters begin and end with questions, which are there to test your pre- and post-knowledge. A range of learning resources are included at the end of the chapters, such as word searches, 'fill in the blanks', crosswords, and label the diagram activities. A list of further resources that you may wish to access with the intention of increasing and advancing your learning is provided at the end of each chapter. Each chapter also has a glossary of terms.

Pathophysiology is concerned with the cellular and organ changes that take place when disease is present, and the effects that these changes have on a person's ability to function. When something happens that interrupts the normal physiological functioning of the body, for example, disease, it becomes a pathophysiological issue. It must always be acknowledged that normal health is not and cannot be exactly the same in any two children, and thus when the term 'normal' is used, it must be treated with caution. An understanding of pathophysiology 'normal' and 'abnormal' can assist the healthcare student in helping the child and family in a kind, sensitive, compassionate, caring, safe and holistic way.

This text is a foundation text providing support to the reader as you grow personally and professionally in relation to the provision of care. The text is primarily intended for nursing students who come into contact with children who may have a number of physically related healthcare problems, in the hospital and community setting. Illness and disease are discussed explicitly, highlighting the fact that children do become ill and they experience disease.

It is not imagined that you will read the text from cover to cover – we would encourage you to dip in and out of it. However, it may assist in your learning if you first read Chapter 1 (The cell and body tissue) and Chapter 2 (Genetics), as these provide a good starting point – they set the scene. The aim is to entice and encourage you, to whet your appetite, and inspire you to read further, and in so doing we hope to instill a sense of curiosity in you.

Reference

Nursing & Midwifery Council (NMC) (2015). *The Code. Professional standards of practice and behaviour for nurses and midwives*. Available at: https://www.nmc.org.uk/globalassets/sitedocuments/nmc-publications/nmc-code.pdf (last accessed April 2018).

Liz Gormley-Fleming, Hertfordshire
Ian Peate, Gibraltar

Acknowledgements

I would like to thank my family, Kieran my husband and my girls, Kate and Eilis. Thank you all for being you and providing me with real-life case studies.

Liz Gormley-Fleming

I would like to thank my partner Jussi Lahtinen for his support and encouragement and Mrs Frances Cohen who, without hesitation, provides me with her help and inspiration.

Ian Peate

About the companion website

This book is accompanied by a companion website:

www.wileyfundamentalseries.com/childpathophysiology

The website includes:

- Multiple-choice questions
- Further resources
- Word-search exercises
- Glossaries
- Crosswords
- 'Fill in the blanks' exercises
- True or false questions

How to use your textbook

Features contained within your textbook

Learning outcome boxes give a summary of the topics covered in a chapter.

Learning outcomes

On completion of this chapter, the reader will be able to:

- Outline the structure and function of a human cell.
- Name and describe the functions of the organelles.
- Explain the cellular transport system.
- Describe the structures and functions of the various tissues of the body, namely: epithelial, connective, muscle and nervous tissues.

Keyword boxes give a summary of the keywords covered in a chapter.

Keywords

- heart
- circulation
- congenital
- acquired
- disorders
- heart failure

Every chapter contains '**Test your prior knowledge**' questions.

Test your prior knowledge

1. Name three different treatment approaches for childhood cancer.
2. Name the most common form of childhood cancer.
3. What percentage of children with cancer are now cured? (a) >60%, (b) >70%, or (c) >80%.
4. What is the difference between a malignant tumour and a benign tumour?
5. What are the differences between chemotherapy and radiotherapy?

Case studies give an up-close, in-depth, and detailed examination of a subject.

Case Study 1

Sophie is 11 and is admitted to hospital for the first time in her life with abdominal pain. Her Mum is with her and is understandably anxious to find out what is causing Sophie's pain. She cannot stay long as she has to get back to nursery to collect Sophie's younger brother, Danny. She will come back later after taking Danny to her estranged husband's flat.

1. What pain tools are appropriate to help to assess Sophie's pain?
2. What other factors would need to be considered?
3. What non-pharmacological methods could used to help Sophie?

Red flags provide quick summaries of alert signs and symptoms.

 ### Red Flag

Nursing considerations

Because this is a potentially fatal condition nurses need to be alert to older children presenting with a more chronic picture of diarrhoea, anorexia, weight loss, periodic pain and vomiting.

How to use your textbook

Your textbook is full of **illustrations and tables**.

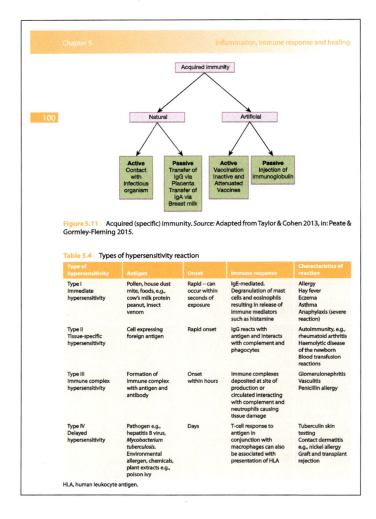

Chapter 1
The cell and body tissue
Peter S. Vickers

Aim

The aim of this chapter is to introduce the reader to the various cells and tissues of the body in order to develop their insight and understanding.

Learning outcomes

On completion of this chapter, the reader will be able to:

- Outline the structure and function of a human cell.
- Name and describe the functions of the organelles.
- Explain the cellular transport system.
- Describe the structures and functions of the various tissues of the body, namely: epithelial, connective, muscle and nervous tissues.

Keywords

- cytoplasm
- plasma membrane
- organelles
- nucleus
- passive transport
- active transport
- epithelial tissue
- muscle tissue
- connective tissue
- mitochondria

Fundamentals of Children's Applied Pathophysiology: An Essential Guide for Nursing and Healthcare Students, First Edition.
Edited by Elizabeth Gormley-Fleming and Ian Peate.
© 2019 John Wiley & Sons Ltd. Published 2019 by John Wiley & Sons Ltd.
Companion website: www.wileyfundamentalseries.com/childpathophysiology

Test your prior knowledge

1. What are the characteristics of human cells?
2. Describe the ways in which substances can pass through the cell membrane.
3. What is the role of the cell nucleus?
4. What are the four main roles of connective tissue?
5. How many different types of muscle tissue are there?
6. Where is epithelial tissue to be found within the body?

CELLS
Introduction

What is a cell? Put simply, a cell is a building block for the formation of all life and, particularly in this case, for the formation and development of the human body. There are many different types of cells and they play different roles in both the structure and functioning of the body. For example, certain cells come together to form skin (a tissue), which acts as a cover and protector for our internal organs (tissues). Other cells combine to form bone (tissue) and hence our skeleton. Then there are other different cells which combine to make up the brain and neurological tissue (nerves). Outside the cells that form our structure are the cells that help to keep us functioning, for example, the cardiac cells, which combine to make the heart (tissue), which in turn keeps blood (cells and a tissue) flowing around our body carrying nutrients to all our cells and tissues and removing waste products from them. Some cells are involved in protecting us from infectious organisms, whilst others form muscles (tissues) which allow us to work and move. So, it can be seen that cells are the basic building blocks of our bodies – indeed, our very 'being'.

All these different types of cells are actually produced from just two cells – ovum and sperm – which fuse together at the moment of conception. Within those two cells are all the plans and schemata for producing the number and diversity of cells that make a human body – truly a miracle! Once they fuse together at conception, they begin to multiply and divide into the different types of cells. This manufacture and diversification of cells is dictated by the genes carried in all of our cells (see Chapter 2, Genetics).

This chapter will give a brief overview of the structure of cells and their roles within the body. In addition, it will discuss some of the problems that can occur and how these can affect the working and health of the body, commencing with the common characteristics of cells (Fig. 1.1).

Characteristics of cells

- Cells are active – carrying out specific functions.
- Cells require nutrition to survive and function. They use a system known as endocytosis in order to catch and consume nutrients – they surround and absorb organisms such as bacteria and then absorb their nutrients. These nutrients are used for the storage and release of energy, as well as for growth and for repairing any damage to themselves.
- Cells can reproduce themselves by means of asexual reproduction in which they first develop double the number of organelles (the organs of a cell) and then divide, with the same number and types of organelle and structure present in each half. This is known as simple fission.
- Cells excrete waste products.

The cell and body tissue — Chapter 1

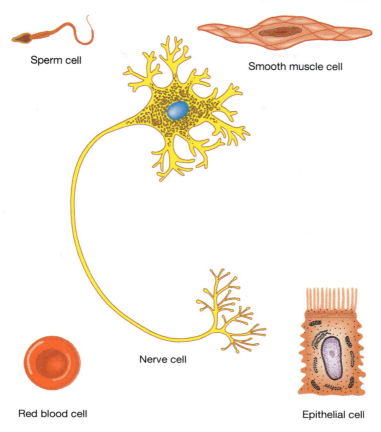

Figure 1.1 Examples of different types of cells in the body. *Source:* Tortora & Derrickson 2009, in: Peate & Gormley-Fleming 2015. Reproduced with permission of Wiley.

- Cells react to things that irritate or stimulate them – for example, in response to threats from chemicals and viruses.

The structure of the cell

There are four main compartments of the cell:

- cell membrane
- cytoplasm
- nucleus
- nucleoplasm.

Within these compartments are many organelles (or small organs). These organelles perform numerous roles to keep cells alive and functioning.

The cell membrane

As can be seen in Fig. 1.2, the various structures of the cell are contained within a cell membrane (also known as the plasma membrane). This cell membrane is a semi-permeable biological membrane separating the interior of the cell from the outside environment, and protecting the cell from its surrounding environment. It is semi-permeable because it allows only certain substances to pass through it for the benefit of the cell itself. For example,

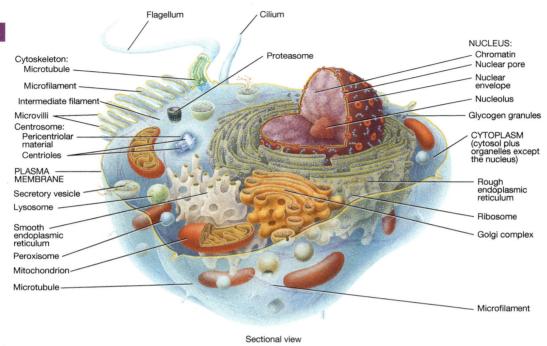

Figure 1.2 Structure of the cell. *Source:* Tortora & Derrickson 2009, in: Peate & Gormley-Fleming 2015. Reproduced with permission of Wiley.

it is selectively permeable to certain ions and molecules (Alberts *et al.*, 2014). Inside the cells are the cytoplasm and the organelles, which include, for example, the lysosomes, mitochondria, and the nucleus of the cell.

The cell membrane, which can vary in thickness from 7.5 nm (nanometres) to 10 nm (Vickers, 2009) is made up of a self-sealing double layer (bilayer) of phospholipid molecules with protein molecules interspersed amongst them (Fig. 1.3). A phospholipid molecule consists of a polar 'head', which is hydrophilic (mixes with water), and a tail that is made up of non-polar fatty acids, which are hydrophobic (repel water). In the bilayer of the cell membrane, all the heads of each phospholipid molecule are situated on the outer and inner surfaces of the cell facing outwards, whilst the tails point into the cell membrane; it is this central part of the cell membrane consisting of hydrophobic tails that makes the cell impermeable to water-soluble molecules (Marieb, 2014). In addition to the phospholipid molecules, the cell membrane contains a variety of molecules, mainly proteins and lipids, and these are involved in many different cellular functions, such as communication and transport. The proteins inserted within the cell membrane are known as plasma member proteins (PMPs), which can be either integral or peripheral. Integral PMPs are embedded amongst the phospholipid tails whilst others completely penetrate the cell membrane. Some of these integral PMPs form channels for the transportation of materials into and out of the cell, others bind to carbohydrates and form receptor sites (e.g., attaching bacteria to the cell so they can be destroyed). Other examples of integral PMPs include those that transfer potassium ions in and out of cells, receptors for insulin, and types of neurotransmitters (Vickers, 2015). On the other hand, peripheral PMPs bind loosely to the membrane surface, and so can be easily separated from it. The reversible attachment of proteins to cell membranes has been shown to regulate cell signalling, as well as acting as enzymes to catalyse cellular reactions through a variety of mechanisms (Cafiso, 2005).

The cell and body tissue Chapter 1

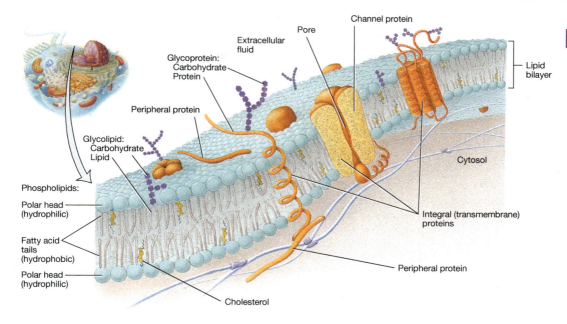

Figure 1.3 Cell membrane. *Source:* Tortora & Derrickson 2009, in: Peate & Gormley-Fleming 2015. Reproduced with permission of Wiley.

Functions of the cell membrane

Briefly, the two major physiological functions of the cell membrane are endocytosis and exocytosis. These are both concerned with the transport of fluids and other essential particulates and waste matter into and out of the cell.

- **Endocytosis** is the passing of fluids and small particles into the cell. There are three types of endocytosis, namely:
  - **Phagocytosis** – the ingestion of large particulates, such as microbial cells
  - **Pinocytosis** – the ingestion of small particulates and fluids
  - **Receptor-mediated** – involving large particulates, such as protein. It is also highly selective as to which particulates are taken up.

Endocytosis involves part of the cell membrane being drawn into the cell interior, along with particulates or fluid, in order to facilitate their ingestion. This part of the membrane is then 'pinched off' to form a vesicle within the cell. At the same time, the cell membrane reseals itself. Once inside the cell, the fate of this vesicle depends upon the type of endocytosis involved and the material that is contained within the cell membrane surrounding it. In some cases, the vesicle may ultimately fuse with a lysosome (an organelle), following which the ingested material can be processed. Endocytosis is also the means by which many simple organisms – such as amoeba – obtain their nutrients.

The cell membrane and transport

Selective permeability, as mentioned in the previous section, is very important to the process of transporting materials into and out of the cell, allowing certain materials to pass through the membrane, whilst preventing others that could harm the cell. This process depends upon the hydrophobicity of some of its molecules (as mentioned earlier). Because the phospholipid molecule tails are composed of hydrophobic fatty acid chains, it is difficult for hydrophilic (water-soluble) molecules to penetrate the membrane. Hence it forms an effective barrier for these types of molecules, which can only be penetrated by means of specific transport systems that control what can enter or leave the cell. For example, the membrane controls the process of metabolism by restricting the flow of glucose and other water-soluble metabolites into and out of cells – as well as between subcellular compartments. In addition, the cell stores energy in the form of transmembrane ion gradients by allowing high concentrations of particular ions to accumulate on one side of the membrane. Ions can pass through the membrane from inside the cell to the outside – or vice versa – so that there are more supplies of these ions just outside the cell or inside it. The membrane controls the speed/rate at which these ions pass through the membrane. The controlled release of such ions on the gradients can be used for:

- extracting nutrients from the fluids around the cells
- passing electrical messages (nerve excitability)
- controlling the volume of the cell.

Cell membrane permeability

There are four factors involved in the degree of permeability of a cell membrane, namely:

1. The size of molecules – large molecules cannot pass through the integral membrane proteins, whilst small molecules (e.g., water, amino acids) can.
2. Solubility in lipids (fats) – substances that easily dissolve in lipids (e.g., oxygen, carbon dioxide, steroid hormones) can pass through the membrane more easily than non-lipid soluble substances can.
3. If an ion has an electrical charge that is the opposite of that found in the membrane, then it is attracted to the membrane and so can more easily pass through it.
4. Carrier integral proteins can bind to substances and carry them across the membrane, regardless of the three processes above, i.e., size, ability to dissolve in lipids, or membrane electrical charge.

Movement of substances across the membrane

There are two ways for this to occur, namely, passive and active.

Passive processes

A passive process is one in which the substances move under their own volition down a concentration gradient from an area of high concentration to an area of lower concentration. In this process, the cell expends little energy on the process (like rolling down a hill).

There are four types of passive transport processes, namely:

- diffusion
- facilitated diffusion
- osmosis
- filtration.

Diffusion is the most common form of passive transport. A substance in an area of higher concentration moves to an area of lower concentration (Colbert et al., 2012). The difference seen between areas of different concentrations is known as the concentration gradient. This particular passive transport process is essential for respiration. It is through diffusion that oxygen is transported from the lungs to the blood and carbon dioxide from the blood into the lungs.

Although similar to diffusion, facilitated diffusion differs from it by the use of a substance (a facilitator) to help in the process (see Fig. 1.4). As an example, glucose is moved

The cell and body tissue   Chapter 1

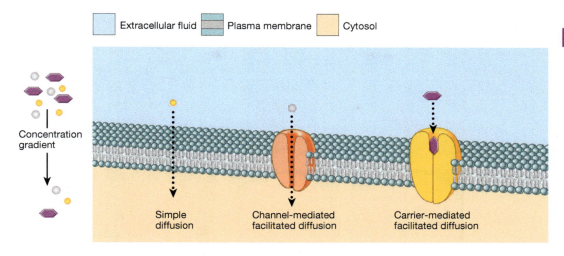

Figure 1.4 Facilitated diffusion. *Source:* Tortora & Derrickson 2009, in: Peate & Gormley-Fleming 2015. Reproduced with permission of Wiley.

using this process. To be able to pass through a membrane, glucose needs to attach itself to a carrier/transport protein (McCance & Huether, 2014).

Osmosis is the process by which water travels through a selectively permeable membrane so that concentrations of a solute (a substance that is soluble in water) are equal on both sides of the membrane. This gives rise to osmotic pressure. The higher the concentration of the solute on one side of the membrane, the higher the osmotic pressure available for the movement of water (Colbert et al., 2012).

If osmotic pressure rises too much, then it can cause damage to the cell membrane, so the body attempts to ensure that there is always a reasonable constant pressure between the cell's internal and external environments. We can see the possible damage if, for example, a red blood cell is placed in a low concentrated solute, then it will undergo haemolysis. On the other hand, if it is placed in a highly concentrated solute, the result will be a crenulated cell. If the red blood cell is placed in a solution with a relatively constant osmotic pressure, it will not be affected because the net movement of water in and out of the red blood cell is minimal.

Filtration is similar to osmosis, with the exception that physical pressure is used in order to push water and solutes across a cell membrane. This is seen in renal filtration, where the heart beating exerts pressure as it pushes blood into the kidneys, where filtration of the blood can then take place to remove any impurities (Colbert et al., 2012).

Active processes
Active processes are:

- active transport pumps
- endocytosis
- exocytosis.

An active process is one in which substances move against a concentration gradient from an area of lower to higher concentration. In order for this to happen, the cell must expend energy, which is released by the splitting of adenosine triphosphate (ATP) into adenosine diphosphate (ADP) and phosphate.

ATP is a compound of a base, a sugar and three phosphate groups (triphosphate), and is held together by phosphate bonds, which release a high level of energy when they are

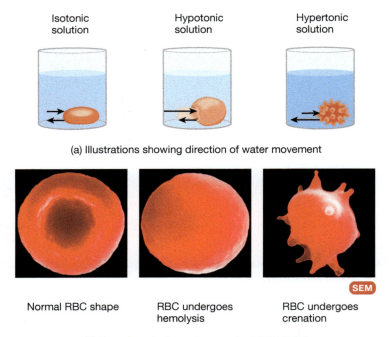

Figure 1.5 Effect of solute concentration on a red blood cell. *Source:* Tortora & Derrickson 2009, in: Peate & Gormley-Fleming 2015. Reproduced with permission of Wiley.

broken. Once one of the phosphate bonds is broken and phosphate has been released, that compound then becomes ADP. The 'spare' phosphate will then join another ADP group, so forming ATP (with energy stored in the phosphate bond). This process is continually recurring within the body.

Active transport pumps need energy to be able to function. This energy occurs as a result of the reaction mentioned earlier. It is necessary when the body is attempting to move an area that already has a high concentration of that substance. The higher the concentration already present, the more energy is required to move further molecules of that substance into that area. Fig. 1.5 demonstrates the effect of solute concentration on a red blood cell.

The organelles

These are rather like small 'organs' within the cells. The following sections give a brief overview of the many cell organelles and their functions.

Cytoplasm

Although, not strictly speaking, an organelle, the cytoplasm is a very important and integral part of the cell interior. Cytoplasm is ground substance (a 'matrix') in which various cellular components are found. It forms part of the protoplasm of the cell (protoplasm is the collective name for everything within a cell). Cytoplasm is a thick, semi-transparent, elastic fluid containing suspended particles along with the cytoskeleton (the cell framework). The cytoskeleton provides support and shape to the cell and is involved in the movement of structures within the cytoplasm – for example, phagocytic cells. Chemically, cytoplasm is made up of 75–90% water along with solid compounds, particularly carbohydrates, lipids and inorganic substances.

The cell and body tissue

The role of the cytoplasm

- Cytoplasm is the substance within the cell in which chemical reactions occur.
- It receives raw materials from the external environment (e.g., from digested food) and converts them/breaks them down into usable energy by means of decomposition reactions.
- It is the site where new substances are synthesised (produced), which can then be used by the cell for its various functions.
- It is the place where various essential chemicals are packaged either for use by itself or transported out for other cells of the body to use.
- The cytoplasm is also the place where various chemicals help with the excretion of waste materials.

The nucleus (see Fig. 1.2)

The cell nucleus is the control centre of a family of cells known as eukaryotes. Eukaryotic cells are found in animals (including humans) and plants. These cells include the prokaryotic cells that are very typical of bacteria – these cells tend to be less complex and often smaller than eukaryotic cells. However, not all human cells have a nucleus. A good example is the red blood cell. The mature red blood cell has lost its nucleus and consequently is concave in shape because it has 'collapsed in' on itself. There are also some human cells (some muscle fibre cells) that have more than one nucleus (see Fig. 1.1).

Some facts about the nucleus

- The nucleus is the largest structure in a human cell.
- It is surrounded by a nuclear membrane (just as the cell is surrounded by a cell membrane).
- It has its own protoplasm, although rather than 'cytoplasm' it is called 'nucleoplasm'.
- The nucleus is responsible for the reproduction of the cell and for making us what we are (see later) – it is where the processes of meiosis and mitosis take place.
- Within the nucleus is found all our genetic material, including DNA leading to chromosomes.
- In humans, there are normally 23 pairs of chromosomes in each cell that contains a chromosome, apart from sperms and ova, which only have 23 single chromosomes (see Chapter 2).

Cell reproduction

In order for the body to grow and also for the replacement of body cells that die or are damaged, our cells must be able to reproduce themselves. In order that the genetic information contained in the cells of the body is not lost, this must be achieved accurately.

As mentioned earlier, in humans there are a total of 23 pairs of chromosomes in each human cell that contains a nucleus. Cells reproduce by means of two processes: mitosis and meiosis, with most cells being reproduced by mitosis, whilst meiosis is restricted to the gender cells, namely the spermatozoa and the ova.

The majority of the cells that are reproduced by mitosis are exact replicas of the parent cells, and contain the full complement of 23 pairs of chromosomes, whilst those cells reproduced by meiosis are totally different in that they only contain one of each of the 23 chromosomes.

To ensure that all the genetic information is passed on accurately, in mitosis, the chromosomes reproduce themselves and then the cell divides into two, ensuring that one pair of each of the chromosomes is found in each new cell. Meiosis, however, is different in that, although initially the process is the same as in mitosis, the cells then undergo other procedures so that the end product is cells with only one copy of each chromosome. This is essential for the reproduction, not of cells, but of humans, as explained briefly in the following paragraph.

During the reproduction of humans, an egg (ovum) is penetrated by a sperm (spermatozoa), which then releases its chromosomes containing DNA which will then combine with the DNA of the egg. Because these two cells (ovum and spermatozoa) only contain one copy of each chromosome rather than the two carried by all other cells of the body, the ovum will only have two copies of each chromosome containing DNA. If the process of meiosis did not take place and the egg and sperm were like all the other cells in the body and had the normal two copies of each chromosome, then the resulting embryo would end up with four copies of each chromosome. If this process was repeated, then the next generation would end up with eight copies of each chromosome, and the following generation with 16 copies …, and so on. This is obviously not practical, which is why the ova and spermatozoa undergo meiosis to ensure that only two copies of the chromosomes are present in each succeeding generation. This will be explored more fully in Chapter 2.

Other organelles

All cells contain many organelles, and these are discussed in the following sections.

Endoplasmic reticulum

The endoplasmic reticulum (ER) consists of membranes that form a series of channels known as cisternae (see Fig. 1.6). These divide the cytoplasm into compartments. There are two types of cisternae:

1. granular ER (rough), which is associated with ribosomes (see Chapter 2)
2. agranular ER (smooth), which is free of ribosomes.

Ribosomes include tiny particles of RNA – these are formed in the cell nuclei and are associated with the synthesis of proteins need by the cell.

- The membranes of the ER contain many enzymes that speed up chemical reactions within the cells.
- ER consists of a series of channels (cisternae), which are concerned with the transport of materials – particularly proteins.
- ER contains a number of enzymes that are important for cell metabolism – such as digestive enzymes, enzymes that are involved in the synthesis (production) of steroids, and enzymes that lead to the removal of toxic substances from the cell (McCance & Huether, 2014).
- The alteration/addition of proteins exported from the cell also occurs in the cisternae.
- ER is also present in liver cells, where it has a role to play in drug detoxification.
- Granular ER is particularly found in cells that actively synthesise and export proteins.
- Agranular ER is found in steroid hormone-secreting cells, such as the cells of the adrenal cortex or, in males, the testes.

Golgi complex (Fig. 1.2)

The Golgi complex (also known a Golgi apparatus) is a collection of membranous tubes and elongated sacs. These are actually flattened cisternae that are stacked together. The Golgi complex has two major roles:

1. Helping to concentrate and package some of the substances that are made in the cell itself, for example, lysozymal enzymes.

The cell and body tissue   Chapter 1

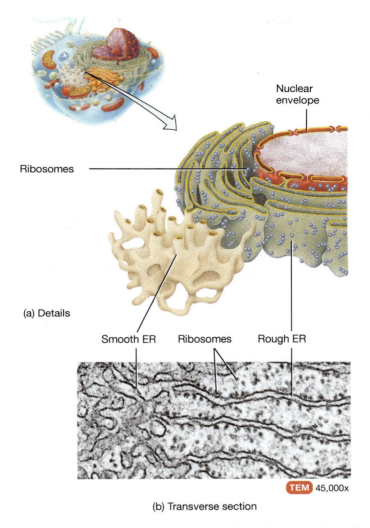

(a) Details

(b) Transverse section

Figure 1.6 Endoplasmic reticulum. *Source:* Tortora & Derrickson 2009, in: Peate & Gormley-Fleming 2015. Reproduced with permission of Wiley.

> 2. Helping with the assembly of substances for secretion outside of the cell. Secretory cells (such as those found in the mucus membrane) have many Golgi stacks, whilst non-secretory cells have few Golgi stacks per cell.

> Proteins for export from the cell are, first of all, synthesised on the ribosomes. They then travel through the ER to the Golgi vesicles (a vesicle is a fluid-filled sac). The vesicles leaving the Golgi complex then fuse with the cell membrane by the process of exocytosis. This allows the contents of the vesicles to be exported out of the cell.
> In addition, the Golgi complex is itself involved in the formation of glycoproteins.

Lysosomes (Fig. 1.2)

Lysosomes are organelles that are bound to the cell membrane and they contain a variety of enzymes. They have a number of functions:

- They are responsible for the digestion of material (e.g., pathogenic organisms) taken up by the process of endocytosis.
- They can break down components within the cell when they are not needed. For example, during the development of a human embryo, the fingers and toes of the embryo are webbed and the lysosomal enzymes remove the cells making up the webbing from between the digits.
- After the baby's birth, the uterus (which can weigh around 2 kg at full term) is invaded by phagocytic cells that are rich in lysosomes. These then reduce the uterus to its non-pregnant weight of approximately 50 g within about 9 days.
- In normal cells, some of the synthesised proteins may be faulty, and so, consequently, it is the lysosomes that are responsible for their removal and destruction.

It is crucially important that lysosomes do not rupture and release their contents inside living cells that we need to function, otherwise the lysosomal enzymes would start to digest and destroy the cell that is needed. If this occurs, the results can be seen in certain degenerative diseases, such as rheumatoid arthritis. The rupturing and breaking down of lysosomes from macrophages causing the release of lysosomal enzymes may be a significant factor in the attacking and destruction of essential living cells and tissues.

Lysosomes also contribute to the production of hormones, such as thyroxine. Thyroxine is a hormone that affects a wide range of physiological activities, such as the rate of metabolism throughout the body.

Peroxisomes (Fig. 1.2)

Peroxisomes are organelles that are similar in structure to lysosomes. However, they are much smaller. These organelles are particularly abundant in the cells of the liver, and they contain several enzymes that are toxic to cells of the body.

The role of peroxisomes in cells appears to be one of detoxification of harmful substances – such as alcohol and formaldehyde – within the cell. Importantly, they also neutralise dangerous free radicals. Free radicals are highly reactive chemicals that contain electrons that have not been 'paired off', and so are 'free' to disrupt the structure of molecules (Marieb, 2014).

Mitochondria (Fig. 1.2)

Mitochondria (mitochondrion, singular) are often thought of as the 'power houses' of the cell because they generate most of the cell's supply of adenosine triphosphate (ATP), used as a source of energy. The mitochondria are often found concentrated in regions of the cell associated with intense metabolic activity.

Anatomically, mitochondria consist of two membranes (an inner and an outer) and an intermembrane space.

The inner membrane has many folds (cristae) that increase the surface area available for chemical reactions to occur, such as the production of ATP (adenosine triphosphate – a coenzyme used as an energy carrier in the cells of all known organisms, which is responsible for the process in which energy is moved throughout the cell). This process is collectively known as internal respiration. The inner membrane is of the same thickness as the outer membrane and is responsible for oxidative phosphorylation.

The mitochondrial matrix is the name given to the space that is surrounded by the inner membrane. It contains enzymes of the tricarboxylic acid (TCA) cycle, as well as those enzymes involved in fatty acid oxidation. About two-thirds of the total protein is found in mitochondria, and, with the inner membrane, they play an important role in the production of ATP, and contain a very concentrated mixture of hundreds of enzymes.

The intermembrane space: Because the outer membrane is freely permeable to small molecules, there is a high concentration of small molecules, such as ions and sugars. However, larger molecules cannot enter this space unless they possess a specific signalling code that allows them to be able to pass through the outer membrane.

The outer mitochondrial membrane encloses the entire organelle. It contains large numbers of integral membrane proteins, known as porins, which form channels in the membrane to allow small molecules to diffuse easily from outside the mitochondria to the intermembrane space, and vice versa. Any disruption of the outer membrane allows proteins in the intermembrane space to leak into the intercellular fluid in the cell (cytosol), leading to certain cell death.

By using ATP, the mitochondria are able to generate the energy needed by the cell for it to be able to function by converting the chemical energy contained in molecules of food. The production of ATP, therefore, requires the breakdown of food molecules, and it occurs in several stages, each requiring the appropriate enzyme. Note that an enzyme is a protein that can initiate and speed up a chemical reaction (it acts as a catalyst). The enzymes in the mitochondria are stored in the membranes in the required order so that the chemical reactions occur in the correct sequence. This mechanism is very important, as it would be disastrous if the chemical reactions occurred out of sequence.

Mitochondria are self-replicating, in that, although most of a cell's DNA is contained in the cell nucleus (see Chapter 2), the mitochondrion has its own independent genetic organisation that is really quite similar to that of bacteria. DNA that is incorporated into the mitochondrial structure controls its own replication system.

The cytoskeleton

The cytoskeleton is a lattice-like collection of fibres and fine tubes and these are found in the cytoplasm of the cell. It is involved with the cell's ability to maintain and alter its shape as required (see Fig. 1.7).

There are three components that make up the cytoskeleton:

- microfilaments
- microtubules
- intermediate filaments.

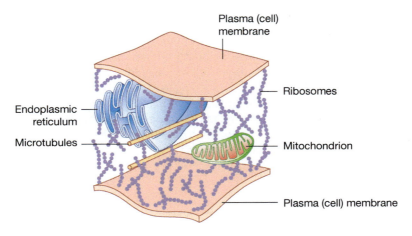

Figure 1.7 The cytoskeleton. *Source:* Peate & Gormley-Fleming 2015. Reproduced with permission of Wiley.

Microfilaments

Microfilaments are rod-like structures that are approximately 6 nanometres (6 nm) in diameter and are made of a protein called actin. In muscles, both actin (which is thick) and another protein – myosin (which is thin) combine together to allow the contraction of muscle fibres. In non-muscle cells, microfilaments help to provide support and shape to the cell. Microfilaments also assist in the movement of the cells themselves, as well as movement within the cells.

Microtubules

Microtubules are relatively straight, slender cylindrical tubules that range in diameter from 18 to 30 nm. They consist of another protein – tubulin.

- Microtubules and microfilaments help to provide shape and support for cells.
- They provide conducting channels – like tunnels – through which various substances can move through the cytoplasm.
- They also assist in the movement of pseudopodia (false arms/legs) – temporary projections of eukaryotic cell membranes. The functions of pseudopodia include locomotion (movement) and the capturing of prey. Pseudopodia sense prey that can then be engulfed. The engulfing pseudopodia are used by phagocytic white cells.

Intermediate filaments

These help to determine the shape of a cell, and range in size from 8 to 12 nm. Examples of intermediate filaments are neurofilaments, which are found in nerves.

Centrioles

These cylindrical structures are found in most animal cells, and are composed of nine sets of microtubule cylinders arranged in a circular pattern. They are particularly involved in cell reproduction. Centrioles are involved in the organisation of the mitotic spindle (see Chapter 2).

Cilia and flagella

These 'hair-like' structures extend from the surface of some cells. They possess the facility to bend, which causes the cells to move.

In humans, cilia generally have the function of moving fluid or particulates over the surface of the cells. However, ciliated cells of the respiratory tract have a very important role to play in our immune and respiratory system in that they are able to move mucus that has trapped foreign particles, including bacteria and viruses, over the surface of respiratory tissues and towards the mouth or nose, thus preventing them from causing illness.

A flagellum (singular of flagella) is usually a much larger structure than a cilium (singular of cilia), and it is often used like a fish's tail to propel the cell forward. The only example of a human cell with a flagellum is a spermatozoon, where the flagellum acts as a tail and propels the spermatozoon towards an ovum.

Conclusion

This ends the section on cells; an understanding of them and their roles in the anatomy and physiology of bodies is of utmost importance in allowing us to understand how the human body functions. The next section in this chapter will look at the various structures and organs of our bodies – all of which are made up of billions of cells.

TISSUES
Introduction

Each of us, as humans, began life as a single cell – a fertilised egg. As soon as fertilisation takes place, the egg divides continuously into many cells by division, leading to the development of an embryo, then a fetus, and finally to a baby (see Chapter 2). However, these cells do not just divide endlessly and haphazardly. Rather, they divide and grow together in such a way that they become specialised and form, for example, muscle cells, skin cells, blood cells, and so on. These specialised cells then group together to become tissues, which themselves join with other tissues to form a human being. So tissues are simply groups of cells that are similar in structure and generally perform the same functions (McCance & Huether, 2014).

There are four primary types of tissues:

- epithelial
- connective
- muscle
- nervous.

These four primary tissue types then interweave to form the fabric of the body (Marieb, 2014). Each of the four types of tissue has a specific role to perform within the body. In simple terms:

- Epithelial tissue is concerned with covering and/or lining the body, both internally and externally.
- Connective tissue is concerned with supporting the body and the tissues and organs that make up the body.
- Muscle tissue is concerned with movement – both of the body and within the body.
- Nervous tissue is concerned with the control of the body – both internally and externally (Marieb, 2014).

These specialist cells form themselves into tissues in one of two ways.

1. The first way is by means of a process known as 'mitosis' (see Chapter 2, for a description of the process of mitosis). Cells formed as a result of the process of mitosis are clones of the original cell. Therefore, if one cell with a specialised function undergoes mitosis, and subsequent generations of daughter cells continue to undergo mitosis, then the resulting hundreds and thousands of cells will all be identical and of the same type, meaning that they will all have the same function. If these identical cells join together, they will become a specialised tissue. So, for example, epithelial cell sheets (such as skin) are formed as a result of mitosis (McCance & Huether, 2014).
2. The second way is by migrating to the site of tissue formation and assembling with other cells to form a tissue. This is particularly seen during the development of the embryo when, for example, cells migrate to sites in the embryo where they differentiate and assemble into a variety of tissues (McCance & Huether, 2014). This movement of cells is known as 'chemotaxis'. Chemotaxis is the movement of cells along a chemical gradient caused by chemical attraction (McCance & Huether, 2014).

Types of tissues
Epithelial tissue

Epithelial tissue lines and covers areas of the body – both outside and inside, as well as forming the glandular tissue of the body. Thus, the exterior of the body (i.e., skin) is covered by one type of epithelial tissue whilst other types of epithelial tissue line digestive organs, such as the stomach and the small intestines, along with the kidneys, and so on. So it can be seen that epithelial tissue covers or lines most of the internal and external surfaces of the body.

Classification

Epithelial tissue is classified in two ways:

1. The number of cell layers:
   - simple – where the epithelium is formed by a single layer of cells (Fig. 1.8)
   - stratified – where the epithelium has two or more layers of cells (Fig. 1.9)
2. Shape:
   - squamous
   - cuboidal
   - columnar.

Simple epithelial tissue is most concerned with absorption, secretion and filtration of fluids and particulates. However, because this tissue is usually very thin, it is not involved in protection.

Simple squamous epithelium rests on a basal layer known as the 'basement membrane'. This is composed of a structural material that is secreted by the cells themselves (Marieb, 2014). The basement membranes provide a layer of cells that supports and separates epithelial tissue from the underlying connective tissue (Fig. 1.10). The squamous epithelial cells fit very closely together to give a thin sheet forming the tissue. This type of epithelial tissue is found in the alveoli of the lungs as well as in the walls of capillaries. It is this very thin tissue that easily allows for rapid diffusion into and out of the cell, thus facilitating oxygen and carbon dioxide exchange through the epithelial tissue that is lining the alveoli of the lungs, and allowing nutrients and gases to pass easily through the epithelial tissue from the cells into the capillaries – and vice versa.

Simple squamous epithelial cells also form the serous membranes that line certain body cavities and organs.

Simple cuboidal epithelial tissue consists of one layer of cells resting on a basement membrane (Fig. 1.11). However, because cuboidal epithelial cells are thicker than squamous epithelial cells, they are found in different places within the body and also perform

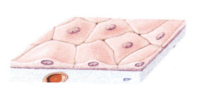

Figure 1.8 Simple epithelium. *Source:* Nair & Peate 2013, in: Peate & Gormley-Fleming 2015. Reproduced with permission of Wiley.

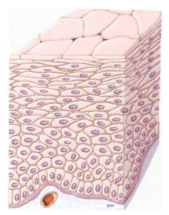

Figure 1.9 Stratified epithelium. *Source:* Nair & Peate 2013, in: Peate & Gormley-Fleming 2015. Reproduced with permission of Wiley.

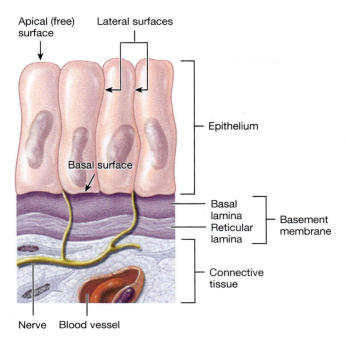

Figure 1.10 Connective tissue reinforces epithelial tissue. *Source:* Tortora & Derrickson 2009, in: Peate & Gormley-Fleming 2015. Reproduced with permission of Wiley.

different functions. This type of epithelial tissue is to be found in glands, such as the salivary glands and the pancreas. In addition, they form the walls of the kidney tubules as well as covering the surface of the ovaries (Marieb, 2014).

Simple columnar epithelium (Fig. 1.12) is the third type of simple epithelial tissue. Like the other types of simple epithelium, it is composed of a single layer of cells, although these cells are relatively tall. However, similar to the other types, they still fit closely together. It is this type of epithelial tissue, which also contains goblet cells, that lines the entire length of the digestive tract from the stomach to the anus. Goblet cells produce mucus, and so, consequently, the simple columnar epithelial tissues that line all the body cavities that are open to the exterior of the body are known as mucous membranes (Marieb, 2014).

Stratified epithelial tissue, unlike simple epithelial tissue, consists of two or more cell layers – so they lie in strata (hence the name). Because these stratified epithelial tissues

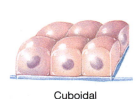

Cuboidal

Figure 1.11 Simple cuboidal. *Source:* Tortora & Derrickson 2009, in: Peate & Gormley-Fleming 2015. Reproduced with permission of Wiley.

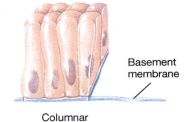

Columnar

Figure 1.12 Simple columnar. *Source:* Tortora & Derrickson 2009, in: Peate & Gormley-Fleming 2015. Reproduced with permission of Wiley.

have more than one layer of cells, they are stronger and hardier than simple epithelia. As a consequence, a primary function of stratified epithelia is protection.

Stratified squamous epithelial tissue consists of several layers of cells and is the most common stratified epithelium found within the human body (Marieb, 2014). Despite being called 'squamous epithelium', it is not composed entirely of squamous cells. Only the cells at the free edges of the epithelial tissue are squamous cells, while those cells that are close to the basement membrane are made up of either cuboidal or columnar cells. This tissue is to be found in parts of the body that are most at risk of everyday damage, such as the oesophagus, the mouth, and the outer layer of the skin.

Stratified cuboidal epithelial tissue has just two layers of cells and is only found in the ducts of large glands, such as the sweat glands, mammary glands, and salivary glands where its role is to protect the ducts of these glands.

Stratified columnar epithelial tissue is also found only in a few particular places in the body, such as in the conjunctiva of the eye, parts of the pharynx and anus, the uterus, and the male urethra and vas deferens. It is also to be found in ducts located within the salivary glands.

Transitional epithelium is a highly modified stratified squamous epithelium and forms the lining of just a few organs and other structures – all of which form part of the urinary system, namely the urinary bladder, the ureters, and part of the urethra. This tissue has been modified so that it can cope with the considerable stretching that takes place within these organs. When one of these organs/structures is *not* being stretched, the tissue is seen to have many layers, with the superficial cells (i.e., those in the top layer) having a rounded appearance like domes. However, when one of these organs/structures is distended with urine, then the epithelium becomes thinner as the surface cells flatten and become just like normal squamous cells. These transitional cells are able to slide past one another and change their shape, thus allowing the wall of the ureters, for example, to stretch as a greater volume of urine flows through it. This type of 'elastic' epithelium allows for more urine to be stored in the bladder, until micturition takes place.

Case Study Epidermolysis bullosa (EB)

Thomas, aged 6 months, was admitted to hospital because his skin was constantly blistering after even the smallest amount of friction. Unfortunately, the parents were not with Thomas as they were being investigated by Social Services for suspected child abuse and neglect.

Fortunately, Thomas was seen by an experienced child dermatologist who recognised the blistering as a medical condition known as junctional epidermolysis bullosa (EB) rather than because of parental abuse. EB occurs as a result of a rare genetic mutation, which can either be dominantly or recessively inherited (see Chapter 2) – although sometimes it can occur as a result of a new genetic mutation in the child's DNA.

Human skin consists of two layers: an outer layer – the epidermis, and beneath that a second layer – the basement membrane, also known as the dermis. These two layers are connected and held together by protein filaments that anchor them to each other. The anchors prevent the two layers from moving independently of each other – known as 'shearing'. In EB, there is a defect in certain genes that are responsible for coding for these anchoring filaments. As a consequence, the skin is extremely fragile and easily damaged by very minor trauma, such as rubbing or pressure. This will cause the layers of the skin to separate and form blisters and intensely painful sores. In addition, there is an increased risk of malignancies (cancers) developing. In severe cases of EB, it is not only the skin that can develop blisters, other membranes, such as those found in the mouth, oesophagus, and digestive tract, can also be affected.

There are three main types of EB, with EB simplex – the least serious – making up over 90% of those born with the condition. Approximately 1% of people with EB have junctional EB – like Thomas. Research is ongoing to find a cure or better treatment for this condition, with bone marrow transplants as a possible cure, and using the patient's own immune system to reduce the effects of the disorder.

Once this diagnosis had been confirmed, the parents were cleared of any ill treatment of Thomas and were able to be with him in hospital to learn about the disorder and, more particularly, how to help care for him.

It was vitally important for the parents to receive psychosocial counselling and support after their ordeal and to help them face the future with Thomas. They will also require genetic counselling in case they wish to have other children. The counselling offered will depend upon the mode of transmission of Thomas's type of EB. Above all, they will need the support of the nurses who are looking after Thomas so that they will learn how to care for him.

Unfortunately, at the present time there is no cure for EB, so palliative care and prevention of complications is essential. In addition, as Thomas grows and develops, he will face further challenges, not only medical, but also physical and psychosocial challenges, which will have to be met not just by his parents and nursing and medical staff (in hospital and the community), but also by social workers, psychologists, educational staff and schoolteachers, along with patient and parent support groups. All these people and groups will require education in dealing with children who have this rare disorder, as well as much support themselves.

Red Flag

Because of the rareness of this condition, many social workers are contacted by GPs and non-specialist doctors and nurses in general hospitals who see the blistering and the damaged skin and assume parental abuse to be the cause. This can lead to the parents being falsely accused of child neglect and cruelty. Thus, once their child has been finally diagnosed with EB, parents can be very guarded and 'difficult' when faced with any authority, including the nurses looking after their child. Consequently, the nurse has to gain their trust and respect by being totally honest, caring and compassionate – not just with the child, but also with the parents and any relatives.

Investigations

To confirm the diagnosis of EB, in addition to the signs and symptoms and medical history, skin biopsies will be necessary to make a definitive diagnosis. Two skin biopsies will be required:

1. One of the intact blisters will need to be excised for histology, which if EB is present, will show a sub-epidermal blister, with infiltration of neutrophils.
2. A biopsy of peri-lesional skin (within 2 cm of the blister) will also need to be taken for direct immunofluorescence (DIF). The sample is put on plain gauze soaked in normal saline and must be examined on the day it is taken. If EB is present, then DIF may show deposits of IgG, IgM and IgA.

Great care must be taken when obtaining these specimens, particularly to prevent infection occurring, and also to prevent further pain and discomfort – thus a local anaesthetic will be injected into the area before obtaining the samples.

Glandular epithelium

Glandular epithelial tissue is to be found within the glands. According to Marieb (2014), a gland consists of several cells that make and secrete a particular product.

There are two major types of glands developed from sheets of epithelial cells:

- exocrine glands
- endocrine glands.

Exocrine glands have ducts leading away from them, and their secretions empty through these ducts to the surface of the epithelium. Examples of exocrine glands include the sweat gland, the liver, and the pancreas.

On the other hand, endocrine glands do not possess ducts. Rather, their secretions diffuse directly into the blood vessels that are found within the glands. All endocrine glands secrete hormones, and include the thyroid, adrenal glands, and the pituitary gland.

Connective tissue

Connective tissue is found everywhere in the body and, as the name suggests, it connects body parts to one another (see Fig. 1.10).

It is the most abundant and widely distributed of all four primary tissue types. Although connective tissues perform many functions and vary considerably in their structure, they all have four main functions:

- protection
- support
- binding together of other tissues (Marieb, 2014)
- acting as storage sites for excess nutrients (McCance & Huether, 2014).

However, the most common structure and function of connective tissue is to act as a framework on which the epithelial cells gather in order to form the organs of the body (McCance & Huether, 2014).

There are several common characteristics of connective tissue, a major one being that there are actually few cells in the tissue. However, these few cells are surrounded by a lot of what is known as 'extracellular matrix'. This extracellular matrix is composed of ground substance and fibres, and it varies in consistency from fluid to a semi-solid gel. The fibres themselves are constructed from fibroblasts. There are three types of fibres in connective tissue:

- collagenous (white) fibres
- elastic (yellow) fibres
- reticular fibres.

The ground substance is composed mainly of water plus some adhesion proteins and large polysaccharide molecules. The adhesion proteins serve as a glue that allows connective tissue cells to attach to fibres. The change of consistency within the ground substance from fluid to a semi-solid gel depends on the number of polysaccharide molecules present; an increase in polysaccharide molecules causes the matrix to change from a fluid to a semi-solid gel. The ground substance can store large amounts of water, and thus acts as a water reservoir for the body.

Collagen fibres have great strength, whilst elastic fibres are able to be stretched and to recoil. The reticular fibres form the internal 'skeleton' of soft organs, such as the spleen.

Connective tissue forms a 'packing' tissue around organs of the body, and so helps to protect them. It is able to bear considerable weight as well as withstand stretching and various traumas, such as abrasions. There is a wide variation in types of connective tissue.

For example, fat tissue is composed mainly of cells and a soft matrix, whilst bone and cartilage have very few cells, but they contain large amounts of hard matrix – which makes them strong.

There are variations in blood supply to the tissue. Although most connective tissues have a good blood supply, there are some types, for example, tendons and ligaments, which have a poor blood supply, while cartilage has no blood supply. This is the reason why these tissues heal slowly when they are damaged. Bone, which has a good blood supply, will heal much quicker than a damaged tendon or ligament (Marieb, 2014).

Types of connective tissue
Bone
Bone is the most rigid of the connective tissues, and it is composed of bone cells surrounded by a very hard matrix containing calcium and large numbers of collagen fibres. Because of their hardness, bones provide protection, support, and muscle attachment.

Cartilage
Cartilage is not as hard as bone, but is more flexible. It is found in only a few places in the body (see Fig 1.13). For example, hyaline cartilage supports the structures of the larynx. It also attaches the ribs to the sternum and covers the ends of bones where they form joints. Another type of cartilage is fibrocartilage, which can be compressed and forms the discs between the spinal and neck vertebrae. Elastic cartilage is found in the external ear, where a degree of elasticity is necessary.

Dense connective tissue
This forms strong, stringy structures such as tendons (which attach skeletal muscles to bones) and the more elastic ligaments (which connect bones to other bones at joints). Dense connective tissue also makes up the lower layers of skin (the dermis). These tissues have collagen fibres as the main matrix element, with many fibroblasts found between the collagen fibres. Fibroblasts are involved in the manufacture of fibres.

Loose connective tissue
These tissues are softer and contain fewer fibres but more cells than other types of connective tissue (with the exception of blood). There are four types of connective tissue:

- areolar tissue
- adipose tissue
- reticular tissue
- blood.

Areolar tissue
Areolar tissue is the most widely distributed connective tissue type in the body. It is a soft tissue that cushions and protects the body organs that it surrounds. It also helps to hold the internal organs together. It has a fluid matrix that contains all types of fibres forming a loose network. This gives it softness and pliability. It also provides a reservoir of water and salts for the surrounding tissues.

All body cells obtain their nutrients from this tissue fluid and they also release their waste into it. It is in this area that, following injury, swelling (oedema) can occur because the areolar tissue soaks up the excess fluid causing it to become puffy (Marieb, 2014).

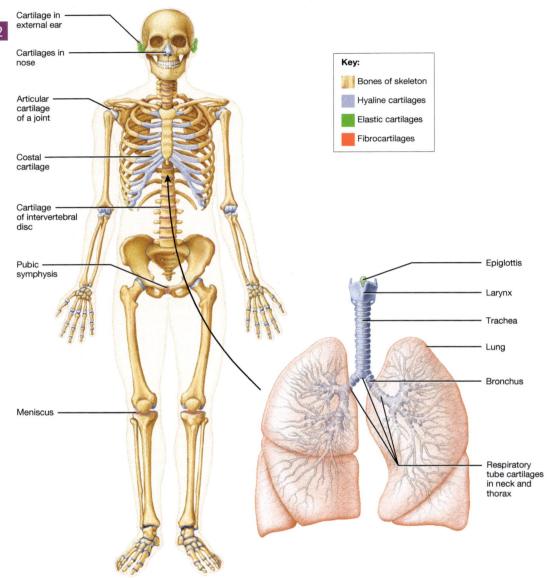

Figure 1.13 Where cartilage is found in the body. *Source:* Jenkins & Tortora 2013, in: Peate & Gormley-Fleming 2015. Reproduced with permission of Wiley.

Adipose tissue

This tissue is commonly known as 'fat'. It is actually adipose tissue in which there is a preponderance of fat cells. This tissue forms the subcutaneous tissue that lies just below the skin, and its role is to insulate the body and protect it from extremes of heat and cold. It also protects some organs such as the kidney and eyeballs.

Reticular connective tissue

This tissue consists of a delicate network of reticular fibres that are associated with reticular cells. It forms an internal framework to support many free blood cells – mainly the lymphocytes – in the lymphoid organs, such as the lymph nodes, spleen, and bone marrow.

Blood

Blood (or vascular tissue) is considered to be a connective tissue. The reason for this is that it is surrounded by a non-living, fluid matrix – blood plasma. Blood is concerned with the transport throughout the body of nutrients, waste materials, gases (oxygen and carbon dioxide), and many other substances.

Muscle tissue

There are three types of muscle tissue. These are responsible for helping the body to move, and for moving substances around the body. The three types of muscle tissue are:

- skeletal muscle
- cardiac muscle
- smooth muscle.

See Figs. 1.14 and 1.15 for examples of skeletal muscle cells and smooth muscle.

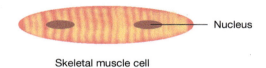

Figure 1.14   Skeletal muscle cells. *Source:* Nair & Peate 2013 in: Peate & Gormley-Fleming 2015. Reproduced with permission of Wiley.

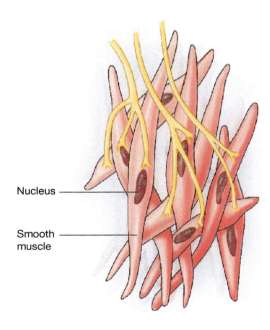

Figure 1.15   Smooth muscle. *Source:* Nair & Peate 2013 in: Peate & Gormley-Fleming 2015. Reproduced with permission of Wiley.

Skeletal muscle

Skeletal muscle is attached to bones and is involved in the movements of the skeleton. These muscles can be controlled voluntarily and form the 'bulk' of the body – the flesh. The cells of skeletal muscles are long, cylindrical, and have several nuclei (Fig. 1.14). In addition, they appear striated (striped). They work by contracting and relaxing, with pairs working antagonistically against each other – i.e., one muscle contracts and the opposite muscle relaxes. So, if the muscles in the front of the arm contract, then the ones at the back relax, which causes the arm to bend.

Cardiac muscle

Cardiac muscle is only found in the heart and its role is to pump blood around the body. It also achieves this by contracting and relaxing. However, unlike skeletal muscles, cardiac muscle works in an involuntary way – the activity cannot be consciously controlled. The cells of the muscle do not have a nucleus.

Smooth muscle

Also known as visceral muscle, smooth muscle is found in the walls of hollow organs – for example, the stomach, bladder, uterus, and blood vessels. Like cardiac muscle, smooth muscle works in an involuntary way. It causes movement in the hollow organs; for example, as smooth muscle contracts, the cavity of the organ constricts – becomes small in volume – and when it relaxes the organ becomes larger in volume (dilates). This allows substances to be propelled through the organ in the right direction, for example, faeces in the intestine. As smooth muscle contracts and relaxes, it forms a wave-like motion (peristalsis) to push the faeces through the intestines to the rectum (see Fig. 1.16).

Nervous tissue

Nervous tissue is concerned with control and communication within the body by means of electrical signals. The neuron (Fig. 1.17) is the main type of cell found in nervous tissue.

All neurons receive and conduct electrochemical impulses around the body. The structure of neurons is very different from other cells. The cytoplasm is found within long processes or extensions – some in the leg are more than a metre long. These neurons receive

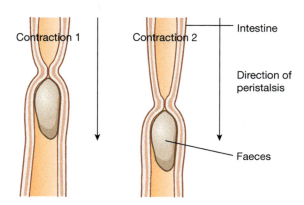

Figure 1.16 Peristalsis. *Source:* Peate & Gormley-Fleming 2015. Reproduced with permission of Wiley.

The cell and body tissue   Chapter 1

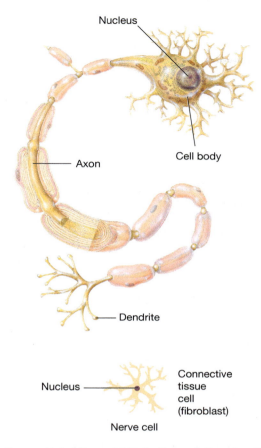

Figure 1.17 Nerve cell. *Source:* Nair & Peate 2013, in: Peate & Gormley-Fleming 2015. Reproduced with permission of Wiley.

and transmit electrical impulses very rapidly from one to the other across junctions (known as synapses). Synapses also allow electric impulses to pass from neurons to muscle cells. The total number of neurons is fixed at birth and cannot be replaced if lost or damaged (McCance & Huether, 2014).

In addition to neurons, nervous tissue includes some cells known as neuroglia (supporting cells). These cells insulate, support and protect the delicate neurons. The neurons and supporting cells comprise the structures of the nervous system, namely:

- brain
- spinal cord
- nerves.

Tissue repair

The many tissues of the body are always at risk of injury or disease. Inflammation is the body's immediate reaction to tissue injury or damage, because when this occurs, it stimulates the body's inflammatory and immune responses to spring into action so that the healing process can begin almost immediately.

Conclusion

This chapter has looked at the building blocks of the human body, namely the cells and tissues. Cells are extremely complicated parts of the body, but an understanding of them and their functions is important to comprehend how the human body itself functions. Cells form tissues, which then form the various structures, systems, and organs of the body. The remainder of this book will look at these systems, structures, and organs – how they function and what can go wrong with them.

Test your knowledge

1. How many primary tissue groups are there?
2. What is the difference between an exocrine and an endocrine gland?
3. What is the function of muscle tissue?
4. Discuss the two main classifications of cells: the prokaryotes and eukaryotes.
5. Each cell is surrounded by a membrane, what is the function of this membrane?

References

Alberts, B., Johnson, A., Lewis, J., *et al.* (2014). *Molecular Biology of the Cell*, 6th edn. Garland Science, New York.

Cafiso, D.S. (2005). Structure and interactions of C2 domains at membrane surfaces. In: Tamm, L.K. (ed.). *Protein–Lipid Interactions: From Membrane Domains to Cellular Networks*. Wiley-VCH, Weinheim.

Colbert, B.J., Ankney, J., Lee, K.T., *et al.* (2012). *Anatomy and Physiology for Nursing and Healthcare Professionals*, 2nd edn. Pearson Education, Harlow.

Gormley-Fleming, E. & Peate, I. (2014). In: Tortora, G.J. & Derrickson, B.H. (eds). *Principles of Anatomy and Physiology*, 14th edn. Wiley, Hoboken, NJ.

Marieb, E.N. (2014). *Essentials of Human Anatomy and Physiology*, 11th edn. Pearson Education, New Jersey.

McCance, K.L. & Huether, S.E. (2014). *Pathophysiology: The Biologic Basis for Disease in Adults and Children*, 7th edn. Mosby, St. Louis.

Vickers, P.S. (2009). Cell and body tissue physiology. In: Nair, M. & Peate, I. (eds). *Fundamentals of Applied Pathophysiology*. Wiley, Oxford.

Vickers, P.S. (2015). The cell. In: Peate, I. & Gormley-Fleming, E. (eds). *Fundamentals of Children's Anatomy and Physiology*, 1st edn. Wiley, Oxford.

Chapter 2

Genetics

Peter S. Vickers

Aim

To introduce the student to the fascinating and very important subject of genetics, so that a knowledge of genetics will enable them to understand many of the illnesses that have a genetic foundation.

Learning outcomes

On completion of this chapter, the reader will be able to:

- Describe the anatomy and functions of a chromosome.
- Understand genes and their importance to our health status.
- Describe the double helix and its bases.
- Identify the differences between DNA and RNA.
- Understand and describe protein synthesis and cell division, and describe their importance.
- Explain the mechanisms involved in inheritance, including Mendelian genetics.
- Explain the modes of inheritance – dominant, recessive and X-linked – and their relevance to some childhood disorders.
- Describe genetic mutations and their potential health and development effects on children.

Keywords

- genes
- chromosomes
- DNA
- RNA
- mutation
- inheritance
- traits
- genetic variation
- genetic disorders

Fundamentals of Children's Applied Pathophysiology: An Essential Guide for Nursing and Healthcare Students, First Edition.
Edited by Elizabeth Gormley-Fleming and Ian Peate.
© 2019 John Wiley & Sons Ltd. Published 2019 by John Wiley & Sons Ltd.
Companion website: www.wileyfundamentalseries.com/childpathophysiology

Test your prior knowledge

1. Which process is involved in genetic knowledge transfer from parents to their offspring?
2. What is the function of a chromosome?
3. Name the components of a chromosome.
4. What is the difference between a genotype and a phenotype?
5. Discuss the differences between autosomal, recessive, and spontaneous mutation with regard to genetic disorders.
6. What is a genetic mutation and how may it affect a child's health and/or development?
7. What are the various stages of mitosis and meiosis?
8. What is Mendelian genetics and what is its importance?
9. What is the function of a gene?

The cell nucleus and DNA

Fig. 2.1 provides an overview of the cell nucleus and DNA.

Introduction

Genetics is an increasingly important field of specialist healthcare about which all nurses need to have knowledge and understanding. Indeed, it is so important that many scientists and doctors are describing this present century as 'the century of genetics' as we learn more about the subject and are able to manipulate human, animal and plant genes in an attempt to eradicate disease and hunger. Clinical genetic services were first established in the United Kingdom in the 1950s, although services for affected families

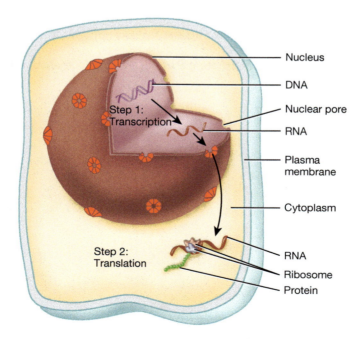

Figure 2.1 The cell nucleus. *Source:* Tortora & Derrickson 2009, in: Peate & Gormley-Fleming 2015. Reproduced with permission of Wiley.

were very limited initially (Patch & Skirton, 2009). It is a very important subject for you to know and understand, because many health problems that you will meet in practice are linked to genes.

Genes

Genes are subdivisions of DNA that are carried within chromosomes. These genes contain sets of instructions related to our bodies and how they function. Almost all the genes that we possess have been inherited from our parents (apart from any spontaneous mutations), who in turn inherited theirs from their parents, and so on.

Here are some technical definitions that will help you to understand this chapter on genetics.

- Deoxyribonucleic acid (DNA) is the essential ingredient of heredity; it comprises the basic units of hereditary material – our genes. The ability of DNA to replicate itself is the basis of hereditary transmission and it organises and produces our genetic code by acting as a template for the synthesis of mRNA.
- RNA and mRNA (ribonucleic acid and messenger ribonucleic acid) determine the amino acid composition of proteins, which in turn determines the function of that protein, and therefore the function of that particular cell.
- Chromosome: a chromosome is a long strand of DNA and protein. Each chromosome is made up of two chromatids joined by a centromere. Each nucleated cell in our body contains, within its genes, all the genetic material to make an entire human being.

The double helix

The double helix was identified in the 1950s by James Watson and Francis Crick (Patch & Skirton, 2009).

The double helix is made up of two strands of DNA and phosphate. It is a spiral-shaped molecule, resembling a corkscrew ladder, whose rungs are pairs of bases. Within the double helix, the genetic information is encoded in a linear sequence of chemical subunits, called nucleotides (see Fig. 2.2).

Deoxyribonucleotides

Deoxyribonucleotides consist of three molecules:

- deoxyribose
- phosphate
- nitrogenous base.

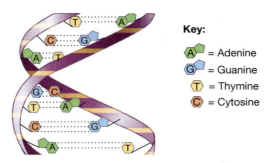

Figure 2.2 A pictorial representation of a portion of the double helix. *Source:* Tortora & Derrickson 2009, in: Peate & Gormley-Fleming 2015. Reproduced with permission of Wiley.

The bases are those elements of the double helix that carry the genetic code. They are arranged in different sequences along the deoxyribose–phosphate strands of the double helix. Each deoxyribonucleotide comprises three parts: a nitrogenous base, a deoxyribose sugar, and one phosphate group.

Bases

There are four different bases found in DNA, namely:

- adenine (A)
- thymine (T)
- guanine (G)
- cytosine (C)

The order in which the bases are organised along the length of the DNA molecule provides the variation that allows for the storage of genetic information.

Look again at the drawing of the double helix; each strand carries different bases. These bases join together and make the molecule stable. However, these bases do not just pair off haphazardly; they can only pair up with bases that match them so that they will fit together (like jigsaw pieces). Because of this, the bases are limited as to which other base they will pair with, and there is a golden rule to remember with this pairing:

- **adenine (A)** always pairs with **thymine (T)**
- **guanine (G)** always pairs with **cytosine (C)**

So, if one half of the DNA has a base sequence

AGGCAGTGC

then the opposite side of the DNA will always have the complementary base sequence

TCCGTCACG

The bases join together by means of hydrogen/polar bonding, and the individual bases are connected to the deoxyribose of the strands by means of covalent bonds. This is important because hydrogen bonds are not as strong as covalent bonds, and thus can separate more easily. The importance of this will become apparent when DNA replication and protein synthesis are discussed (Jorde *et al.*, 2015).

Question 1

If we had a base sequence of CAGTTAC, what would the complementary base sequence be? (Answer after the section on 'Chromosomes')

Chromosomes

A chromosome does not just consist of DNA. Rather, the nuclear DNA (known as nucleic acid) of cells is combined with protein molecules (known as histones). Together, the DNA and histones make up the nucleosomes contained within the cell nucleus. This nucleic acid–histone complex is known as chromatin.

If we unravelled all the chromatin from every cell in a human adult body, its length would be equivalent to nearly 70 trips from the Earth to the Sun and back, and, on average, a single human chromosome consists of a DNA molecule that is almost 5 cm in length (Cell, 1966). We only manage to package that amount of DNA and histone molecules in our bodies because they are so neatly folded that they fit into each cell of the body. The chromatin cannot just be pushed into the cell haphazardly – it would never fit and there would be a high possibility of things going wrong (Vickers, 2011). Consequently, the chromosomes twist on one another before being arranged into loops and superloops, until they assume the shape that is recognisable as a chromosome – i.e., the X-shape that can be seen in a human cell (Fig. 2.3) (Jorde et al., 2015).

Each chromosome is made up of two chromatids joined by a centromere to make an 'X' shape. Each half of the chromosome is a chromatid, and where they join near the top of the X, that is the centromere (Fig. 2.3).

In most humans, each nucleated body cell (i.e., each body cell with a nucleus) has 46 chromosomes, arranged in 23 pairs. Of those 23 pairs, one pair determines the gender of the person. These sex chromosomes are designated as X and Y chromosomes (all the others have numbers from 1 to 22), as can be seen in Fig. 2.4.

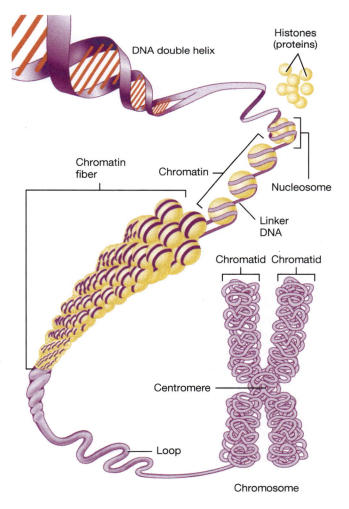

Figure 2.3 DNA from double helix to chromosome. *Source:* Tortora & Derrickson 2009, in: Peate & Gormley-Fleming 2015. Reproduced with permission of Wiley.

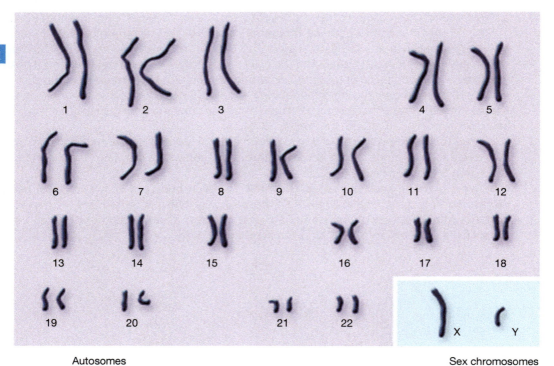

Figure 2.4   Male human chromosomes. *Source:* US National Library of Medicine. Genetics Home Reference. Lister Hill National Center for Biomedical Communications (2010), p. 16; http://ghr.nlm.nih.gov/handbook/basics/howmanychromosomes.

- Females have a matched homologous (similar) pair of X chromosomes, i.e., XX.
- Males have an unmatched heterologous (different) pair – one X and one Y chromosome.
- The remaining 22 pairs of chromosomes are known as autosomes. In biology, the word 'some' means body, so autosome means 'self body'.
- Autosomes determine physical/body characteristics – in other words, all characteristics of a person that are not connected with gender.

One of each pair of a chromosome that we inherit comes from our mother and one comes from our father, and the position a gene occupies on a chromosome is called a locus. There are different loci for colour, height, hair, etc. Think of the locus as the address of that particular gene on Chromosome Street – just like your address signifies that that is where you live.

Genes that occupy corresponding loci and code for the same characteristic are called alleles. Alleles are found at the same place in each of the two corresponding chromatids, and an allele determines an alternative form of the same characteristic, whether it be hair colour, eye colour, or propensity for certain diseases, and so forth.

Example:
Look at the colour of a person's hair – the gene that determines hair colour is found at the same place on each of the two chromatids of one particular chromosome. One gene will come from the father and the other from the mother. If parents of a child have different coloured hair from each other – perhaps the mother has red hair and the father brown hair, the child may have red or brown hair, depending upon factors that will be discussed later in this chapter.

This principle applies to each of a person's characteristics, for example, eye colour, or height. A person with a pair of identical alleles for a particular gene locus is said to be homozygous for that gene, whilst someone with a dissimilar pair is said to be heterozygous for that gene.

There are two other very important facts to mention about genes: some genes are 'recessive' and some genes are 'dominant'.

- A dominant gene is one that exerts its effect when it is present on only one of the chromosomes. (The name 'genotype' is given to the type of genes found in the body, whilst the name 'phenotype' is given to any gene that is manifested in the person.)
- A recessive gene (genotype), however, has to be present on both inherited chromosomes in order to manifest itself (phenotype).

This is a very important concept to grasp because of the significance that it brings to bear on hereditary disorders.

Answer to Question 1

The complementary base sequence would be:

GTCGACGT

From DNA to proteins

Returning to the biology of genetics, as was explained earlier in this chapter, nuclear acids are components of DNA and they have two major functions:

1. The direction of all protein synthesis (i.e., the production of protein);
2. The accurate transmission of this information from one generation to the next (from parents to their children), and, within the body, from one cell to its daughter cells.

Protein synthesis

Synthesis means 'production', for example, the production of protein from raw materials. All the genetic instructions for making proteins are found in DNA, but in order to synthesise these proteins, the genetic information encoded in the DNA has first to be translated into RNA and then into a protein.

Initially, all of the genetic information in a region of DNA has to be copied in order to produce a specific molecule of RNA (ribonucleic acid).

Then, through a complex series of procedures, the information contained in RNA is translated into a corresponding specific sequence of amino acids in a newly produced protein molecule.

There are two parts to this procedure: transcription and translation.

Transcription

In transcription, the DNA has to be transcribed into RNA because protein cannot be synthesised (produced) directly from DNA. By using a specific portion of the cell's DNA as a template, the genetic information stored in the sequence of bases of that DNA is rewritten so that the same information appears in the bases of RNA. To do this, the two strands of the DNA first have to separate (Fig. 2.5), and the bases that are attached to each strand then pair up with bases that are attached to strands of RNA.

It is important to note here that, while there is only one form of DNA, there are three types of RNA: mRNA (messenger RNA), tRNA (transfer RNA), and rRNA (ribosomal RNA). Each of these plays a different role in the synthesis of genetic material.

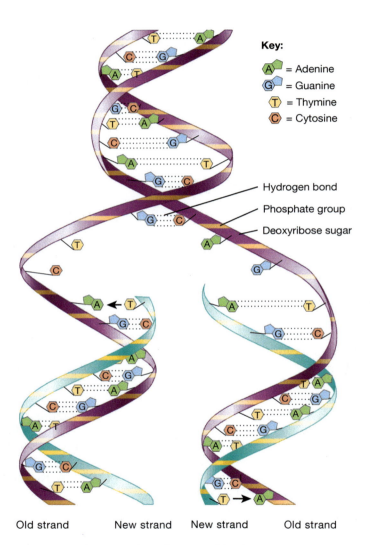

Figure 2.5 The separation of DNA and production of further DNA. *Source:* Tortora & Derrickson 2009, in: Peate & Gormley-Fleming 2015. Reproduced with permission of Wiley.

As with the two strands of DNA, the bases of DNA can only join up with a specific base of mRNA. As with DNA, guanine can only join up with cytosine in RNA, but in RNA, the adenine in DNA can only join to uracil (U) in the RNA, because there is no thymine in RNA:

Genetics Chapter 2

DNA		mRNA
guanine (G)	–	cytosine (C)
cytosine (C)	–	guanine (G)
thymine (T)	–	adenine (A)
adenine (A)	–	uracil (U)

For example,

- if DNA has a base sequence **AGGCAGTGC**
- then mRNA will have a complementary base sequence **UCCGUCACG**

Fig. 2.5 shows how the DNA separates and makes more DNA. This same process occurs during transcription, except that the new strand with its bases is RNA rather than DNA.

Question 2

In the DNA sequence below, what should the RNA bases be?

C A G C T G C A

(Answer at the end of this section)

Thus, DNA acts as a template for mRNA (Vickers, 2011). However, in addition to serving as the template for the synthesis of mRNA, DNA also synthesises two other kinds of RNA: rRNA and tRNA.

- rRNA = ribosomal RNA – rRNA, together with ribosomal proteins, makes up the ribosomes.
- tRNA = transfer RNA – this is responsible for matching the code of the mRNA with amino acids.

Once ready, mRNA, rRNA and tRNA leave the nucleus of the cell and in the cytoplasm of the cell commence the next step in protein synthesis, namely translation (Fig. 2.6).

Answer to Question 2

G U C G A C G U

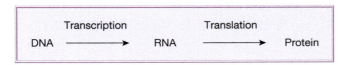

Figure 2.6 Brief summary of protein synthesis. *Source:* Peate & Nair 2011, in: Peate & Gormley-Fleming 2015. Reproduced with permission of Wiley.

Genetic mutations

It is during these stages of transcription, translation and protein synthesis that mistakes (mutations) can occur, due particularly to the extreme speed and complication of the processes. The mistakes can lead either to cell death or to a malfunctioning gene, which, in turn, can have varying effects on health and development. The effect on the body of these mutations depends on where they occur and whether they alter the function of essential proteins (US National Library of Medicine, 2016).

The DNA sequence of a gene can be changed in several different ways, of which a few are discussed in the following sections.

Missense mutation

This occurs when there is a change in one DNA base pair, which leads to the replacement of one amino acid for another in the protein for which that gene is an important component.

DNA bases	T A G	T T C	A G C	T A G
Amino acids	1	2	3	1

If, in the above gene sequence, one of the nucleotides is altered so that the sequence becomes:

DNA bases	T A G	T G C	A G C	T A G
Amino acids	1	4	3	1

Then that change in the sequence causes that triplet to code for a different amino acid, and hence a different protein is formed. So the gene does not make sense – hence 'missense'.

An example of a genetic disorder caused by a missense mutation is sickle cell anaemia.

Nonsense mutation

When a nonsense mutation occurs, there is also a change in one DNA pair. However, rather than substituting one DNA base pair for another, this type of mutation sends a signal for the sequence to be prematurely concluded. This leads to a shortened protein which may, or may not, function properly, or even may not function at all.

DNA bases	T A G	T T C	A G C	T A G
Amino acids	1	2	3	1

If, in the above gene sequence, one of the nucleotides is altered so that the sequence becomes:

DNA bases	T A G	T G C	A G C	T A T
Amino acids	1	2	3	end

Then the sequence for this gene is altered in such a way that the production of the protein is terminated prematurely. The subsequent resulting shortened protein may not function as it should or may not even function at all.

Cystic fibrosis is an example of a disease caused by a nonsense mutation.

Deletion

A deletion mutation occurs when the numbers of DNA bases are reduced by the removal of a piece of DNA. The resultant problems may occur as a result of just one or two base pairs within a gene or the removal of a complete gene or even several genes. When this occurs, the function of the resulting protein (or proteins) may be altered.

22q11.2 deletion syndrome is one such disease caused by this mutation. It is caused by the deletion of just a small section of chromosome 22. There are many health problems with this deletion mutation including cleft palate, heart defects, autoimmune disorders, to name just a few. The symptoms vary considerably from child to child, but they can also be accompanied by learning disabilities and mental illness.

Other problems caused by genes occur following:

- **Insertion** – where the number of DNA bases are increased by adding a piece of DNA to the sequence. Examples of diseases caused by this mutation include Fragile X syndrome and Huntington's disease.
- **Frameshift mutation** – this is a mutation that is caused by an insertion or deletion of a nucleotide, which causes a shift in the translational reading frame (the groups of three nucleotide bases that each code for one amino acid). This results in the moving of one nucleotide forward or back within one triplet, so that the resultant triplets are out of synchronisation. This usually results in a non-functioning protein – hence the body is missing that protein. Crohn's disease and Tay–Sachs disease are just two of the diseases caused by frameshift mutations, which are also a factor in some cancers.
- **Duplication** – sometimes a mutation can occur when a piece of DNA is copied wrongly, so that there is more than one copy of it. This can lead to altered functioning in the resulting protein. One such disease caused as a result of duplication is Charcot–Marie–Tooth disease type 1, which leads to disorders of the peripheral nervous system, which causes progressive loss of muscle tissue and loss of touch sensation.

Red Flag

Most of the clinical application of genetics in health/ill health is, currently and for the foreseeable future, the responsibility of doctors and genetic scientists. However, one extremely important aspect of genetics in ill health comes very much into the nurse's role, and that is **support** and **counselling**. This role particularly applies to paediatric nurses because most genetic health problems manifest during infancy and childhood.

Most hospitals now have genetic counsellors, but they can only give limited time to the family and child, while nurses will see them throughout their stay in hospital, and possibly in the community if the child is being cared for at home. So, whilst the primary contact with the family (and child, if old enough) regarding the genetic foundation of the child's condition may be with the genetic counsellor, the long-term support will come from the nurse. As a consequence, the nurse needs to have not only knowledge of the child's condition, but also of the genetics underpinning it, in order to be able to confidently support the family and child as they come to terms with the diagnosis of the genetic medical condition and its long-term ramifications. However, above all, the paediatric nurse will need to show empathy and have good listening skills, particularly if the genetic condition is inherited, because the nurse then not only has to help the family and child come to terms with the diagnosis, but also to cope with the devastating guilt that many, if not most, parents feel about being responsible for their child's condition. In addition, if it is an inherited genetic condition, the nurse's support will be needed to back up the genetic counsellor's discussions with the parents regarding future children.

So, in what ways can the paediatric nurse support the family and child, and also the genetic counsellor's initial and subsequent consultations with the family?

- Ensure that you have a knowledge and understanding of the child's condition and the genetics underpinning it, and also of the possible treatments, the long-term prognosis,

and how it will affect, not only the child's future life, but also that of the parents, any brothers and sisters, and the extended family.
- Be empathetic at all times, but also be completely honest. Children, particularly, are able to cope with total honesty, while the parents may find it harder to accept, but will rely on you to be honest with them.
- Always explain (often more than once) what has happened, is happening, will happen in terms appropriate for the family, the child and any siblings (who also have a vested interest in this, because it may impinge upon their present and future lives).
- Along with the genetic counsellor, help the child/family to make informed and independent decisions concerning the present and future implications of the genetic condition.
- While always trying to be 'there' for the patient (at the same time not neglecting other patients in your care), also give them time (and perhaps a space if they are on a multi-bedded ward) to grieve, and to try to come to terms with what they have been told.
- Always be truthful about potential consequences of the genetic disorder and the future, but, at the same time, try to emphasise any positives over negatives. For example, if a couple have a child with an autosomal recessive disorder, such as cystic fibrosis – which means that both parents are carriers, explain that while that means that there is a 1 in 4 chance that any subsequent children will also have cystic fibrosis, that actually means that there is a 3 in 4 chance that any future children will not have the disease. Also stress, as the genetic counsellor will have done, that these odds apply to every pregnancy, so, for example, the couple could have four further children and all have, in our example, cystic fibrosis, or they could have four further children and none of them will have cystic fibrosis. As an example, the author has known of one family where all four of their children were affected by a particular autosomal recessive genetic disorder, and another family in which the first four children were fit and well, but the fifth child had the disorder.
- Above all – and this cannot be stressed enough – just be prepared to listen empathetically while all involved try to come to terms with the diagnosis.

Finally, be aware that caring for families who have just been told that their child has a potentially, or actual, fatal genetic disorder can also be traumatic and psychologically exhausting for the nurse, so the nurse must ensure that s/he has her/his own support system.

For more information on gene mutations, the US National Human Genome Research Institute has a very good website (https://www.genome.gov/glossary).

The transference of genes
Introduction
Genetic information is transferred from cells to new cells, as well as from parents to their children. In order for the body to grow, and also for the replacement of body cells that die, while ensuring that genetic information is not lost, the cells must be able to reproduce themselves accurately. The process of transference of genes (or reproduction of cells carrying genetic information) is divided into two stages: mitosis and meiosis.

Mitosis
Cell reproduction takes place by mitosis, in which the number of chromosomes in the daughter cells has to be the same as in the original parent cell.

Genetics Chapter 2

Mitosis can be divided into four stages:

- prophase
- metaphase
- anaphase
- telophase.

Before and after it has divided, the cell enters a stage known as interphase.

Interphase

Mitosis begins with interphase – during this period the cell is actually very busy as it gets ready for replication (Fig. 2.7). During interphase, the cell is producing two of everything, not just DNA, but all the other organelles in the cell, such as the mitochondria. The cell obtains and digests nutrition so that it has the raw materials for this duplication, and also for the energy that will power the various functions of the cell.

During interphase, the chromosomes in the nucleus of the cell are present in the form of long threads so that they can be duplicated. During the process of duplication, the cells ensure that there will be sufficient genetic material for each of the two daughter cells. The strands of DNA separate and reattach to new strands of DNA. Because of the selectivity of the base to base necessary contact, an exact replication of the DNA will occur (Fig. 2.5).

In addition, extra cell organelles are manufactured by the replication of existing organelles, and the cell builds up a store of energy, which will be required for the process of division.

Prophase

The chromosomes become shorter, fatter and more easily visible. Each chromosome now consists of two chromatids, each containing the same genetic information. These two chromatids are joined together at the centromere. The two centrosomes move to opposite

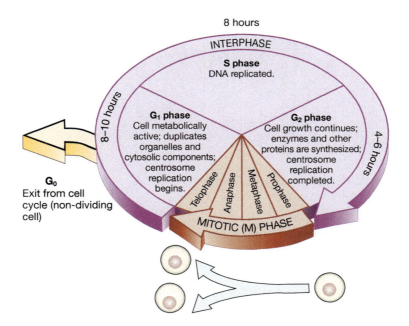

Figure 2.7 The cell cycle. *Source:* Tortora & Derrickson 2009, in: Peate & Gormley-Fleming 2015. Reproduced with permission of Wiley.

Chapter 2

Genetics

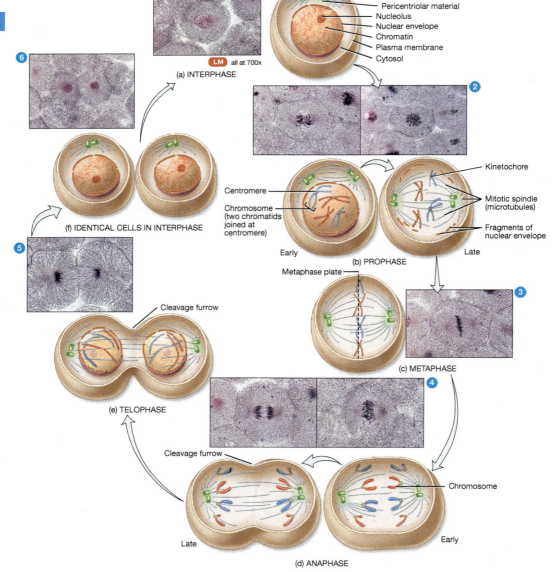

Figure 2.8 Mitosis. *Source:* Tortora & Derrickson 2009, in: Peate & Gormley-Fleming 2015. Reproduced with permission of Wiley.

ends of the cell (the poles) and are joined together by the nuclear spindle, which stretches from pole to pole of the cell. Finally, the nucleolus and nuclear membrane disappear, leaving the chromosomes in the cytoplasm (Fig. 2.8).

Metaphase

The 46 chromosomes (two of each of the 23 chromosomes), consisting of two chromatids, move to the centre of the nuclear spindle, and here they become attached to the spindle fibres (Fig. 2.8).

Anaphase
The chromatids in each chromosome are separated, and one chromatid from each chromosome then moves towards each pole (Fig. 2.8).

Telophase
There are now 46 chromatids at each pole, and these will form the chromosomes of the daughter cells. The cell divides to form two daughter cells. The nuclear spindle disappears, and a nuclear membrane forms around the chromosomes in each of the daughter cells. The chromosomes become long and threadlike again (Fig. 2.8).

Cell division
Cell division is now complete (Fig. 2.8), and the daughter cells themselves enter the interphase stage in order to prepare for their replication and division. This process of cell division explains how we grow by producing new cells as well as replacing old, damaged and dead cells.

Meiosis
Whilst mitosis is concerned with the reproduction of individual cells, meiosis is concerned with the development of whole organisms – for example, human beings.

The reproduction of humans depends upon the fusion of reproductive cells (known as gametes) from each of the parents. These gametes are:

- spermatozoa (sperm) from the male
- ova (eggs) from the female.

Each cell of the human body contains 23 pairs of chromosomes (i.e., 46 in total). It is very important that during the process of human reproduction, the cell formed when the gametes fuse has the correct number of chromosomes for a human being (23 pairs). Therefore, each gamete must possess only 23 single chromosomes because when gametes fuse during reproduction, all their chromosomes remain intact in the new life form. If each gamete had a full complement of 46 chromosomes, the resulting fused cell would possess 92 chromosomes – or four copies of each chromosome. To prevent this, the gametes only possess one copy of each chromosome, so that the resulting cell would have 46 chromosomes.

- **A diploid cell** is a cell with a full complement of 46 chromosomes (23 pairs).
- **A haploid cell** is a cell with only half that number of chromosomes (23 single chromosomes).

Gametes are therefore haploid cells, because they only possess one copy of each chromosome, whilst all other cells of the body are diploid cells.

Gametes develop from cells with 46 chromosomes, and it is through the process of meiosis that they end up with just 23 chromosomes. During meiosis, the cells divide twice, without the replication of DNA occurring again before the second division.

Meiosis can be divided into eight stages (not four as in mitosis), and consists of two meiotic divisions each with four stages. However, they have the same names, but are given either the number I or II. As with mitosis, these stages are continuous with one another.

First meiotic stage

- prophase I
- metaphase I
- anaphase I
- telophase I

Second meiotic stage

- prophase II
- metaphase II
- anaphase II
- telophase II

First meiotic division

Prophase I

Prophase I is similar to the stage of prophase in mitosis. However, instead of being scattered randomly, the chromosomes (consisting of two chromatids) are arranged in pairs – 23 in all. For example, the two chromosome 1 s will pair up, as will the two chromosome 2 s, and so on. Within each pair of chromosomes, genetic material may be exchanged between the two chromosomes, and it is these exchanges that are partly responsible for the differences between children of the same parents. This process is called 'gene crossover' (Fig. 2.9). Remember that the DNA is not replicated during the first meiotic division.

Metaphase I

The chromosomes become arranged on the spindles at the equator. However, they remain in pairs.

Anaphase I

One chromosome from each pair moves to each pole, so that there are now 23 chromosomes at each end of the spindle

Telophase I

The cell membrane now divides the cell into two halves. Each daughter cell now has half the number of chromosomes that each parent cell had.

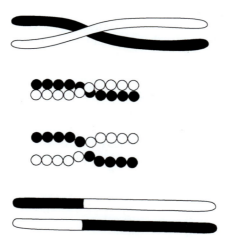

Figure 2.9 Gene crossover. *Source:* Peate & Nair 2011, in: Peate & Gormley-Fleming 2015. Reproduced with permission of Wiley.

Second meiotic division

During the second meiotic division, both of the cells produced by the first meiotic division now divide again.

Prophase II, metaphase II, anaphase II, and telophase II are all similar to their equivalent stage in mitosis, with the exception that the chromosomes are not replicated, before prophase II, so there are only 23 single chromosomes in each of the 'granddaughter' cells. That way, when the gametes fuse during reproduction, there are still only 23 pairs of chromosomes per human cell.

Of the 23 pairs of chromosomes, 22 pairs are autosomal and one pair consists of the sex chromosomes. Autosomal means 'self body'. So, autosomal chromosomes are concerned with the body. On the other hand, the sex chromosomes determine the gender of a person. Male sex chromosomes are designated by the letter Y, and female chromosomes are designated by the letter X. A male will carry the chromosomes XY (an X chromosome from the mother and a Y chromosome from the father), whilst a female will carry the chromosomes XX (an X chromosome from both the father and the mother).

Mendelian genetics: the role of genetics in inheritance

There are two definitions:

1. **Genotype** = the actual genetic make-up of a person (full heredity information).
2. **Phenotype** = the actual observed characteristics, such as physical properties and development/behaviour (although environment also plays a large part in these). Mendel demonstrated that members of a pair of alleles separate clearly during meiosis. We all have a pair of genes (alleles) at each locus, but because of the process of meiosis we can only pass one of those pairs of genes to our child.

Fig. 2.10 will make things clearer.

At the same locus on a chromosome, the father has the two alleles Aa and the mother has the two alleles Bb. When they reproduce, the father can pass either gene A or gene a (both are at the same locus and are therefore alleles) and the mother can pass on either gene B or gene b. However, each child can only inherit one of gene A or gene a from the father and one of gene B or gene b from the mother. Note that dominant genes are usually given capital letters, whilst recessive genes are usually given lower case letters.

What the child cannot do is inherit both gene A and gene a or gene B and gene b. Only one allele from each parent can be inherited by a child. This is known as Mendel's first law.

What are the statistical chances of a child inheriting any one of those sets of genes from the parents AB, Ab, aB, ab? The answer is 1 in 4 (or 1 : 4). So, there is a 25% chance that any child will inherit one of those pairs of genes from its parents.

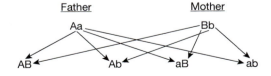

Figure 2.10 Genetic inheritance. *Source:* Peate & Nair 2011, in: Peate & Gormley-Fleming 2015. Reproduced with permission of Wiley.

Mendel's second law asserts that different pairs of alleles sort independently of each other during gametogenesis (the production of gametes), and each member of a pair of alleles may occur randomly with either member of another pair of alleles. Gametogenesis is the production of haploid sex cells so each carries one-half of the genetic make-up of the parents.

This now brings us to the concept of dominant and recessive genes, which is important in many health disorders that we may encounter, as well as determining such characteristics as eye colour and hair colour, and so forth.

Dominant genes and recessive genes

Remember that at each locus, the two alleles can be either dominant or recessive.

Look again at Fig. 2.10: suppose two parents had four children and they all had different genotypes, so that they each were represented by one of the pairs of genes. How many of the offspring would carry at least one dominant gene, and how many would carry only recessive genes at this locus?

The answer is that three out of the four children (75%) would carry at least one dominant gene, and one out of the four children (25%) would carry both recessive genes. Of course, in real life, all four children may inherit the same pair of genes at this locus, or maybe two will inherit the same genes. So there is a 1 in 4 chance at each pregnancy that the children will carry a certain genotype.

Example:

A man with red hair married a woman with brown hair. As time goes by, they have several children, all of whom have brown hair. Which is the dominant gene for hair colour and who carries it?

The gene for brown hair carried by the mother was the dominant gene in this instance.

Autosomal dominant inheritance and ill health

If the dominant gene of one of the parents is the one that causes a medical disorder, for example, Huntingdon's disease or neurofibromatosis, what will be the risk of any child of those parents having the disease?

The answer is 50% or a 1 in 2 risk of a child having an autosomal dominant disorder.

Why is this? Look back at Fig. 2.10, and assume that the father (genes **A** and **a**) carries the mutant gene on gene **A**. As a dominant gene is always expressed in the phenotype, then statistically there will be a 50% chance of any child having the disease, because the child could inherit gene **a**. Of course, any child who carries gene **A** will have a 100% chance of having the disease, there is no escaping it.

Autosomal recessive inheritance and ill health

Autosomal recessive diseases occur when both parents are carrying the same defect on a recessive gene at the same locus. Both parents have to carry the defective gene otherwise the child cannot be affected by the disease.

In autosomal recessive diseases, if the child (or parent) only carried the defect on one gene, then s/he is a carrier of that disease, and can pass that defective gene on to his (or her) children. They in turn could pass it on to their children, who, if they inherit it, would also be carriers, and this situation could continue through many generations until the carrier has children with someone who is also a carrier of that mutant gene. There is then a risk of their children being either a carrier, or having the disorder.

So then, what are the risks of:

- a child being a carrier of the recessive gene?
- a child having the disease caused by this mutated/abnormal gene?

To work it out, look again at Fig. 2.10. In this case, the small case letter '**a**' represents the abnormal recessive gene. In this scenario, both parents carry this abnormal gene, for example, for cystic fibrosis – this is a well-known disease that is inherited as an autosomal recessive disorder.

If one of the two recessive genes (a) that code for cystic fibrosis is carried by each of the parents, then the chances at each pregnancy of:

- having an affected child are 1 in 4 (or 25%)
- having a child who is a carrier are 2 in 4 (or 50%)
- having a child who is neither affected nor a carrier is 1 in 4 (or 25%).

Why is this so? Look at Fig. 2.10 again.

- Only one child possesses two affected genes (aa), and because both affected genes have to be present in order for the disease to appear, then this is one child out of four, or 25%.
- Only one child does not possess an affected gene (a), and so the disease cannot occur, neither can the child be a carrier, because there is no affected gene to be carried, so this is one child out of four, or 25%.
- Two children possess an affected gene, but they also contain an unaffected dominant gene, so they are both carriers.

Whenever there is a dominant gene, then the affected recessive gene cannot be expressed in the phenotype – the dominant gene blocks the action of the affected recessive gene, so two out of four children (or 50%) could be carriers. However, always remember that children who are carriers can pass the affected gene onto their children.

It is important to remember – and stress – that these odds occur for each pregnancy, so you could have four children and have:

- 1 affected
- 2 carriers and 1 unaffected
- 4 carriers
- 3 affected and 1 carrier
- and so on.

Remember that the odds are the same for each child born to those parents (LeMone & Burke, 2008)!

Morbidity and mortality of dominant versus recessive disorders

Autosomal dominant disorders are generally less severe than recessive disorders because if someone carries the affected gene they would have that disorder, whereas with autosomal recessive disorders a person can be a carrier but not have the disease. If autosomal dominant disorders were as severe and fatal as many autosomal recessive disorders, then the disease would die out as all the people with an affected autosomal dominant gene would normally die before being old enough to pass it on to their offspring.

An exception is Huntington's disease, which is a fatal autosomal dominant disorder, but it survives because the symptoms do not usually become apparent until the affected person is in their 30s, by which time they could have passed on the affected gene to their children.

X-linked recessive disorders

As well as autosomal inheritance, we can also inherit disorders via the sex chromosomes. The main role of these chromosomes is to determine the gender of the baby.

- **XX = girl**
- **XY = boy**

First, look at the possibilities of having a boy or a girl when you decide to have a baby. From Fig. 2.11, it can be seen that the chances for each pregnancy of a boy or a girl are 50%. Some disorders are only passed on via the X chromosome. Examples are haemophilia and Duchene muscular dystrophy. With these disorders, only the boys can be affected, and only girls may be carriers but unaffected.

If we assume that the small case '**x**' is the affected gene for haemophilia, then what is going to happen with our family in Figure 2.11?

- The first child is a girl who does not carry the affected gene, but rather two normal genes, so she is neither a carrier nor affected.
- The second child carries a normal X and a Y, so he is a boy who does not carry the abnormal gene – consequently he is neither a carrier nor affected.
- The third child is a girl who carries the abnormal gene, but the action of that gene is blocked by the other normal X gene, so she is not affected, but is a carrier.
- The fourth child is a boy who carries an abnormal X gene and a normal Y gene. Unfortunately, the Y gene is unable to block the action of the abnormal gene, so he is a carrier and is also affected.

Consequently, we can say that there is a chance that:

- 1 out of 2 girls (50%) will be a carrier
- 1 out of 2 boys (50%) will be affected.

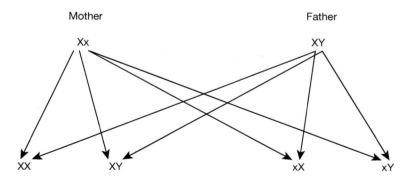

Figure 2.11 X-linked inheritance. *Source:* Peate & Nair 2011, in: Peate & Gormley-Fleming 2015. Reproduced with permission of Wiley.

But remember that in real life, all or no girls could be carriers, and if no girl in a family is a carrier, then the abnormal gene cannot be inherited by future generations – the disease will 'die out' in that family.

Case Study Sunburn

William, aged 13, is a lively, pale-skinned boy who loves playing outdoors whenever he can, particularly when the sun is shining. However, one late summer afternoon, accompanied by his mother, he arrived in the children's emergency admission unit at his local hospital complaining of painful skin on his face, arms, torso and legs, as well as a severe headache and nausea. His skin was so painful that he could not bear anyone to touch it, or even wear clothes. According to his mother he had been playing all afternoon in the garden and paddling pool wearing just swimming trunks. Although his mother had put sun cream on him after lunch, by playing in the paddling pool the sun cream had been washed away quite early on, and then he had tired himself out and fallen asleep on the grass where there was no shade. When he woke up, he was in such pain and so unwell that his mother quickly drove him to the hospital.

William was first seen by the specialist nurse on duty who gently took his vital signs and reassured both his mother and William. William had a raised temperature and pulse, while his blood pressure was quite low (see PEWS Fig. 2.12). The nurse immediately alerted the doctor on duty, because it was apparent that this could be more serious than a straightforward case of sunburn, and that he may have heatstroke. The doctor agreed with the nurse's initial diagnosis of severe sunburn and, following the insertion of an intravenous (IV) catheter and the commencement of IV fluids and pain relief, arranged for William to be admitted onto the children's ward as he was deemed too ill to go home.

🚩 Red Flag

When a young child is admitted into hospital as an emergency, there has been no time for the family to prepare, so the nurse has to be aware of the actual and potential disturbance to the family. Thus it is important to be aware of the needs of the whole family, for example, checking whether there are any other young children in the family, and who will be able to look after them if one of the parents is with the child in hospital. Also, if the admitting parent has to leave for any reason, it is important to reassure that parent that their sick child will be well looked after and that the nurse will contact the parent if there is any change in the child's condition. This is particularly important if a parent is unable to stay with the sick child because of other family or work commitments.

Spontaneous mutation

Now to briefly mention another way in which an unusual or abnormal gene can occur in an individual and cause genetic disorders. This is known as spontaneous mutation. Because of the great speed and precision needed at each replication of DNA in the germ cells, and of protein synthesis, it is possible for mistakes to occur, and so genetic mutations arise. Finally, there are also the problems of chemical/trauma mutations to consider, all of which could potentially cause disorders to arise in genes – for example, cancers.

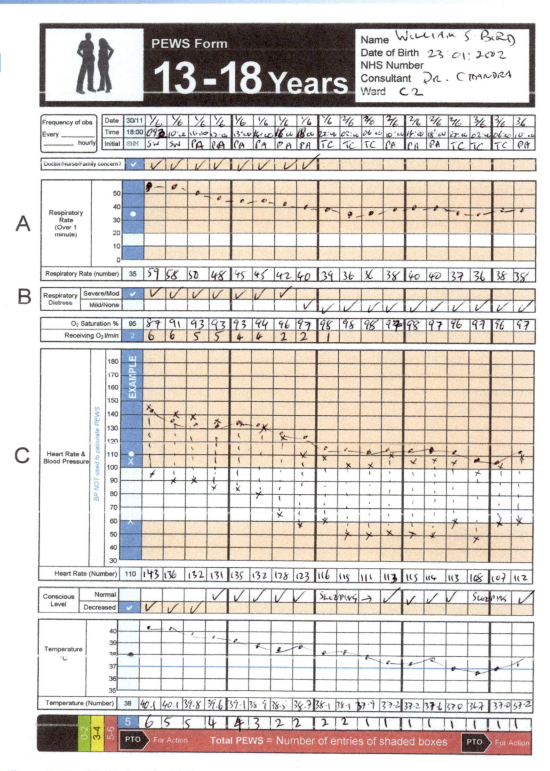

Figure 2.12 PEWS chart for William.

Conclusion

This introduction to genetics has demonstrated just how important it is for you to understand the subject, because not only do our genes make us what we are, but they can also leave us susceptible to certain diseases and affect how we respond to treatment for diseases, and indeed, how we live our lives, work, develop relationships, and survive in the world. Paediatric nurses often come across patients who have a genetic disease (because many of the most serious conditions manifest at a very early age, if not at birth); consequently, throughout your career as a nurse, you will need to explain things, not only to children diagnosed with a genetic disease, but also to their families as they struggle to come to terms not only with their child being ill, but maybe also their guilt as they realise that their child is ill because of their genes.

Finally, in recent years, there has been much interest in using genetic therapy to treat illnesses, with varying levels of success. However, probably the most exciting and, to date, successful gene therapy is that used to treat a very few of the many primary immunodeficiency diseases, which, unlike secondary immunodeficiencies (see Chapter 5, Inflammation, immune response and healing), have a genetic cause. In the early 2000s, the first successful replacement of a faulty gene in a child with adenosine deaminase (ADA) deficiency – a rapidly fatal disorder – took place (Hacein-Bey-Abina et al., 2002; Rosen, 2002). Since then this treatment has been used successfully in children with this disorder, and occasionally on children with other severe immune disorders, and research continues to try and improve this technique for other genetic disorders.

Importantly, in June 2016, it was widely reported that, within the next 10 years, scientists plan to recreate entire human cells from scratch. The aim is to make chemically accurate versions of all the six billion or so building blocks (adenine, thymine, cytosine and guanine) of human DNA (i.e., the human genome), which will then be implanted into a living cell, which, it is hoped will start to divide. This could then be a major step in creating a whole new range of medical treatments and cures for genetic diseases. However, the ethical, legal and social implications of this research will need to be assessed and deliberated upon.

In the meantime, we are already manipulating the human genome to treat and even permanently cure human genetic disorders as mentioned in this chapter, such as the work of treating children with ADA SCID, and this type of treatment will become more widespread over the next 20 years or so. Consequently, it is important that nurses become familiar with this subject because, within their working life, they are likely to be involved in caring for children undergoing gene therapy.

References

Cell (1996). In: *The World Book Encyclopedia*. Field Enterprises, Chicago.

Hacein-Bey-Abina, S., Le Diest, F., Carlier, F., et al. (2002). Sustained correction of X-linked severe combined immunodeficiency by ex vivo gene therapy. *New England Journal of Medicine* 346(16), 1185–1193.

Jorde, L.B., Carey, J.C. & Bamshad, M.J. (2015). *Medical Genetics*, 5th edn. Elsevier Health Sciences, Cambridge, MA.

LeMone, P. & Burke, K. (2008). *Medical-Surgical Nursing: Critical Thinking in Client Care*, 4th edn. Pearson Prentice Hall, New Jersey.

Patch, S. & Skirton, H. (2009). *Genetics for the Health Sciences*, 2nd edn. Scion Publishing, Banbury.

Peate, I. & Gormley-Fleming, E. (eds) (2015). *Fundamentals of Children's Anatomy and Physiology*, 1st edn. Wiley, Oxford.

Peate, I. & Nair, M. (eds) (2011). *Fundamentals of Anatomy and Physiology for Student Nurses*. Wiley, Oxford.

Rosen, F. (2002). Successful gene therapy for severe combined immunodeficiency. *New England Journal of Medicine* 346(16), 1241–1242.

Tortora, G.J. & Derrickson, B.H. (2009). *Principles of Anatomy and Physiology*, 12th edn. Wiley, Hoboken, NJ.

US National Library of Medicine (2016). Genetics Home Reference: Your Guide to Understanding Genetic Conditions. [online] Available at: https://ghr.nlm.nih.gov/(accessed 16 May 2016).

Vickers, P.S. (2011). Genetics. In: *Peate, I.* & Nair, M. (eds). *Fundamentals of Anatomy and Physiology for Student Nurses*. Wiley, Oxford, pp. 550–584.

Chapter 3

Cancer

Tanya Urquhart-Kelly

Aim

The aim of this chapter is to introduce the reader to the basic principles that are associated with cancer; understanding these principles can help the reader provide care that is evidence-based, compassionate and competent.

Learning outcomes

On completion of this chapter, the reader will be able to:

- Identify the most common childhood cancers.
- List the different treatment approaches used for childhood cancer and their potential side effects.
- Describe the common presenting symptoms of childhood cancer and what causes them.
- Discuss the psychological impact of childhood cancer on the child and family.
- Be aware of some important specific care needs for children receiving treatment for cancer.

Keywords

- cancer
- neoplasm
- malignant
- tumour
- haematology
- oncology
- chemotherapy
- radiotherapy
- trials
- late effects
- surgery

Fundamentals of Children's Applied Pathophysiology: An Essential Guide for Nursing and Healthcare Students, First Edition.
Edited by Elizabeth Gormley-Fleming and Ian Peate.
© 2019 John Wiley & Sons Ltd. Published 2019 by John Wiley & Sons Ltd.
Companion website: www.wileyfundamentalseries.com/childpathophysiology

Test your prior knowledge

1. Name three different treatment approaches for childhood cancer.
2. Name the most common form of childhood cancer.
3. What percentage of children with cancer are now cured? (a) >60%, (b) >70%, or (c) >80%.
4. What is the difference between a malignant tumour and a benign tumour?
5. What are the differences between chemotherapy and radiotherapy?

Introduction

In the United Kingdom, more than 350 000 patients are diagnosed annually with cancer (Cancer Research United Kingdom [CRUK], 2016a). Of these, childhood cancer accounts for only 0.5%, indicating that cancer is relatively rare in children. Approximately 1750 children are diagnosed with cancer per annum in the UK, that is 31 children every week (CRUK, 2016b). Around 1 in 500 children in Great Britain will develop some form of cancer by 14 years of age (CRUK, 2016b).

Despite its rarity, cancer remains the most common single cause of death in the 1–14-year age group, accounting for 20% of all deaths (Smith & Phillips, 2012). There have, however, been significant improvements in cancer treatments over the last 50 years meaning that more children than ever are being cured (Children's Cancer and Leukaemia Group [CCLG], 2016). Continuing research informs improved treatments with reduced side effects. Given the poor prognosis, treatments in the early 1960s and 1970s were designed to obtain 'cure at any cost'. Refinement of treatment through clinical trials, has not only improved cure rates to over 82%, compared to less than 30% in the 1960s, but also reduced the associated burden of morbidity and mortality from treatment side effects.

Biology of cancer

Childhood cancers differ from adult cancers as they are histologically very diverse (Stiller, 2004), whereas most adult cancers are carcinomas. Acute lymphoblastic leukaemia is the most common form of childhood cancer, accounting for approximately 25–30% of new cases annually (Vora, 2016). This is followed by tumours of the central nervous system (CNS) and lymphomas. Fig. 3.1 shows the incidence rates for childhood cancer.

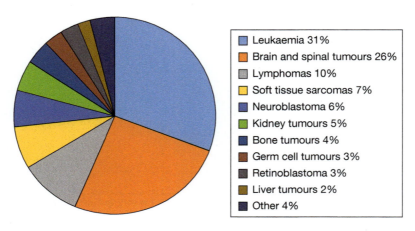

Figure 3.1   Incidence rates for childhood cancer.

Pathogenesis of cancers

Cells reproduce to grow in number or replace those that die off naturally. The process by which a cell reproduces is known as mitosis. Mitosis involves the DNA in the nucleus of a cell condensing and packing itself into the 23 pairs of identical chromosomes. These then self-replicate at which point the cell splits into two leaving each daughter cell with 23 chromosomes, which duplicate to create identical pairs. Mitosis is controlled by a number of master regulatory genes which tell cells to either continue to divide or stop.

Genes

All cancers arise when a cell is genetically altered and unable to control its own growth and proliferation. Over the last decade there have been significant advances made in understanding the molecular genetics of several childhood cancers (Pritchard-Jones, 1996). There are three known major classes of cancer genes: (1) *Oncogenes* – mutated forms of normal cellular genes that have become cancer causing. They increase the speed of cell division (proliferation), block differentiation and act in a dominant manner, i.e., mutation in only one of the pair of genes is sufficient for pathogenicity; (2) *Tumour suppressor genes* – whose function is to inhibit cell division, survival and associated properties of cancer cells (e.g., p53, see next section); (3) *Deoxyribonucleic acid (DNA) processing genes* – whose normal function is to regulate DNA replication and when mutated, allow rapid accumulation of mutations in other cancer-causing genes. Chronological mutation of all three of these cancer genes may be involved in the development and progression of a single cancer.

p53

The most important tumour suppressor gene in human cells is p53, which expresses a protein that controls cell division and survival. The protein is mutated or inactivated in about 60% of cancer cases; it is found in increased amounts in a wide variety of transformed cells.

Aetiology of cancers
Genetic predisposition

Inherited variants in p53 cause a familial cancer syndrome called Li-Fraumeni syndrome; in these families, the affected relatives develop a diverse set of malignancies including leukaemia, breast carcinomas, sarcomas (bone tumours), and brain tumours at unusually early ages.

There are other known genetic predispositions for some cancers, for example, children with Down syndrome are known to have a higher risk of developing leukaemia (Siegel, Naishadham & Jemal, 2013). However, some solid tumours occur less frequently than expected in Down syndrome, specifically there is a complete absence of neuroblastoma and Wilms tumour (nephroblastoma) (Satgé, Sasco & Lacour, 2003). It is therefore likely that there are genes on chromosome 21 that increase the risk of some cancers while others have an opposite effect. Furthermore, children who have hereditary retinoblastoma (RBS) (a rare tumour of the eye) have an increased risk of developing osteosarcoma. This is a classic example of a cancer resulting from an inherited genetic abnormality. It is not unusual for families to contain more than one affected member and in more than one generation. In most familial cases, both eyes are affected, indeed heritable RBS is usually defined as any case with bilateral tumours or a family history (Stiller, 2004a).

Table 3.1 Examples of congenital factors associated with childhood cancer

Factor	Associated childhood cancer
Chromosomal abnormality	
Down syndrome (trisomy 21)	Acute leukaemia
13q syndrome	Retinoblastoma
Genetic syndrome	
Beckwith–Wiedemann syndrome	Wilms tumour
Inherited immunodeficiency	
Fanconi anaemia	AML, hepatoma
Familial neoplastic syndromes	
Li-Fraumeni syndrome	Soft tissue carcinoma and adrenocortical carcinoma
Familial retinoblastoma	Retinoblastoma and osteosarcoma
Neurofibromatosis type 1	Astrocytoma, ALL and rhabdomyosarcoma

The familial aggregation of childhood cancer is widely studied. Often a familial link for childhood cancer will only come to light following the diagnosis of a second sibling. Table 3.1 lists examples of congenital factors associated with childhood cancer, which give rise to an increased risk of childhood cancer.

Environmental factors

Despite numerous literature reviews of environmental or exogenous exposures, there is little evidence of these being firmly established as risk factors for childhood cancer (Stiller, 2004b). They include: neonatal administration of vitamin K, parental use of medications and drugs, proximity to electromagnetic fields, parental employment and exposure to potential mutagens (Vora, 2016).

Ionising radiation (IR)

IR has been implicated in the induction of leukaemia (Vora, 2016). Research also shows that cells can detect and respond epigenetically, altering gene expression after low doses of IR (Jones *et al.*, 2010). More than 67 years ago, a correlation between antenatal obstetric diagnostic X-rays and cancer in the offspring were discovered (Stewart *et al.*, 1958). At that time it was thought that 5% of all childhood cancers were as a result of in utero irradiation. However, this number has reduced and is attributable to significantly lower numbers of women being exposed to irradiation in pregnancy.

Viruses

There is an association with Epstein–Barr virus (EBV) and both paediatric Hodgkin and Burkitt lymphomas (Paola & Preciado, 2013). International variations in the incidence of childhood lymphoma are therefore apparent (Stiller, 2004a).

Hormones

The hormone diethylstilboestrol (DES) is the only established trans-placental carcinogen; it was administered to pregnant women threatening abortion >40 years ago (Giusti *et al.*, 1995). This drug is no longer used and thus DES-related clear-cell adenocarcinoma of the vagina or cervix in young women should cease.

Signs and symptoms

There are no early warning signs or screening tests for cancer in children. Presenting symptoms vary widely depending on the type and site of the cancer, i.e., abdomen, bone, brain, kidney and blood. Commonly seen symptoms in leukaemia and lymphoma include:

- Tiredness, breathlessness and pale skin (due to anaemia and reduction in red blood cells)
- Chronic fatigue
- Tiny red spots on the skin (petechiae)
- Abnormal bleeding of the gums and epistaxis
- Bone pain and muscle aches
- Abdominal pain due to enlarged spleen and/or liver
- Swollen lymph glands in the groin, neck and under the arms
- Weight loss.

Solid tumours may present with a mass of increasing size (more evident with weight loss), pain, malaise and abnormalities of the central nervous system (particularly headaches, early morning vomiting, altered eye appearances and disturbed vision). All of which should be viewed as early warning signs. It is common for these generic symptoms to be attributed to other common childhood diseases. See Fig. 3.2 for the possible signs and symptoms of solid and CNS tumours.

Staging cancers

The stage of a cancer is often used to describe its size and whether it is found in only one part of the body (localised disease) or if it has spread beyond its original site (metastatic disease).

Although cancer 'staging' is not applied in acute leukaemia, the presenting clinical features, leukaemia cytogenetics and early response to treatment are powerful predictors of cure. Combinations of these are used for risk stratification purposes to determine the intensity of treatment a particular patient should receive. Table 3.2 lists the current UK risk stratification approach.

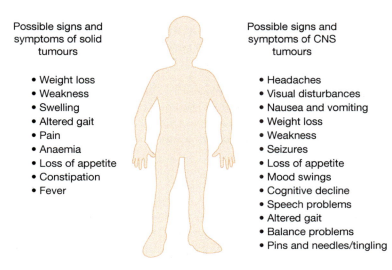

Figure 3.2   Possible signs and symptoms of solid and CNS tumours.

Table 3.2 UK risk stratification to the treatment of acute lymphoblastic leukaemia (ALL)

Risk	Definition
Standard	<10 yrs of age WCC < 50 × 10^9/L
Intermediate	>10 yrs of age WCC > 50 × 10^9/L
High	Any patient with a cytogenetic abnormality. Failure to remit at Day 29.

Historically, it was evidenced that the prognosis for acute leukaemia was worse for boys than girls. However, this is no longer evident from contemporary studies (Vora, 2016). Patients who show slow clearance of blast cells from their blood or bone marrow following induction therapy are associated with a higher risk of relapse than those who do not. Today, minimal residual disease monitoring (MRD) is a more sophisticated and sensitive measure that identifies patients who will or will not relapse.

Staging occurs following the cancer diagnosis and can be helpful in giving an indication of the prognosis. Staging can be decided on following other investigations such as blood tests and imaging. Knowing the particular type and stage of a cancer helps in decision making regarding the most appropriate treatment. Thus it is common that childhood neoplasms are classified according to histology rather than the primary site.

The standard classification scheme is the *International Classification of Diseases for Oncology* (ICD-O) (WHO, 2013), which has been used for nearly 35 years, principally in tumour or cancer registries, for coding the site (topography) and the histology (morphology) of the neoplasm, usually obtained from a pathology report.

The ICD-O comprises 12 major groups: leukaemias, lymphomas, brain and spinal tumours, sympathetic nervous system tumours, retinoblastoma, kidney tumours, liver tumours, bone tumours, soft tissue sarcomas, gonadal and germ cell tumours, epithelial tumours and other unspecified malignant neoplasms.

Central nervous system tumour staging

Astrocytic tumours, medulloblastoma and ependymoma account for about 80% of all paediatric central nervous system (CNS) tumours. Extent of disease is an important prognostic factor in determining the intensity of therapy and predicting the outcome for many CNS malignancies, including medulloblastoma, other embryonal CNS tumours (pineoblastoma, primitive neuroectodermal tumour, atypical teratoid rhabdoid tumour), and ependymomas (Louis et al., 2007). Extent of disease is classified according to the M stage. In the absence of visible disease beyond the primary on imaging (MRI brain and spine) and of malignant cells in the cerebrospinal fluid, M0 applies. M1 codes positive tumour cells in the cerebrospinal fluid, M2 visible metastases in brain, M3 visible metastases in spine, and M4 metastases outside the CNS (Harisiadis & Chang, 1977).

Some pathologists also grade the tumours, but practice varies widely around the world, with the majority not grading tumours at all. The codes in Table 3.3 for histologic grading and differentiation may be added as a 6th digit to the classification code.

Differentiation describes how much or how little a tumour resembles the normal tissue from which it arose. If a code is not used, the following adverbs may be used by pathologists: 'well', 'moderately', and 'poorly' to indicate degrees of differentiation. These approximate to grades I, II, and III. 'Undifferentiated' and 'anaplastic' usually correspond to grade IV.

Table 3.3 Tumour grades

Code	Grade	Description
1	I	Well differentiated/Differentiated, NOS
2	II	Moderately differentiated/Moderately well differentiated/Intermediate differentiation
3	III	Poorly differentiated
4	IV	Undifferentiated/Anaplastic
9	NA	Grade or differentiation not determined, not stated or not applicable

Treatment of cancer

Treatments for childhood cancer vary widely and are specific to the site, stage and type of cancer. A combination of treatment modalities is often used, namely chemotherapy, radiotherapy, and surgery. A multidisciplinary approach to treatments is also paramount. This includes consultant medical staff, junior doctors, neurosurgeons, sonographers and radiologists, nursing staff, specialist oncology outreach nurses, oncology pharmacist, psychology, CLIC Sargent social workers, occupational therapist, clinical oncologist, laboratory staff, oncology surgeon, physiotherapist, speech and language therapist, hospital play specialists (HPS), and housekeepers. Additionally, the laboratory, medical and radiology teams inform diagnosis and treatment whilst the HPS, psychologists, nursing staff and CLIC Sargent workers prepare the child and family for coping with the physical and emotional burden of treatment. There are newer treatment modalities including targeted therapies, which are mentioned later in this chapter.

Treatment can be complex and is delivered with the goal of cure, improving survival while minimizing toxicity and preserving quality of life (Wills-Alcoser & Rodgers, 2003). Adjuvant therapies are known to enhance these factors. Surgical intervention combined with chemotherapy is known to increase and improve the survival in children with solid tumours such as Wilms and osteosarcoma. Likewise low-dose radiation therapy and adjuvant chemotherapy in patients with Hodgkin lymphoma who show an inadequate response to first-line chemotherapy (EuroNet, 2013).

Treatment for childhood cancers in the UK involves the use of multicentre trials and following guidelines refined and informed from previous trials. The main body in the UK responsible for clinical trials is the National Cancer Research Institute (NCRI, 2016) Children's Cancer & Leukaemia Clinical Studies Group (NCRI CCL CSG, 2015). The treatment is delivered by a network of primary treatment centres (PTCs). A professional organisation, the Children's Cancer & Leukaemia Group (CCLG), constituted by members representing all disciplines involved in the care of children with cancer based in, or linked to, PTCs across the UK and Ireland, is responsible for guidelines and advocacy (CCLG, 2017).

Red Flag

If a healthcare professional has a suspicion that a child may have malignant disease they should be referred directly and without hesitation to the appropriate lead physician in the nearest PTC. Several investigations are common to all malignant disease but others are specific for the disease in question. Many children require numerous blood tests, which should be co-ordinated to limit repeated venepuncture. Table 3.4 shows the mandatory investigations for all new suspected cases of malignancy.

Table 3.4 Mandatory investigations for all new suspected cases of malignancy

Haematology	FBC, group and save, and serum
Biochemistry	U&Es, creatinine, calcium, magnesium, phosphate and LFTs
Virology	Serology for varicella, measles and CMV should be sent prior to any transfusions
Auxology	Accurate height and weight

Drug therapy

Chemotherapy agents play a significant role in the treatment of childhood cancer and act in a variety of ways to contain tumour cell proliferation and survival. Without chemotherapy, just 30% compared to the current >85% of children would be cured (English, 2009). Cells are most vulnerable and sensitive to chemotherapy while actively dividing. Some agents act at specific points in the cell cycle while others do not rely on a specific phase of a cycle.

Chemotherapy works by either inducing cell death through apoptosis (cytotoxic) or to prevent cell division (cytostatic). Thus cytotoxic chemotherapy has the ability to reduce tumour burden while cytostatic agents generally prevent further growth of the cancer. Chemotherapy is usually given in combinations and in cycles of treatment. These cycles are spaced so as to allow for recovery of blood counts and healthy cells while at the same time prevent significant cancer cell re-growth (MacDonald, 2010). Chemotherapy cannot distinguish between a cancerous and a normal cell. Thus once a course of chemotherapy is complete, pancytopenia follows due to transient bone marrow failure. Pancytopenia (pan = all, cyto = cells, penia = lack of/deficiency) is a deficiency of all types of blood cells, including white blood cells, red blood cells, and platelets. Another important reason cycles of treatment are used is to ensure the cancer cells are targeted in an active growth phase.

Chemotherapy is given in doses that achieve maximal effect with minimal and manageable toxicity. Modalities of administration also differ depending on whether a drug is cell-cycle specific. Continuous infusions or prolonged 'maintenance' treatment ensure maximum exposure to the tumour cells at the required point of the cell cycle and are used in tumours that are slow growing.

⚑ Red Flag

Chemotherapy should always be prescribed by an appropriately trained and qualified doctor. The same rule applies to the administration of chemotherapy. Certain agents can only be administered by a doctor, specifically chemotherapy, which is administered via the intrathecal (IT) route.

Only nursing staff who have been trained appropriately and deemed competent, and whose name appears on the Trust intrathecal register can second-check the intrathecal chemotherapy with the designated doctor.

The second-checker nurse should verify that the doctor performing the intrathecal chemotherapy administration appears on the Trust's intrathecal register prior to the procedure.

Before the oncology/haematology lumbar puncture theatre list can begin, all bolus chemotherapy MUST be removed from the ward fridge and returned to the pharmacy department until the theatre list is complete. This is to ensure that vincristine (which is an intravenous bolus drug) is not administered via the intrathecal route. To do so would be fatal to the patient. Paralysis occurs followed by death.

National Patient Safety Alerts (NPSA) have dictated that all connections associated with lumbar punctures and the administration of IT drugs have different connectors to intravenous cannulas and bungs. This is another safety mechanism to avoid incorrect drugs being administered via an incorrect route. Intrathecal equipment, drug kardex charts, drugs and labelling should be distinctly different from all other packaging and colour coded. The font on the drugs should be large, bold and clear. These will vary per PTC.

Corticosteroids are a class of steroid hormone. Since their early introduction into treatment protocols as early as 1950, corticosteroids have revolutionised leukaemia and lymphoma practice. Like the natural hormones, these synthetic compounds have glucocorticoid (GC) and/or mineralocorticoid properties. Mineralocorticoids affect ion transport in the epithelial cells of the renal tubules and are primarily involved in the regulation of electrolyte and water balance. GCs, on the other hand, are predominantly involved in carbohydrate, fat and protein metabolism, and have anti-inflammatory, immunosuppressive, anti-proliferative, and vasoconstrictive effects (Liu et al., 2013). The glucocorticosteroids prednisone and dexamethasone bind intracellularly to the glucocorticoid receptor (GR) and are able to cause cell death by apoptosis (Thompson, 1994); however, the mechanism for this remains poorly understood. Studies have demonstrated that a persistent therapeutic plasma concentration of GC is more effective than a peak plasma concentration (Estlin, 2000). They are used in three phases of acute lymphoblastic leukaemia therapy: induction, intensification and consolidation.

Serious side effects of GC are known to occur in prolonged use and in high doses. These include: osteoporosis, adrenal suppression, hyperglycaemia, dyslipidaemia, cardiovascular disease, Cushing's syndrome, psychiatric disturbances and immunosuppression. Many of these are transient in children undergoing treatment for cancer. However, osteonecrosis is particularly debilitating and thus early diagnosis and a low threshold for evaluating joint pain and mobility is paramount. Treatment involves non-weight-bearing mobilisation or bed rest combined with appropriate analgesia, predominantly non-steroidal anti-inflammatory drugs (NSAID). Research also suggests that intravenous bisphosphonates, in particular pamidronate, are beneficial to this patient population (Leblicq et al., 2013). Awareness of these side effects ensures where possible that GC are prescribed and administered at the lowest possible dose and for the shortest time to achieve the required health outcome.

⚑ Red Flag

Where a patient has been exposed to large doses of steroids and/or for a prolonged period of time, their cortisol levels should be monitored closely. Rather than immediate withdrawal of such medication, it is safer to presume adrenal insufficiency and commence these patients on replacement hydrocortisone therapy. This should include sick-day rules and training in the administration of an emergency intramuscular (IM) hydrocortisone injection to be used in the event of sudden illness/acute injury.

The delivery of replacement steroids usually allows for adrenal recovery (in the absence of other pathology or known risks) and 9 a.m. fasted cortisol levels can be checked at intervals (omitting the morning dose until after testing) to assess adrenal recovery and adrenal reserve. Once an improving and appropriate 9 a.m. cortisol level is achieved then a 'gold standard' synacthen test should be performed to accurately assess adrenal response. It is only following the results of this that any replacement hydrocortisone therapy may be withdrawn.

Radiation therapy (radiotherapy)

Radioactive substances give out radiation all of the time. There are three types of nuclear radiation: alpha, beta, and gamma. Alpha is the least penetrating, while gamma is the most penetrating. Nonetheless, all three are ionising radiation (IR). IR occurs in two forms: waves or particles. Radiotherapy treats cancer by using high-energy rays to destroy cancer cells in a particular part of the body, while doing as little harm as possible to normal cells. This is achieved by the IR exposing its energy to the cells within the treatment field causing molecular damage, particularly to the DNA. As a result of this exposure, the cancer cells will either be killed or damaged sufficiently so as to lead to self-destruction. The treatment is usually given in a specialist hospital radiotherapy department as a series of short daily sessions over a few weeks. The number of sessions required and administered are referred to as fractions and may be abbreviated in medical notes and care plans with the symbol #.

Longer wave length, lower frequency waves (heat and radio) have less energy than shorter wave length, higher frequency waves (X- and gamma rays). Not all electromagnetic (EM) radiation is ionizing. Only the high-frequency portion of the electromagnetic spectrum, which includes X-rays and gamma rays, is ionizing.

The international (SI) unit of measure for absorbed dose is the gray (Gy), which is defined as 1 joule of energy deposited in 1 kilogram of mass. The old unit of measure for this is the rad, which stands for 'radiation absorbed dose' – 1 Gy = 100 rad. Documenting the cumulative IR dose in Gy is imperative for the survivor of childhood cancer, as although IR is used in the treatment of cancer, it can as a long-term consequence cause the development of a new cancer many years from receipt and completion of initial and primary disease treatment. Like chemotherapy, IR cannot distinguish between cancerous and normal cells. Thus, following treatment with IR and depending on the site and field of treatment, localised swelling, erythema, and bone marrow suppression may occur. Other significant longer term consequences of IR can affect childhood cancer survivors, such as problems with growth and puberty, fertility, heart function, and respiratory function (Urquhart & Collin, 2016). Historically, very young children who were deemed to be unable to lie still and tolerate radiotherapy while awake were given full general anaesthetics (GA) in close succession. These were sometimes twice a day but usually Monday to Friday for up to 6 weeks. However, with the increase of Health Play Specialist (HPS) roles, preparatory work for this group of patients to avoid multiple GAs has advanced significantly. Now, children as young as 3 years of age can tolerate their therapy thanks to the efforts of the HPS. Moulds for ensuring the child does not move can be made embellished with a favourite superhero design; likewise a smaller mask can be made for their favourite toy. Even something as simple as holding the end of a reel of ribbon with their parent or significant other at the other end outside the treatment room offering a gentle collaborative tug, offers sufficient reassurance (Cooper, 2015).

🚩 Red Flag

As eluded to earlier, IR can cause swelling to local tissues and organs involved in the radiation field. Thus patients who are in receipt of IR to their brain are required to remain as an inpatient for the first week of treatment to allow for close observation of any symptoms associated with intracranial swelling. This is achieved by undertaking 4-hourly neurological observations. These are guidance timings and local policy should always be followed.

Surgery

Before the discovery of chemotherapy and IR, surgery was the principle treatment for solid cancers of childhood (Wills-Alcoser & Rodgers, 2003). Today, however, surgery may be used as one of a triad of treatment approaches. Diseases such as osteosarcoma can only be cured with the use of surgery. This is followed by chemotherapy to treat any residual disease and prevent metastasis or local relapse. A patient with ALL, however, will probably only require the insertion of a central venous catheter (CVC). A paediatric oncology surgeon is another key member of the multidisciplinary team. The need for surgery depends on the diagnosis, and surgical interventions vary widely. That said, surgery can be central to the diagnostic process: biopsy, excision and/or resection of a neoplasm. The majority of children and young people will require the insertion and removal of a CVC, i.e., a patient requiring HSCT will benefit from a double lumen Hickman line to allow for the multiple intravenous drugs and parenteral nutrition to be administered over the required period. Furthermore these long-term catheters can be used for blood sampling, blood and platelet transfusions, and antibiotics and antifungals during febrile and neutropenic episodes.

Haematopoietic stem cell transplantation (HSCT)

HSCT, formerly referred to as bone marrow transplantation, has been used as a treatment for cancer since the late 1960s. Transplantation comprises the use of both allogeneic (donor cells) and autologous (own cells). HSCT involves administration of chemotherapy and/or IR to eradicate disease and render the bone marrow empty. Harvested stem cells are then infused into the patient allowing for recovery of healthy bone marrow. The increase of bone marrow registries, such as Anthony Nolan (2017), means that those without a sibling now have the opportunity to receive a matched unrelated donor transplant. The wider benefits of the use of peripheral blood stem cells for transplantation demonstrated patients with chronic myeloid leukaemia could be reconstituted with autologous peripheral blood cells (Brito-Babapulle *et al.*, 1989). This in turn has reduced the need for a donor to undergo a general anaesthetic for marrow harvest; instead the introduction and use of granulocyte colony-stimulating factor (GCSF) allowed for peripheral blood stem cell (PBSC) mobilisation to replace the use of bone marrow for transplantation. The first successful cord blood stem cell transplant occurred in 1988 and since that time it has increased in popularity as a mode of transplantation (Gluckman *et al.*, 1989).

The following decade demonstrated a proliferation of HSCT combined with increased understanding of this treatment. Likewise there is escalating use of autologous HSCT in the treatment of lymphomas (Cairo, Woessmann & Pagel, 2013) and solid tumours (Elborai *et al.*, 2015). Improvements in supportive therapies have also played a part in the success of HSCT; namely anti-infectious agents including antifungals and antiviral drugs (Remberger *et al.*, 2011).

Targeted therapies

Targeted therapies such as monoclonal antibody drugs (mAbs) have been established in adult cancer treatment for >10 years and are now more commonly embedded in the treatment of some paediatric malignancies. The benefit of such biologics is that the agents are uniquely or partially tumour-specific rather than indiscriminately cytotoxic (MacDonald, 2010). These mAbs can bind to an antigen which is either only or differentially expressed on the tumour cell surface, and either marks that cell for destruction by the patient's immune system or carries a toxin or radionuclide capable of killing the cell directly.

Bispecific antibodies, are a new class of mAbs. Blinatumomab is an example and is able to recognize two distinct antigenic targets. Blinatumomab targets CD19 on B-cell malignancies (and normal B cells) and CD3 on normal T cells. By aligning the CD19-expressing cancer with a T cell, and simultaneously activating the T cell through its CD3 molecule, the T cell recognizes the cancer and eliminates it. Patients with a high burden of disease are now experiencing dramatic remissions compared with previously (Handgretinger et al., 2011).

Prevention of cancer

Adult cancers can be associated with lifestyle factors, such as being overweight, eating an unhealthy diet, not getting enough exercise, and habits like smoking and drinking alcohol. Lifestyle factors usually take many years to influence cancer risk, thus they are not thought to play much of a role in childhood cancers. We know that most childhood cancers are not caused by inherited DNA changes but the reasons for the few that are, are not known.

Promoting healthy lifestyles to families with children is of upmost importance, particularly to instil good role modelling at an early age. Targeting teenagers and young adults regarding the risks of developing cancer from smoking and poor sexual behaviours is also essential. Indeed, teenagers who are survivors of childhood cancer are encouraged to accept the human papillomavirus (HPV) vaccine as it is known to be highly effective at preventing HPV infections (Wentzensen et al., 2015). It is particularly important to this patient cohort, as their risk of developing a cancer later in life is slightly greater than that of the general population.

Examples of cancers

Case Study   Acute lymphoblastic leukaemia

Adam is a 13 year old who lives at home with his mother, stepfather, and his two half-siblings, Emma age 2 and Ted 5. Mother is a primary school teacher and stepfather is employed by a local engineering company and works shifts. Adam's biological father is believed to be unemployed and was last known to live >2 hours away; he has had decreasing contact with Adam over the previous 5 years with no contact in the past 2. The family have their own car and both maternal and paternal grandparents live >1 hour away by car. Paternal grandparents are in poor health and maternal grandparents both work. Adam presented to his GP 2 weeks ago with malaise, fever and bruising of unknown cause. He has been admitted to his local district general hospital and is on the children's ward. A series of screening bloods have been taken: full blood count (FBC) including blood film, urea and electrolytes (U&Es), liver function tests (LFTs), and chest X-ray. A FBC demonstrates a low haemoglobin (Hb), elevated white cell count (WCC), low platelets, neutrophils and blast cells. This raises suspicion of a blood cancer and he will need further investigation in a specialist children's hospital with a primary treatment centre (PTC) for paediatric cancer. The nearest one for Adam's family is 45 minutes away by car. Understandably the family are devastated but they have been involved with telling Adam what may be wrong with him.

Investigation	Results	Reference range
Hb g/dL	56 g/dL	130–160
White cell count 10^9/L	66	4.5–14.5
Platelets 10^9/L	21	150–450
Neutrophils 10^9/L	1.2	1.8–8.0
Blasts	70%	0

Think about the information presented and then consider the following points:

- Consider the social history and list some factors that will have a significant impact on the family if Adam is confirmed to have a blood cancer.
- What professionals will be required to support the family?

Adam is transferred that evening to the PTC and receives further diagnostic testing including a bone marrow (BM) aspirate under general anaesthetic. He recovers well from the anaesthetic but he continues to ooze blood from his iliac crest where the bilateral BM aspirates were performed. The BM confirms a diagnosis of acute lymphoblastic leukaemia (ALL). He has no poor risk cytogenetics identified from his BM. The family receive a specific plan of treatment from Adam's treating consultant haematologist. They are aware that Adam will receive 3 years of treatment, which is further broken down into courses comprising: induction, intensification, and maintenance. The induction and intensification courses are delivered primarily as an inpatient with some treatment being given in the community. Maintenance therapy is delivered as an outpatient with clinic visits either weekly or once every 2 weeks, and a day-case theatre visit once every 12 weeks for a lumbar puncture (LP) and administration of intrathecal (IT) chemotherapy. As discussed earlier, the drug therapy will cause pancytopenia (anaemia, neutropenia, and thrombocytopenia). IT chemotherapy allows for penetration of the blood–brain barrier, which is not possible by the systemic chemotherapy agents. This route of administration is necessary to prevent relapse of CNS disease. Historically, CNS disease was treated using cranial irradiation, but long-term side effects of this treatment have been identified, specifically memory and learning problems. These are reduced with IT therapy while still achieving remission. Adam should NOT receive any live vaccines while he is receiving active cancer treatment.

Medicines Management

Children receiving cytotoxic drugs are at risk of infection, particularly bacterial. The risk is greatest in children undergoing intensive treatment such as HSCT, high-dose chemotherapy with stem cell support, or during leukaemia induction treatment.

Children with solid tumours can also become severely pancytopenic. Blood count nadir usually occurs 1–14 days after a course of treatment and recovery by day 21.

Prophylactic antibiotics are given to children who are expected to have a prolonged period of neutropenia. Neutropenia is classed as an actual neutrophil count (ANC) $\leq 0.5 \times 10^9$/L. Febrile neutropenia is classed as a single temperature $\geq 38.5\,°C$ or $>38\,°C$ on two occasions more than 1 hour apart. If N are between 0.5 and $<1.0 \times 10^9$/L, management is determined by the overall condition of the child and also whether the WCC is likely to still be falling or is expected to rise soon. Any child receiving chemotherapy who appears unwell but is not febrile or neutropenic may still require treatment with antibiotics. If in any doubt about whether antibiotics are needed, it is preferable to err on the side of caution and give them. Always refer to local policy and discuss with a senior colleague.

Now you have this additional treatment information and reflecting back to your earlier reading in this chapter:

- Consider and add to your earlier list, new factors that will have an impact on Adam and his family.
- What treatment group will Adam have been risk stratified into? Why?

Red Flag

Live vaccines should never be given to children receiving chemotherapy or within 6 months following completion of chemotherapy. Chemotherapy suppresses the immune response to vaccinations, potentially resulting in an attenuated response.

Inactivated influenza is the only exception to this rule and should be given during treatment and for those still within 6 months of completion of chemotherapy, unless the patient is less than 6 months of age, has an egg allergy or known history of an allergy to the specific vaccine.

- Thinking about Adam's age, what other aspects of his care should be considered by the multi-professional team?
- What further surgical procedure will Adam require?
- What are some of the other short-term effects Adam may experience from his cancer treatments?

Outcomes and survivorship

One in 1000 adults in the UK is a survivor of childhood cancer (CRUK, 2016b). This means that more than 26 000 young adults living in the UK are survivors of childhood cancer, meaning they are more than 5 years from the end of active treatment and remain disease free (CRUK, 2015).

As discussed earlier in this chapter, the action of cancer therapies means healthy cells, as well as cancerous cells, will be destroyed; the consequence of these cytotoxic effects on maturing tissues may only become apparent many years following completion of treatment and with subsequent development, hence the term 'late effects' (LE) (Bicheno, 2004). In comparison, short-term side effects of cancer treatments – such as alopecia, nausea and vomiting, and pancytopenia – are observed at the time of treatment. LE of treatment are different to side effects. A LE is the term used to describe any physical, psychological, or social consequence of the disease itself or the disease treatment.

The most common effect of these treatments is on growth, endocrine function, fertility, neuropsychology, and the cardiac systems. Two-thirds of childhood cancer survivors will experience at least one LE and the endocrine system is commonly involved. Another third of patients will develop two or more LE, which may be severe or life threatening (Oeffinger et al., 2006).

These occur more commonly in patients who receive increasing cumulative doses of both drug agents and IR, for example, a patient with ALL risk stratified as high risk goes on to suffer a relapse requiring a HSCT. More chemotherapy would be administered to achieve a further remission followed by total body irradiation (TBI) as conditioning before return of the stem cells. Another example is a patient with a medulloblastoma (malignant brain tumour). Treatment is prolonged, aggressive and involves chemotherapy often with adjuvant cranial IR, or even craniospinal IR. Patients such as these who receive high doses of IR experience significant neuropsychological late effects. The impact and burden of these is often life changing and impact significantly on the wider family unit.

Conclusion

Childhood cancer brings with it many challenges for the child, the family and those providing care. This chapter has provided an introduction to some childhood cancers. The chapter emphasises the need to ensure that the patient is safe and care delivered is appropriate and responsive to needs.

Children's cancers often differ from cancers that affect adults; they tend to occur in different parts of the body to adult cancers. When analysed under the microscope (histology), they also look different and respond differently to treatment.

Cure rates for children are much higher than for most adult cancers. Since the 1960s, the survival rate for children's cancer has more than doubled. On average, 82% (over 8 in 10) of all children can now be completely cured. For certain types of children's cancer, the cure rate is much higher than this.

It is important that those who are offering care to children and their families understand the pathophysiological changes that occur as well as the impact cancer can have on the child and family; holistic patient- and family-centred care is needed ensuring that all times the patient is at the centre of everything that is done. A competent and confident approach is required.

References

Anthony Nolan (2017). [online] Available at: https://www.anthonynolan.org/?gclid=Cj0KEQiAzNfDBRD2xKrO4pSnnOkBEiQAbzzeQcMzaLqUJ_XiFEYESyzFCv2xNezzNs0ybEaaHNG9zEIaAqDz8P8HAQ (accessed January 2017).

Bicheno, S. (2004). Childhood survivors. *Cancer Nursing Practice* 3(1), 12–14.

Brito-Babapulle, F., Bowcock, S.J., Marcus, R.E., et al. (1989). Autografting for patients with chronic myeloid leukaemia in chronic phase: peripheral blood stem cells may have a finite capacity for maintaining haematopoiesis. *British Journal of Haematology* 73, 76–81.

Cairo, M., Woessmann, D. & Pagel, J. (2013). Advances in hematopoietic stem cell transplantation (HSCT) in childhood and adolescent lymphomas. *Biology of Blood Marrow Transplant* 19(1 Suppl), S38–S43.

Cancer Research UK [CRUK] (2016a). Cancer statistics for the UK. [online] Available at: http://www.cancerresearchuk.org/health-professional/cancer-statistics (accessed December 2016).

Cancer Research UK [CRUK] (2016b). Children's cancer statistics. [online] Available at: http://www.cancerresearchuk.org/health-professional/cancer-statistics/childrens-cancers (accessed December 2016).

Children's Cancer and Leukaemia Group [CCLG] (2015). [online] Available at: http://www.cclg.org.uk/Survival-rates (accessed December 2016).

Children's Cancer and Leukaemia Group [CCLG] (2017) [online] Available at: http://www.cclg.org.uk/About-Us (accessed January 2017).

Cooper, C. (2015). Play works. Empowering children undergoing radiotherapy treatment at Sheffield Children's Hospital. *The Journal of the National Association of Health Play Specialists* 2(56), 8–12.

Elborai, Y., Hafez, H., Moussa, E.A., et al. (2016). Comparison of toxicity following different conditioning regimens for advanced stage neuroblastoma: experience of two transplant centers. *Pediatric Transplant* 20, 284–289.

English, M. (2009). Principles of chemotherapy. *Paediatrics and Child Health* 20(3), 123–128.

Estlin, E. (2000). The clinical and cellular pharmacology of vincristine, corticosteroids, L-asparaginase, anthracyclines and cyclophosphamide in relation to childhood acute lymphoblastic leukaemia. *British Journal of Haematology* 110, 780–790.

EuroNet-Paediatric Hodgkin Lymphoma Study Group (2013). Recommendations for the diagnostics and treatment of children and adolescents with a classical Hodgkin's lymphoma during the interim phase between the end of the EuroNet-PHL-C1 Study and the start of the EuroNet-PHL-C2 Study. [online] Available at: https://www.skion.nl/workspace/uploads/EuroNet-PHL-Interim-Treatment-Guidelines-2012-12-3v0-2.pdf (accessed January 2017).

Giusti, R.M., Iwamoto, K. & Hatch, E.E. (1995). *Annals of International Medicine* 122, 778–788.

Gluckman, E., Broxmeyer, H., Auerbach, A.D., et al. (1989). Hematopoietic reconstitution in a patient with Fanconi's anemia by means of umbilical cord blood from an HLA-identical sibling. *New England Journal of Medicine* 321, 1174–1178.

Handgretinger, R., Zugmaier, G., Henze, G., et al. (2011). Complete remission after blinatumomab-induced donor T-cell activation in three pediatric patients with post-transplant relapsed acute lymphoblastic leukemia. *Leukemia* 25(1), 181–184.

Harisiadis, L. & Chang, C.H. (1977). Medulloblastoma in children: a correlation between staging and results of treatment. *International Journal of Radiation Oncology • Biology • Physics* 2, 833–841.

Jones, J., Casey, R. & Karovia, F. (2010). Ionising radiation as a carcinogen. In: McQueen, C.A. (ed.). *Comprehensive Toxicology*. Elsevier, St. Louis.

Leblicq, C., Laverdie, C., Décarie, J., et al. (2013). Effectiveness of pamidronate as treatment of symptomatic osteonecrosis occurring in children treated for acute lymphoblastic leukemia. *Pediatric Blood Cancer* 60, 741–747.

Liu, D., Ahmet, A., Ward, L., et al. (2013). A practical guide to the monitoring and management of the complications of systemic corticosteroid therapy. *Allergy, Asthma & Clinical Immunology* 9(1), 30.

Louis, D.N., Ohgaki, H., Wiestler, O.D. & Cavenee, W.K. (eds). (2007). *WHO Classification of Tumours of the Central Nervous System*, 4th edn. International Agency for Research on Cancer, Lyon, France.

MacDonald, T. (2010). Paediatric cancer: a comprehensive review. Part II: Chemotherapy, monoclonal antibodies and tyrosine kinase inhibitors. *Canadian Pharmacist's Journal* 143(4), 240–247.

National Cancer Research Institute. Children's Cancer & Leukaemia Clinical Studies Group (NCRI CCL CSG) (2016). [online] Available at: http://csg.ncri.org.uk/groups/clinical-studies-groups/childrens-cancer-and-leukaemia/(accessed January 2017).

National Cancer Research Institute (NCRI) (2016). [online] Available at: http://www.ncri.org.uk/ (accessed January 2017).

Oeffinger, K., Mertens, A., Sklar, C., et al. (2006). Chronic health conditions in adult survivors of childhood cancer. *New England Journal of Medicine* 355, 1572–1582.

Paola, A.C. & Preciado, M.V. (2013). EBV primary infection in childhood and its relation to B-cell lymphoma development: a mini-review from a developing region. *International Journal of Cancer* 133, 1286–1292.

Pritchard-Jones, K. (1996). Genetics of childhood cancer. *British Medical Bulletin* 52(4), 704–723.

Remberger, M., Ackefors, M., Berglund, S., et al. (2011). Improved survival after allogeneic hematopoietic stem cell transplantation in recent years. *Biology of Blood and Marrow Transplantation* 17(11), 1688–1697.

Satgé, D., Sasco, A.J. & Lacour, B. (2003). Are solid tumours different in children with Down's syndrome? *International Journal of Cancer* 106(2), 297–298.

Siegel, R., Naishadham, D. & Jemal, A. (2013). Cancer statistics 2013. *Cancer Journal for Clinicians* 63, 71–81.

Smith, H. & Phillips, B. (2012). Childhood cancer. *innovAiT* 5(10), 595–603.

Stewart, A., Webb, J. & Hewitt, D. (1958). A survey of childhood malignancies. *British Medical Journal* 1495–1508.

Stiller, C.A. (2004a). Epidemiology and genetics of childhood cancer. *Oncogene* 23, 6429–6444.

Stiller, C.A. (2004b). In: Pinkerton, C.R., Plowman, P.N. & Pieters, R. (eds). *Paediatric Oncology*, 3rd edn. Arnold, London, pp. 3–24.

Thompson, E.B. (1994). Apoptosis and steroid hormones. *Molecular Endocrinology* 8(6), 665–673.

Urquhart, T. & Collin, J. (2016). Understanding the endocrinopathies associated with the treatment of childhood cancer: Part 2. *Nursing Children and Young People* 28(9), 36–41.

Vora, A. (2016). Childhood acute lymphoblastic leukaemia. In: Hoffbrand, V., Higgs, D., Keeling, D. & Mehta, A. (eds). *Postgraduate Haematology*, 7th edn. Wiley, Oxford.

Wentzensena, N., Schiffmana, M., Palmer, T. & Arbync, M. (2015). Triage of HPV positive women in cervical cancer screening. *Journal of Clinical Virology* 76, S49–55.

Wills-Alcoser, P. & Rodgers, C. (2003). Treatment strategies in childhood cancer. *Journal of Paediatric Nursing* 18(2), 103–112.

World Health Organization (2013). *International Classification of Diseases for Oncology*, 3rd edn. [online] Available at: http://apps.who.int/iris/bitstream/10665/96612/1/9789241548496_eng.pdf?ua=1 (accessed January 2017).

Chapter 4

Homeostasis

Mary Brady

Aim

The aim of this chapter is to help you to further develop and apply your understanding of homeostatic mechanisms within the body related to children and young people (0–18 years of age), to enable you to provide high-quality, safe and effective informed care.

This chapter will build on the learning gained in Chapters 2, 10, 11 and 13 in Peate and Gormley-Fleming (2015).

Learning outcomes

On completion of this chapter, the reader will be able to:

- Revisit homeostasis.
- Describe the impact of dehydration homeostasis.
- Describe the impact of respiratory illness on homeostasis.
- Describe the impact of renal disease on homeostasis.
- Describe the impact of diabetes on homeostasis.
- Describe how any changes in the child's condition should be escalated to senior staff.

Keywords

- homeostatic regulation
- internal and external environments
- feedback systems
- compensatory systems
- metabolism
- hormones
- pituitary gland
- hypothalamus
- nervous system
- electrolytes
- homeostatic disorders

Fundamentals of Children's Applied Pathophysiology: An Essential Guide for Nursing and Healthcare Students, First Edition.
Edited by Elizabeth Gormley-Fleming and Ian Peate.
© 2019 John Wiley & Sons Ltd. Published 2019 by John Wiley & Sons Ltd.
Companion website: www.wileyfundamentalseries.com/childpathophysiology

Test your prior knowledge

1. What is homeostasis?
2. What conditions affect hydration of the body?
3. How do acute and chronic respiratory illnesses affect the body?
4. How do acute and chronic renal illnesses affect the body?
5. What effect does diabetes have on homeostasis?
6. How should the nurse escalate his or her concerns to senior staff?

Introduction

The World Health Organization (WHO, 2016) revealed that 5.9 million children under the age of 5 died in 2015; children living in sub-Saharan Africa are more than 14 times more likely to die before they reach their 5th birthday. Leading causes are preterm birth, pneumonia, birth asphyxia, diarrhoea and malaria. WHO noted that of the deaths recorded, more than half could have been prevented or treated with simple interventions.

As described in Brady (2015), the cells of the human body function within a narrow range of parameters and there are various mechanisms that operate to enable this balance to be maintained. Much of this book will address the imbalance due to illness and this chapter will focus on the pathophysiology that disrupts normal homeostatic control.

Children's nurses will often care for children and young people whose ability to maintain homeostasis will be severely impaired and in such situations, it becomes imperative that the nurse can detect subtle changes indicating altered homeostasis, initiate appropriate emergency care, and escalate his/her concerns appropriately to other members of the multidisciplinary team, to instigate the best evidence-based care. Integral to this is the ability to clearly communicate the changes in the child/young person to their family or carers and to be able to explain any treatments provided.

This chapter will use the term 'child' to refer to those in the 0–18-year age range, except where specific information is provided for neonates and premature infants.

Dehydration

Children are more prone to dehydration due to their large surface area to volume ratio and higher percentage of water volume ranging between 60% and 80% (Kanneh, 2010) depending on their age. Fluid loss due to acute gastroenteritis accounts for about 1.7 million cases globally of which 760 000 deaths per year occurred in children under 5 years old (WHO, 2013).

Dehydration due to gastrointestinal fluid loss

Please revisit Chapter 12, Outerridge (2015).

Babies under 1 year are particularly susceptible to dehydration because of their large surface area and immature kidneys that are unable to concentrate urine (Gormley-Fleming, 2015).

Babies are also more susceptible to gastrointestinal infections that cause diarrhoea and vomiting because of reduced hydrochloric acid in their stomach and an immature immune system, especially if the baby was born prematurely. At birth, the stomach contents are less acidic with a neutral pH of 7 due to the amniotic fluid that has been swallowed while in utero (Chamley et al., 2005). Gradually with the introduction of feeding, especially breast feeding, *Lactobacillus bifidus* proliferates and this helps to increase the acidity within the stomach. Furthermore, Westerbeek et al.'s (2006) review of the literature clearly identified the beneficial effects of breast feeding in preterm babies due to the presence of bifidobacteria and lactobacilli, which suppress the growth of potentially pathogenic bacteria. By about 10 years of age, gastric secretions have reached adult levels; thus, children are vulnerable to gastrointestinal infections during the early part of their life and this is a relatively common problem seen in both the developed and developing world.

When a child loses fluid through vomiting and diarrhoea, s/he can quickly become dehydrated and experience medical 'shock', where the volume of circulating fluids is insufficient to perfuse the organs. Normally, with the onset of dehydration, receptors in the anterior hypothalamus detect changes in the osmolality and volume of the extracellular fluid (in the interstitial spaces and plasma) triggering messages of thirst in the individual, who can address this need; however, very young children are unable to verbalise this except through crying to alert their parent or carer who in turn provides the necessary fluids.

An unwell child has a reduced blood volume that leads to a decrease in blood pressure, although it is important to note that hypotension is a late sign in children due to their ability to compensate for fluid loss. The reduced circulating blood volume stimulates the kidneys to release the enzyme renin, which acts on angiotensin converting it to angiotensin I, which is converted into angiotensin II by the angiotensin-converting enzyme (ACE) produced by the lungs and nephrons. Angiotensin II causes aldosterone to be produced by the adrenal cortex, which leads to vasoconstriction of the arterioles, which subsequently helps to increase the blood pressure (Fig. 4.1).

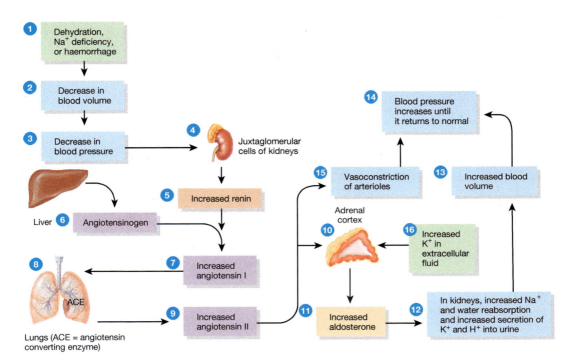

Figure 4.1 Regulation of aldosterone by the renin-angiotensin-aldosterone pathway. *Source:* Tortora & Derrickson 2009, in Peate & Gormley-Fleming 2015. Reproduced with permission of Wiley.

A child who has lost fluid will also have lost weight, so it is important that the child is accurately weighed, enabling an estimation of their weight loss to be calculated and fluid rehydration commenced appropriately. Therefore, all children under 2 years of age should be weighed naked. As a nurse you will also record observations of temperature, pulse, respiratory rate, blood pressure, oxygen saturation, capillary refill time, as well as noting the appearance of their skin and eye turgor, fontanelle depression and urine output (Rudolph, Lee & Levene, 2011).

The fontanelle in infants under 18 months is a useful indicator of their state of hydration, with a depressed fontanelle indicating dehydration. Early signs of shock include restlessness and tachycardia with a weak pulse, pallor and a widening core-peripheral temperature gap. These observations become even more crucial as the child's condition worsens and they become quiet and lethargic. The amount of urine produced will reduce as the body strives to conserve fluid, and kidney perfusion reduces due to hypotension.

To gain a more accurate clinical picture, blood samples are taken promptly, such as blood gas analysis, urea and electrolytes, and blood glucose (Table 4.1) to identify the cause and initiate treatment.

Kanneh (2010) explained that blood tests help to clarify the type of dehydration present (Table 4.2); stating that since normal plasma sodium in a child is greater than 145 mmol/l, symptoms would be apparent when the sodium level was less than 120 mmol/l or above 150 mmol/l. NICE (2015b) guidance exists to guide appropriate fluid rehydration.

Table 4.1 Signs and symptoms of medical shock

Observation	Finding
Temperature	Depends on the underlying cause, may be raised due to infection
Heart rate	Tachycardic
Respiratory rate	Tachypnoea
Colour	Pallor with peripheral mottling or cyanosis
Blood pressure	May be normal or low
Level of consciousness	Restless, confused,
Oxygen saturations	May be normal or low depending on the cause
Capillary refill	More than 2 seconds

Table 4.2 Blood tests used in dehydration

Test	Finding
Blood gas	Anaerobic tissue metabolism
Haemoglobin (Hb)	Reduced due to haemorrhage
Packed cell volume (PCV)	Decreased due to haemorrhage Raised if less than 55% plasma due to hypovolaemia
Urea	Raised urea indicating reduced GFR and kidney excretory capacity due to hypovolaemia
Sodium	Raised if the fluid volume in the blood vessels and cells is reduced giving a higher concentration of solute
Plasma osmolality	Raised if there is less fluid in the blood vessels giving a concentrated plasma
Blood glucose	Hypoglycaemia
Electrocardiogram	Cardiac arrhythmia due to abnormal potassium levels
Central venous pressure (CVP)	Low in severe dehydration. A CVP line will monitor fluid replacement

About 70% of dehydrated children have isonatraemic dehydration with plasma sodium levels between 135–145 mmol/l and normal plasma osmolality of 275–295 mOsm/kg H_2O. This is usually due to diarrhoea and vomiting and in this situation the amount of sodium and water loss is equal and the kidneys facilitate equilibrium by compensating; however, the extracellular fluid in the blood vessels and interstitial space is reduced with the ensuing hypotension.

About 10% of dehydration is hyponatraemic where more sodium is lost via micturition and usually arises due to severe burns or vomiting and diarrhoea. Intravenous fluids may be given or the child could be encouraged, if well enough, to drink large quantities of sugary drinks, thereby counteracting the fluid loss as the cells take in the glucose and leave the water in the extracellular spaces. Careful monitoring is required to ensure the correct diagnosis, since the imbalance could be due to water intoxication where too much water has been consumed or where the cause is due to inappropriate ADH syndrome.

Twenty percent of children will have hypernatraemic dehydration with plasma sodium levels greater than 145 mmol/l and plasma osmolality greater than 295 mOsm/kg H_2O. In this situation, more water is lost than sodium and it is a manifestation of conditions such as diabetes insipidus, hyperpyrexia and hyperventilation with loss of fluids due to increased insensible loss. Another reason could be the accidental administration of hypertonic intravenous fluids. In an effort to dilute the plasma, fluid in the cells passes into the circulatory system. A similar situation arises with diabetes mellitus, where there is hyperglycaemia instead of hypernatraemia. The end result is a reduced volume in the circulatory system and in the interstitial spaces.

Dehydration due to blood loss

Children may suffer haemorrhage following surgery or trauma; the cause needs to be ascertained promptly and investigations commenced as per Table 4.1, plus obtaining a full blood count (FBC) where the haemoglobin (Hb) and packed cell volume levels (PCV) will be decreased due to haemorrhage. As well as administering intravenous fluids (0.9% saline), a blood transfusion may also be given depending on the severity of the blood loss. Drugs to strengthen cardiac function (inotropes) may also be required.

The child requiring surgery

In the past, concern has been raised regarding the possibility of regurgitation and aspiration of acidic gastric contents for all patients undergoing surgery, and to reduce this incidence all patients requiring surgery were fasted overnight prior to undergoing surgery. However, with children this is recognised as dangerous because of the risk of dehydration; it is also unnecessary due to their different physiology, for instance, babies have faster stomach emptying times, especially if fed breast milk (Neill & Knowles, 2004).

The RCN (2005) has provided clear guidance regarding pre-operative fasting for children, which has been further endorsed by Brady *et al.*'s (2009) systematic review. Brady *et al.* (2009) observed that children who were allowed to drink up to 2 hours before surgery were less thirsty and more comfortable than those who were fasted for longer. Current guidance advises that 6 hours prior to surgery, all patients should be advised to stop taking solid food, milk and milk-containing drinks, and should only drink clear fluids until 2 hours prior to their operation, after which they fast. Breast milk can be given up to 4 hours prior to surgery; however, for children who are at a higher risk of regurgitation, individual decisions will be made by the clinical staff in the best interest of the child and this may include commencing intravenous fluids to prevent dehydration (Aker & O'Sullivan, 1998).

The child with respiratory impairment

Respiratory problems are common in childhood, accounting for about 50% of GP consultations (Lissauer & Clayden, 2011). These illnesses can range from upper respiratory tract infections to bronchiolitis, chest infections, asthma, and many more.

When a child's ability to breathe is compromised, the amount of oxygen circulating falls (hypoxia) and carbon dioxide (CO_2) levels increase (hypercapnia). This reaction stimulates chemoreceptors within the aorta and carotid arteries, information is then transmitted via the glossopharyngeal and vagus nerves stimulating the diaphragm and intercostal muscles to contract, thereby increasing the intake of oxygen and exhalation of CO_2. These muscles also receive further impulses via the phrenic and intercostal nerves, as the rising level of CO_2 within the cerebrospinal fluid is detected by chemoreceptors within the medulla oblongata (Figs 4.2 and 4.3).

So the child or young person's respiratory rate becomes faster and deeper to remove the excess CO_2. If the situation continues the CO_2 combines with water to form carbonic acid ($^-HCO_3$), which alters the pH of the circulating blood, as demonstrated in the reversible equation below:

$$CO_2 + H_2O \leftrightarrow H_2CO_3 \leftrightarrow H^+ +^- HCO_3$$

Since the reason for the shift in pH is due to an accumulation of acid and the origin is respiratory, the child or young person is described as having a respiratory acidosis.

Children and young people who have chronic respiratory or cardiac problems, such as cystic fibrosis, tend to tolerate higher than normal CO_2 levels, so their physiology differs, in that the stimulus to breathe depends on a low level of oxygen. It follows that when administering oxygen to a child with a chronic respiratory or cardiac problem and using a pulse

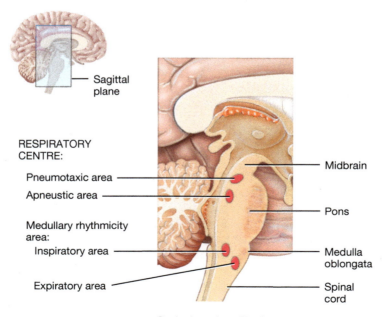

Figure 4.2 Locations of areas of the respiratory centre. *Source:* Tortora & Derrickson 2006, in Peate & Gormley-Fleming 2015. Reproduced with permission of Wiley.

Homeostasis Chapter 4

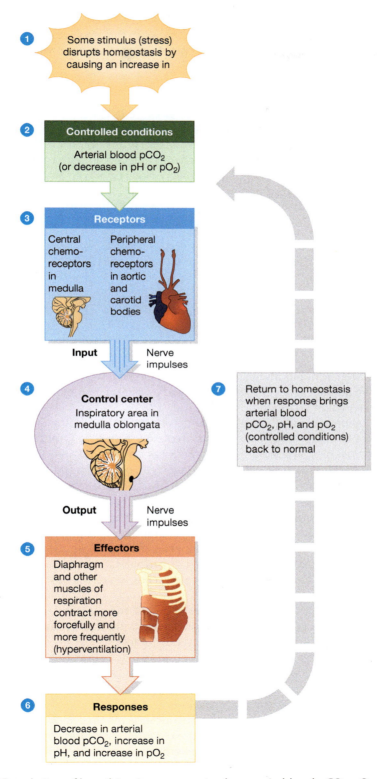

Figure 4.3 Regulation of breathing in response to changes in blood pCO_2, pO_2 and pH (H^+ concentration) via negative feedback control. *Source:* Tortora & Grabowski 2003. Reproduced with permission of Wiley.

oximeter to titrate the amount of oxygen required, it is possible to impede the stimulus to breathe, so agreement needs to be reached between the medical and nursing staff caring for the child/young person regarding acceptable oxygen saturation levels, for example, to keep saturations at 85% rather than above 94%.

The child with renal impairment

Please revisit Chapter 13, Gormley-Fleming (2015).

Chronic kidney disease is a major worldwide public health concern that affects 6–16% of the adult population (Kim *et al.*, 2013). Often the renal impairment may have been acquired in childhood or due to a congenital abnormality. Nowadays, with antenatal screening, congenital abnormalities are detected in 1 in 200–400 births enabling damage limitation interventions to prevent renal scarring that would otherwise affect kidney function (Lissauer & Clayden, 2011). Antenatal screening can detect:

- absent kidney (renal agenesis)
- multicystic dysplastic kidney
- horseshoe kidney
- duplex kidney
- bladder exstrophy
- pelvi-ureteric junction obstruction
- vesico-ureteric junction obstruction
- urethral valves (male infant).

Acquired renal conditions include urinary tract infections and conditions considered to be due to an autoimmune reaction following a bacterial or viral infection, such as nephrotic syndrome and glomerulonephritis.

Inflammation of the nephron at the glomerular region results in a disruption to filtration, which allows protein to leak out of the circulatory system with ensuing water loss and hypoalbuminaemia. Hypoalbuminaemia reduces oncotic pressure that counterbalances hydrostatic pressure causing hypotension leading to oedema, as fluid accumulates outside the circulatory system in the interstitial space. The child, although oedematous, is hypovolaemic due to the shift in fluid location, which leads to sodium retention either by triggering the renin–angiotensin response (Brady, 2015) or in nephrotic syndrome the renal tubule may be affected which means that sodium retention occurs (McFarlane, 2010).

A further complication of hypoalbuminaemia affects the pleural and peritoneal membranes resulting in the movement of fluid into the pleural space resulting in a pleural effusion and into the peritoneal space resulting in ascites, which will have an additional impact on breathing (McFarlane, 2010).

Glomerulonephritis may result in a reduction of the glomerular filtration rate (GFR), which leads to a reduced urine output and the retention of sodium and water with ensuing oedema and hypertension as the water is redistributed.

When hypovolaemia is detected by baroreceptors in the aortic arch and carotid sinus with ensuing slight reduction in blood pressure, the child's body initially compensates by increasing the heart and respiratory rate to maximise oxygen transportation around the body. Additionally, the peripheral circulation vasoconstricts and fluid moves from the interstitial spaces into the intravascular compartments to increase the circulating blood volume and the pulse pressure (difference between systolic and diastolic pressures) reduces as will the capillary refill time. The renin–angiotensin–aldosterone system is also activated, which results in an increase in the blood pressure (Brady, 2015). However, the situation is temporary, because children are able to withstand a loss of 20–25% of their circulating volume (Elliott, Callery & Mould, 2010) and require correction of the fluid loss to avoid hypotension and cell necrosis.

Homeostasis Chapter 4

The child with an infection

Please revisit Chapter 7, Mosenthal (2015).

Infections are a common aspect of childhood and account for the deaths of about 7 million children across the world during their first 5 years of life (Lissauer & Clayden, 2011). At birth, the term baby possesses an immature immune system consisting of immunoglobulins acquired from the mother transplacentally. This innate immune system consists of barriers (such as the skin and mucous membranes), cell-mediated mechanisms and antimicrobial proteins, which provide a humoral defence mechanism (Fig. 4.4).

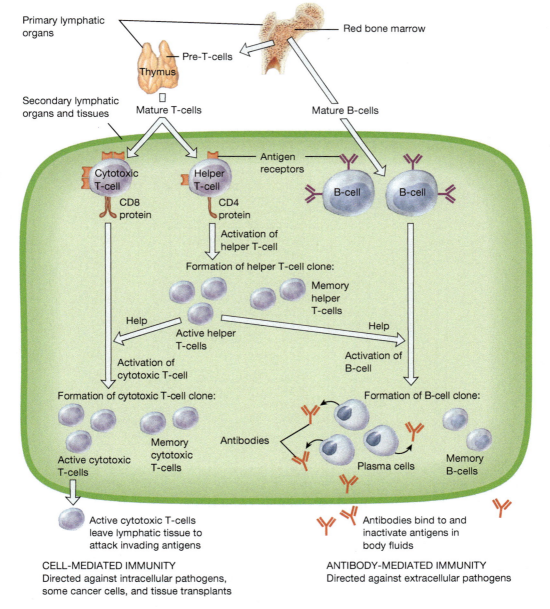

Figure 4.4 Cellular and humoral immune responses. *Source:* Tortora & Derrickson 2009, in Peate & Gormley-Fleming 2015. Reproduced with permission of Wiley.

Over the ensuing few months, these reduce, increasing the baby's vulnerability to infection, but at the same time the body learns to adapt its immune response as it becomes exposed to a variety of pathogens.

If the baby has no immunity to a specific bacterium or virus and this micro-organism gains access to the tissues, where they rapidly reproduce, plasma proteins known as complement are activated, initiating phagocytosis where the invading micro-organism is engulfed in an effort to destroy the infection. The macrophages are derived from monocytes and neutrophils (formed from the bone marrow); however, the neutrophils are short-lived but do have a fast response and ability to create antibactericidal enzymes known as lysozymes, which destroy the bacteria.

Inflammation also occurs and is seen as redness, swelling, heat and pain, for example, with inflamed skin, tonsils, breathing difficulties due to reduced airway lumen. Histamine and serotonin are released causing vasodilation, which enables a greater flow of blood (with plasma proteins) to the affected area to trap and destroy the invading micro-organisms. The accumulated dead cells and micro-organisms form pus, which may be visible at the site of infection, such as in tonsillitis with red, inflamed, pus-producing tonsils. See Fig. 4.5, a flow chart demonstrating inflammatory events.

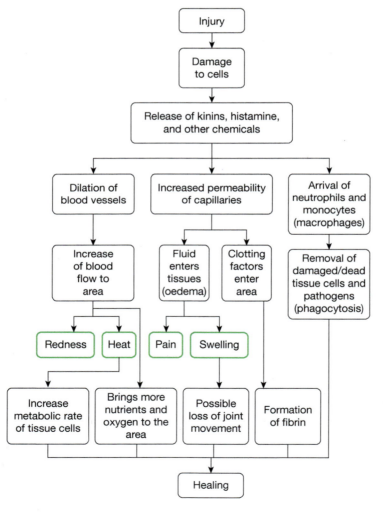

Figure 4.5 Flowchart of inflammatory events. *Source:* Adapted from Marieb 2012.

Prostaglandin and leukotrienes are produced by the cell walls of the affected tissue and are responsible for the pain associated with inflammation. The body temperature increases after the release of cytokines by macrophages which act on the hypothalamus causing a resetting of thermoregulation. The hypothalamus stimulates the sympathetic nervous system to cause vasoconstriction, raising the metabolic rate. To deal with the increased metabolic rate there is an increased demand for oxygen and energy release from glycogen stores. Usually a higher temperature indicates the more pathogens in the body; however, children under 5 have an immature nervous system and thereby immune response, so temperature does not always correlate with the severity of the infection (Neill & Knowles, 2004).

Furthermore, the steep rise in temperature may result in a febrile convulsion as the body reacts to the hyperpyrexia. This is an alarming event for parents who may be concerned that their child will develop epilepsy. Febrile convulsions are usually benign and due to a viral infection but if focal, prolonged or repeated should be investigated for an underlying pathology (Lissauer & Clayden, 2011).

The pyrexia that accompanies an infection is believed to be therapeutic, in that it reduces the availability of iron and zinc in the blood, which are needed by bacteria for growth, and may also create an ambient temperature that renders the bacteria inert. However, the concomitant sweating may cause dehydration, especially since small children have relatively large heads in comparison to their bodies and may lose significant heat and water by evaporation.

The diabetic child

Please revisit Chapter 2, Brady (2015).

Diabetes is a condition where the body's ability to metabolise glucose is impaired resulting in hyperglycaemia. According to Diabetes UK (2016), its incidence in the United Kingdom is estimated to be 24.5 per 100 000; of these, an estimated 95.1% have type 1, 1.9% have type 2, and 2.73% have maturity-onset diabetes of the young (under 25 when diagnosed).

Type 1 diabetes is an autoimmune disease that appears to involve genetic predisposition and environmental triggers (Gan, Albanese-O'Neil & Haller, 2012), whereas type 2 diabetes is related to obesity and appears to be increasing in children/young people.

In diabetes, an autoimmune response leads to the destruction of beta cells with the resultant inability to respond adequately to the need for insulin to release glucose for energy, thus seriously impairing homeostasis.

Insulin and glucagon are hormones that are secreted by the pancreas. Insulin is secreted by beta cells and glucagon by alpha cells. When blood glucose levels rise insulin is secreted and acts on the cell membranes enabling the conversion of glucose into glycogen for storage in the liver and muscles (by glycogenesis) and the storage of fats within adipose tissue. When blood glucose levels fall, glucagon is secreted, which acts on the liver enzyme phosphorylase that enables glycogen to be converted to glucose for release into the blood circulation.

Newly diagnosed children/young people have usually exhibited the symptoms of lethargy, thirst, weight loss and polyuria in the preceding weeks. Their blood results will indicate above normal blood glucose levels and metabolic acidosis. Depending on their blood results the child may need rehydration with 0.9% saline intravenously and correction of acidosis.

Overall management of this challenging condition involves good glycaemic control, measured by frequent blood glucose tests and titration of insulin accordingly, as well as 2–3-monthly glycated haemoglobin A_{1c} (HbA_{1c} levels) to reduce the development of microvascular complications such as retinopathy, nephropathy and neuropathy (NICE, 2015a).

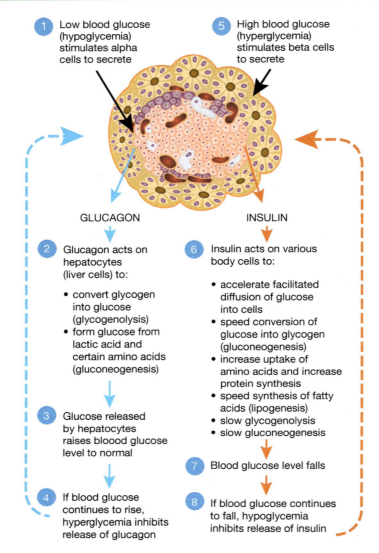

Figure 4.6 Negative feedback regulation of the secretion of glucagon (blue arrows) and insulin (orange arrows). *Source:* Tortora & Derrickson 2011. Reproduced with permission of Wiley.

Technological developments over recent years have enabled improved control with the use of continuous infusion pumps that enable a basal rate of insulin to be infused and additional boluses to be given as required. Home blood testing is also more accessible with user-friendly devices that enable the transfer of data to a computer, which enables tracking of glycaemic control.

At times, extreme levels of hyperglycaemia arise resulting in the potentially fatal condition called diabetic ketoacidosis (DKA). This may be due to illness or non-compliance with insulin injections and results in glycosuria and metabolic acidosis caused by the metabolism of fats and proteins into glucose. The hyperosmolar effect of glycosuria causes the excretion of vast amounts of urine with ensuing dehydration.

An electrolyte imbalance also occurs as potassium is lost in the urine and the higher levels of sodium within the body lead to accumulation of water within the cells, with an associated risk of cerebral oedema as fluid enters the brain cells (Lissauer & Clayden, 2011). Careful fluid rehydration with 0.9% saline, correction of potassium deficits and insulin infusion titrated to blood glucose levels is required. In addition to the usual observations, neurological observations are required to detect any cerebral oedema and subsequent neurological deficit.

Hypoglycaemia is another complication and can be due to a discrepancy between the amount of insulin given, food consumed, and exercise. It occurs when more insulin has been given in comparison to the intake of food. Correction is by addressing the hypoglycaemia with sufficient carbohydrate and adjustment of insulin dosage. The cause needs to be ascertained, for example, concurrent infection or growth spurt and involvement of the Diabetic Specialist Nurse may also be required to help address any underlying reasons.

During puberty, hormonal changes that result in increased growth (and increased insulin requirements), and changes due to cognitive development and the transition towards independence have an impact on diabetic control where glycaemic control may be erratic.

Illness and infection also have a negative impact on glycaemic control; as the body responds to the stress, the adrenal glands produce adrenaline and noradrenaline. The production of adrenaline results in an increased need for glucose with associated need for insulin; however, the diabetic is unable to respond and will therefore rely on the administration of extra insulin via injection or pump mechanism. It follows that during times of illness, the need for vigilance of blood glucose and ketones levels is imperative in ensuring that homeostasis is maintained. Increasing ketone levels indicate that the body has had to metabolise fat and amino acids to facilitate glucose availability.

Escalating your concerns as a nurse

As a nurse, you should be observing for pyrexia, tachycardia, tachypnoea, low saturations, hypotension, pallor, anorexia, tiredness and widening peripheral-core temperature gap. The frequency of these observations will depend on the child's condition and potential for deterioration. Your recordings will be noted on an observation chart to observe for trends and illustrate deterioration. As a nurse it is important that you recognise what observations are age-appropriate and can proactively escalate any deviations to relevant senior staff. Paediatric early warning score charts, alongside the Situation, Background, Assessment, Recommendation (SBAR) tool (https://www.england.nhs.uk/improvement-hub/wp-content/uploads/sites/44/2017/11/SBAR-Implementation-and-Training-Guide.pdf), are now being used increasingly to escalate concerns promptly and with all the relevant information; however, your interpretation and synthesis of data as a nurse are crucial to this activity. As always, accurate documentation of your findings and subsequent actions is fundamental.

Conclusion

During illness, the pathophysiology of homeostasis is a complex process which the body usually manages to return to stability. This chapter has explored some of the common illnesses that disrupt homeostasis. It has also explored the recording and interpretation of patient observations with subsequent analysis of the underlying pathophysiology. Furthermore, the prompt escalation of any concerns has been identified as an integral part of your role as a nurse.

To help consolidate your learning some activities have been included. The answers are at the end of this chapter. To assist with your analysis of the case studies, please use the PEWS (Paediatric Early Warning System) charts available at: http://ihub.scot/spsp/maternity-children-quality-improvement-collaborative-mcqic/pews/.

Case Study 1

Daisy is 9 months old and has been admitted to the emergency department with a 3-day history of diarrhoea and vomiting. It is estimated that she has lost about 10% of her body weight, which has been recorded as 7 kg. Daisy has a sunken fontanelle, looks pale and is rather drowsy and last had a wet nappy about 6 hours previously.

Her observations are:

Heart rate: 155/minute
Respiratory rate: 60/minute
Blood pressure: 90/45
Temperature: 36.5 °C
Oxygen saturation: 92%
Capillary refill: 4 seconds

Access the PEWS chart for 0–11 month olds and plot her observations, then decide on your actions as a nurse.

How would you cascade this data to a senior person?

What possible treatment will she require?

Case Study 2

Zac is a 6-year-old child who has been admitted to the ward. In the emergency department, he received a bronchodilating nebuliser, but remains pale with an audible wheeze, tracheal tug and use of intercostal accessory muscles. On admission his observations are:

Heart rate: 124
Respiratory rate: 30/minute with an audible wheeze
Temperature: 37 °C
Oxygen saturations in air: 91%
Capillary refill: 3–4
Blood pressure: 88/94

Access the PEWS chart for 5–12 year olds and plot Zac's observations, then decide on your actions as a nurse.

How would you cascade this data to a senior person?

What possible treatment will he require?

References

Aker, J. & O'Sullivan, C. (1998). The selection and administration of perioperative intravenous fluids for the pediatric patient. *Journal of PeriAnesthesia Nursing* 13(3), 172–181.

Brady, M. (2015). Homeostasis. In: Peate, I. & Gormley-Fleming, E. (eds). *Fundamentals of Children's Anatomy and Physiology*, 1st edn. Wiley, Oxford, pp. 17–39.

Brady, M.C., Kinn, S., Ness, V., et al. (2009). Preoperative fasting for preventing perioperative complications in children. *Cochrane Database of Systematic Reviews* (4): CD005285.

Chamley, C.A., Carson, P., Randall, D., et al. (2005). *Developmental Anatomy and Physiology of Children: A Practical Approach*. Elsevier, Edinburgh.

Diabetes UK (2016). https://www.diabetes.org.uk/ (last accessed 4 April 2018).

Elliott, B., Callery, P. & Mould, J. (2010). Caring for children with critical illness. In: Glasper, A. & Richardson, J. (eds). *A Textbook of Children and Young People's Nursing*, 2nd edn. Churchill Livingstone Elsevier, Edinburgh, pp. 691–718.

Gan, M.J., Albanese-O'Neil, A. & Haller, M.J. (2012). Type 1 diabetes: current concepts in epidemiology, pathophysiology, clinical care and research. *Current Problems in Pediatric Adolescent Health Care* 42, 269–291.

Gormley-Fleming, E. (2015). The renal system. In: Peate, I. & Gormley-Fleming, E. (eds). *Fundamentals of Children's Anatomy and Physiology*, 1st edn. Wiley, Oxford, pp. 282–304.

Kanneh, A. (2010). Caring for children and young people with body fluid and electrolyte imbalance. In: Glasper, A. & Richardson, J. (eds). *A Textbook of Children and Young People's Nursing*, 2nd edn. Churchill Livingstone Elsevier, London, pp. 353–368.

Kim, J.J., Booth, C.J., Waller, S., et al. (2013). The demographic characteristics of children with chronic kidney disease stages 3–5 in South East England over a 5-year period. *Archives of Disease in Childhood* 98, 189–194.

Lissauer, T. & Clayden, G. (eds) (2011). *Illustrated Textbook of Paediatrics*, 4th edn. Mosby Elsevier, Edinburgh.

Marieb, E.N. (2012). *Essentials of Human Anatomy and Physiology*, 10th edn. Pearson Benjamin Cummings, San Francisco.

McFarlane, K. (2010). Caring for children with genitourinary problems. In: Glasper, A. & Richardson, J. (eds). *A Textbook of Children and Young People's Nursing*, 2nd edn. Churchill Livingstone Elsevier, London, pp. 369–383.

Mosenthal, A. (2015). The immune system. In: Peate, I. & Nair, M. (eds). *Fundamentals of Anatomy and Physiology for Student Nurses*. Wiley, Oxford, pp. 140–166.

Neill, S. & Knowles, H. (2004). *The Biology of Child Health: A Reader in Development and Assessment*. Palgrave Macmillan, Basingstoke.

National Institute for Health and Care Excellence (NICE) (2015a). *Diabetes (type 1 and type 2) in children and young people: diagnosis and management*. NICE Guideline [NG18]. Methods, evidence and recommendations. [online]. Available at: https://www.nice.org.uk/guidance/ng18/resources/diabetes-type-1-and-type-2-in-children-and-young-people-diagnosis-and-management-1837278149317 (last accessed 9 April 2018).

National Institute for Health and Care Excellence (NICE) (2015b). *Intravenous fluid therapy in children and young people in hospital*. [online]. Available at: https://www.nice.org.uk/guidance/ng29/chapter/Recommendations#managing-hyponatraemia-that-develops-during-intravenous-fluid-therapy-2 (accessed 29 May 2018).

Outerridge, J. (2015). The digestive system and nutrition. In: Peate, I. & Gormley-Fleming, E. (eds). *Fundamentals of Children's Anatomy and Physiology*, 1st edn. Wiley, Oxford, pp. 256–281.

Peate, I. & Gormley-Fleming, E. (eds) (2015). *Fundamentals of Children's Anatomy and Physiology*, 1st edn. Wiley, Oxford.

Royal College of Nursing (RCN) (2005). Clinical Practice Guidelines. *Perioperative fasting in adults and children: An RCN guideline for the multidisciplinary team*. [online]. Available at: http://www.rcn.org.uk/_data/assets/pdf_file/0009/78678/002800.pdf (accessed 25 July 2016).

Rudolph, M., Lee, T. & Levene, M. (2011). *Paediatrics and Child Health*, 3rd edn. Wiley, Oxford.

Tortora, G.J. & Derrickson, B.H. (2009). *Principles of Anatomy and Physiology*, 12th edn. Wiley, Hoboken, NJ.

Tortora, G.J. & Derrickson, B.H. (2011). *Principles of Anatomy and Physiology*, 13th edn. Wiley, Hoboken, NJ.

Tortora, G.J. & Grabowski, S.R. (2003). *Principles of Anatomy and Physiology*, 10th edn. Wiley, Hoboken, NJ.

Westerbeek, E.A.M., van den Berg, A., Lafeber, H.N., et al. (2006). The intestinal bacterial colonisation in preterm infants: a review of the literature. *Clinical Nutrition* 25, 361–368.

World Health Organization (2013). Diarrhoeal disease. Fact sheet. [online]. Available at: http://www.who.int/mediacentre/factsheets/fs330/en/(accessed 11 July 2016).

World Health Organization (2016). *Breast feeding*. [online]. Available at: http://www.who.int/mediacentre/events/2016/world-breastfeeding-week/en/(accessed 11 July 2016).

Chapter 5

Inflammation, immune response and healing

Alison Mosenthal

Aim

This chapter provides the reader with an understanding of the complexities associated with inflammation and the immune response. Developing your understanding further can assist you to provide competent care to children and young people and their families.

Learning outcomes

On completion of this chapter, the reader will be able to:

- Describe the role and function of the blood cells, tissues and organs of the immune system.
- Differentiate between innate and adaptive immunity.
- Describe how the body responds to infection.
- Discuss the features of the inflammatory response.
- Describe the processes involved in wound healing.
- Discuss normal and abnormal pathophysiological changes occurring during the immune response.

Keywords

- organs and tissues
- immune system
- blood cells
- pathogens and infection
- inflammatory process
- innate immunity
- acquired immunity
- wound healing

Test your prior knowledge

1. Outline the role and function of the immune system.
2. List the blood cells, tissues and organs of the immune system.
3. Describe the natural barriers to infection.
4. Discuss what is meant by innate and adaptive immunity.
5. Describe the systemic signs of inflammation.
6. Discuss what factors might contribute to impaired immune function in the infant and child.

Introduction

From birth, an individual is exposed to a wide range of potentially harmful microbes such as bacteria, viruses and parasites. The immune system is made up of cells and tissues that resist infection and it is the coordinated reaction of these cells and tissues to an invading pathogen that provides the immune response in order to eliminate it. This defence against invading microbes is provided by two components of the immune system: the innate immune system and the adaptive immune system.

In this chapter these two types of immunity will be discussed and their roles in non-specific and specific immunity explored. As part of their response to infection the innate and adaptive components of the immune system also initiate the inflammatory response, and this will be discussed in relation to wound healing and acute and chronic inflammation.

Two key features of the immune system are its ability to recognise 'self' components from 'non-self' and its ability to react to a known antigen and prevent further infection. The immune system is manipulated to provide immunity with vaccination and to improve the success in organ transplantation. The immune system can also cause disease, however, if it is deficient or unable to make an appropriate immune response. This can occur in allergy, where a powerful immune response is made to a substance that is normally harmless such as pollen. The immune system's ability to self-regulate can also be affected and the body's immune cells can attack the body's own cells resulting in autoimmune diseases such as juvenile idiopathic arthritis. There are times when there is a defect or deficiency in the immune system and this can cause an increased susceptibility to infections, which in some cases can be life threatening. Some aspects of this altered pathophysiology of the immune system will also be discussed.

The immune system

The ability of the individual to defend itself against infection is described as host defence (Macpherson & Austyn, 2012) consisting of two components: innate immune system and adaptive immune system. Innate immunity is non-specific providing the first line of defence against an invading organism. It is an extremely rapid response, usually effective within minutes or hours in preventing and eliminating infection. Adaptive immunity takes longer to respond – usually within a few days – but a feature of this type of immunity is its ability to respond specifically to a known foreign protein (antigen) and its ability to respond rapidly to this known antigen if it encounters it again (immunological memory). Both types of immunity are essential to provide immunity to most types of infection. The innate immune system will activate the response from the adaptive immune system.

The immune system is made up of organs, tissues, cells and molecules that are connected by the blood and lymphatic systems. The coordinated reaction of these cells to infectious microbes is known as the immune response (Abbas, Lichtman & Pillai, 2016), see Fig. 5.1.

Inflammation, immune response and healing   Chapter 5

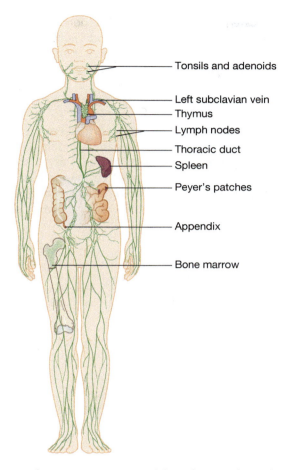

Figure 5.1 Distribution of organs, tissues and lymph vessels and nodes. *Source:* Peate & Gormley-Fleming 2015. Reproduced with permission of Wiley.

The blood cells primarily involved in immune function are the white blood cells (leukocytes) specialised to perform different functions. Those involved within the innate response are:

- neutrophils
- eosinophils
- basophils
- tissue macrophages and monocytes.

Further details regarding the roles of these cells are discussed in Chapter 7 of Peate and Gormley-Fleming (2015).

The other group of cells that play an important part in the innate response are the natural killer (NK) cells. These are able to detect the presence of virally infected cells and are described as cytotoxic (cell-killing) cells, which like the cytotoxic T cells (see later) play an important part in the destruction of virally infected cells.

The white blood cells involved in the adaptive immune response are the lymphocytes, divided into two main groups:

- B lymphocytes
- T lymphocytes.

Both types of cells are produced initially in the bone marrow but the B lymphocytes mature there before being released into the blood. The B lymphocytes have specific surface receptors to a known antigen, and exposure to that antigen stimulates the B cells to grow and multiply rapidly. There are two types of mature B cells: (1) plasma cells, which secrete antibodies that are produced as a response to a specific antigen; and (2) memory cells, which when they come into contact again with the antigen will rapidly start dividing to produce mature plasma cells.

The T lymphocytes migrate as immature lymphocytes to the thymus gland where they undergo a maturation process. They differentiate into different types of cells within the thymus, primarily as regulator and coordinator cells as part of the adaptive immune response, and also as cytotoxic cells that can kill cells (apoptosis) infected with viruses and other microbes. They also learn to recognise the body's own cells and learn to differentiate between self and non-self and develop the ability to combine with a specific antigen, see Fig. 5.2 and Table 5.1.

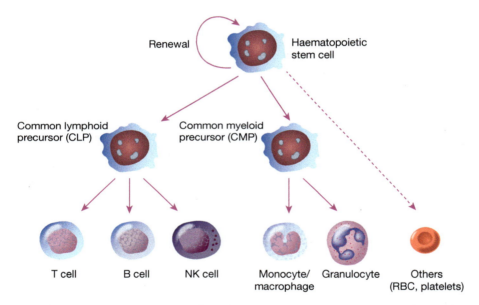

Figure 5.2 Diagram showing development of blood cells. *Source:* Adapted from MacPherson & Austyn 2012, in: Peate & Gormley-Fleming 2015.

Table 5.1 Different types of cells involved in the innate and adaptive immunity

Innate immune system	Function
Neutrophil	Phagocytosis
Macrophage	Phagocytosis, antigen presentation
Tissue mast cells	Release of histamine and other inflammatory mediators
Natural killer cells	Apoptosis of virally infected cells
Adaptive immune system	
B lymphocytes	Produce plasma cells which secrete immunoglobulin
T lymphocytes	Apoptosis of virally infected cells, activated cells release cytokines

Defence against infection

Our bodies are constantly exposed to micro-organisms in our environment and also to infectious agents from affected individuals. The majority of these micro-organisms do not cause disease but those that do can cause serious disease and sometimes death, and are known as pathogens. The major classes of pathogens are viruses, bacteria, protozoa and worms and the nature of a pathogen is to invade the host, reproduce and survive to infect other hosts. These pathogens use different mechanisms to achieve this – viruses and some bacteria and fungi live within the cells and viruses require the host cells to replicate. Other bacteria and fungi are found in extracellular spaces and some of the protozoa are too large to invade cells but can live in body cavities such as intestinal worms (Macpherson & Austyn, 2012). The action of these pathogens will trigger an immune response. The type of response will depend on the invading pathogen – the initial response by the innate immune system, followed by the inflammatory response, and then activation of the adaptive immune system.

Innate immune system (Fig. 5.3)

The innate immune system consists of a range of non-specific defence mechanisms to try and prevent entry by these pathogens and further infection. However, there are natural barriers, which provide a first line of defence before these systems are activated. The skin, and the mucosal surfaces of the respiratory, gastrointestinal and urogenital tracts are the first areas of contact for invading microbes and have specialised protective functions.

The skin

The skin provides a major barrier to the invasion of pathogenic bacteria. Many of the immune responses are initiated within the epithelial and dermal layers of the skin where the mast cells, macrophages and dendritic cells are situated. At birth the skin is sterile but rapidly becomes colonised by micro-organisms. The majority of these are harmless and are called commensal; they have a role in protecting the skin from being colonised

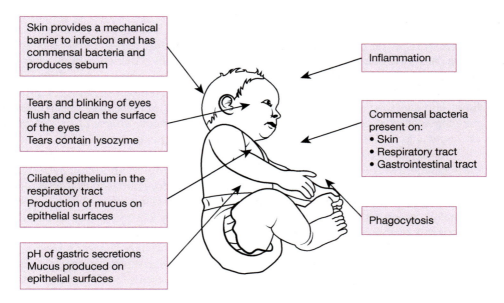

Figure 5.3   Features of the innate immune system.

by potentially pathogenic organisms. However, it is acknowledged that transmission of hospital-acquired infection from the skin of healthcare workers can occur with transfer of organisms to patients and equipment. Good hand hygiene is considered to be the most effective factor in the control of infection (Weston, 2013). Chapter 19 in Peate and Gormley-Fleming (2015) provides further detail on the anatomy and physiology of the skin.

The mucosal surfaces of the body

The epithelial membranes that line the respiratory, gastrointestinal and urogenital tracts contain goblet cells that produce mucus, which provides lubrication of those surfaces and can trap invading pathogens. In the respiratory tract, the cilia that line the tract move the mucus towards the mouth and nose so that inhaled pathogens can be removed by sneezing and coughing. Children with cystic fibrosis have recurrent respiratory tract infections because they are unable to expel the invading microbes. They require nebulised mucolytic drugs to reduce the viscosity of the mucus and daily physiotherapy to assist with its removal.

Apart from providing a physical barrier, the mucosal surfaces also produce chemical substances that are antimicrobial. Lysozyme is an antibacterial enzyme that is present in tears, perspiration and saliva, which can break down some bacterial cell walls. These secretions provide an acidic environment within which most bacteria are unable to survive. In the stomach, hydrochloric acid is secreted and the low pH in conjunction with the bile salts and digestive enzymes helps to destroy ingested pathogens. An individual who is unable to secrete gastric acid may be more susceptible to gastrointestinal infections such as *Salmonella* (Macpherson & Austyn, 2012; Helbert, 2017).

Another barrier to infection is the presence of commensal bacteria that are found on mucosal surfaces in the gastrointestinal tract, respiratory tract and the vagina and epithelial surfaces of the skin. These are micro-organisms that are found normally on these surfaces; they are sometimes referred to as 'friendly' bacteria as they form a barrier and prevent colonisation of pathogenic bacteria. This barrier can be disrupted by antibiotic treatment, which removes the commensal bacteria and the resulting invasion of the pathogenic organisms causes disease.

Phagocytosis

Phagocytosis is the process by which an invading organism is destroyed by phagocytic blood cells – the neutrophils and macrophages. These cells provide the body's first line of cellular defence and engulf, ingest and destroy the organism intracellularly. They are effective in removing small extracellular organisms, such as bacteria, small parasites (protozoa), fungi, and damaged and dead cells (Helbert, 2017). This is a crucial mechanism in the host defence against infection as it ensures that many infectious organisms do not become pathogenic to the individual as they are eliminated very quickly (see Fig. 5.4).

The two types of blood cells that are mainly involved in phagocytosis are neutrophils, and macrophages, which are derived from monocytes. Neutrophils and monocytes are both produced from the same stem cell in the bone marrow, more neutrophils than monocytes are produced on a daily basis. The neutrophils have a short life span (1–2 days) and are not normally present in tissues but, they respond very quickly when an infection occurs. They migrate quickly to the site of infection by a process of chemotaxis, where chemicals released by the invading bacteria and proteins at the site of infection stimulate this response.

The neutrophils have receptors that recognise bacteria and other pathogens (Helbert, 2017). They are essential for the defence against pyogenic (pus-forming) bacteria such as *Staphylococcus* and *Streptococcus*. During an infection the number of neutrophils will increase rapidly and the blood levels of neutrophils will be increased. The rapid production

Inflammation, immune response and healing   Chapter 5

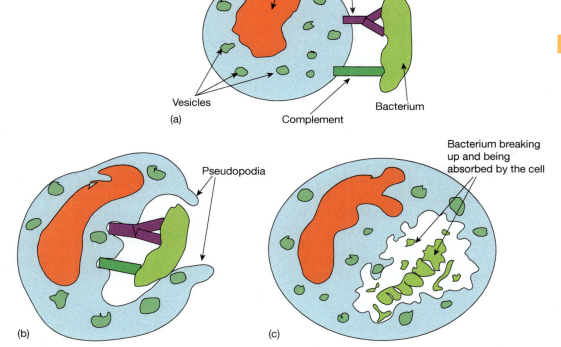

Figure 5.4 Stages of phagocytosis: (a) stage 1, (b) stage 2 and (c) stage 3. *Source:* Peate & Nair 2011, in: Peate & Gormley-Fleming 2015.

of neutrophils by the bone marrow is further stimulated by colony-stimulating factors released by the tissue macrophages. Neutrophils are highly phagocytic and once they have engulfed the invading microbe, antibactericidal enzymes such as lysozyme contained within the cytoplasmic granules are released to destroy it.

Medication Alert

The short life span of neutrophils means that when production of blood cells in the bone marrow is affected as in ionising radiation and in cancer chemotherapy treatment, the number of neutrophils decreases rapidly. Children undergoing stem cell transplant and oncology treatment and those who have a deficiency of neutrophils, such as in congenital neutropaenia, become neutropaenic (low neutrophil count) and are very vulnerable to bacterial and fungal infections.

Treatment for children undergoing stem cell transplant who have neutropaenia can be by subcutaneous injection of recombinant human granulocyte colony-stimulating factor (filgrastim). This can accelerate the production of neutrophils and help to protect a neutropaenic patient from a life-threatening bacterial infection. Common sites for the administration of this drug are the arms, thighs and abdomen. As with other subcutaneous treatments, it is important to ensure that the sites for administration are rotated.

Monocytes enter the tissues where they develop into macrophages. The macrophages are present in most body tissues and form an important part of the innate immune system. They possess receptors that can distinguish between different types of infectious agents, such as viruses, bacteria and fungi. Some of these receptors enable the macrophage to phagocytose the invading organism and others stimulate the release of cytokines. These are small hormone-like enzymes that attract neutrophils to the site of infection and also initiate the adaptive immune response. When an infection occurs, large numbers of monocytes migrate to the site of infection with neutrophils and develop into macrophages that have enhanced phagocytic properties in addition to those of the resident tissue macrophages. These are sometimes known as inflammatory macrophages. Once phagocytosis has occurred further enzyme pathways are activated. This is known as the oxidative burst and toxic molecules are produced to damage the pathogens. Children with a rare immune deficiency called chronic granulomatous disease are unable to initiate this oxidative process and although they present with normal levels of neutrophils that can migrate and initiate phagocytosis, they are unable to kill the invading bacteria. These children will present with an increased incidence of fungal and pyogenic (staphylococcal and streptococcal) infections such as abscesses, ear, nose and throat infections and pneumonia, and their inability to clear these infections can result in the formation of granuloma – a feature of chronic infection (Helbert, 2017).

When the phagocyte dies at the site of inflammation, lysis occurs and the cell releases its contents including the enzymes into the surrounding tissues. This can cause the tissue damage associated with inflammation.

Inflammation

If microbes succeed in getting across these barriers, the innate immune system responds rapidly in an attempt to eliminate them by the process of inflammation and and by antiviral mechanisms (Abbas *et al.*, 2016).

Inflammation is the body's non-specific response to tissue damage or injury and forms an essential part of the innate immune system. The role of inflammation is to localise and minimise the tissue damage and to ensure that the specialised cells and molecules that are required to deal with the infectious agent are transported to the correct place to allow healing to take place (Macpherson & Austyn, 2012).

Causes of inflammation

Any type of tissue damage will stimulate the inflammatory response even if infection is not present. This could be:

- trauma (this includes a cut with a sterile scalpel)
- irritation with chemicals, including extremes of pH
- extreme heat
- infection by pathogens.

Recognition of infection in a peripheral site leads to local inflammation. The characteristic signs of inflammation are redness, heat, swelling and pain. If the infection is of a short duration and the infectious agent is rapidly removed, the response is known as acute inflammation, such as in the case of a skin abscess, an otitis media (ear infection), meningitis and pneumonia.

In cases where the infection is prolonged and the microbes are still present, the inflammatory process continues with much more extensive tissue damage and this is described as chronic inflammation, which can be seen in wound infections, bone infections and deep-seated infections associated with internal organs such as a liver abscess, which can be life threatening. There are also situations where the body is unable to clear the infection such as in tuberculosis. In this case the infective organism is *Mycobacterium tuberculosis*, which may persist for many months or years and lead to the formation of granulomas, which are groups of specialised macrophages that surround the infective organism to wall it off from the rest of the body.

Inflammation at the site of infection can also affect more distant sites and this is known as the systemic effects of infection. This leads to the rise in temperature (pyrexia), loss of appetite and malaise associated with an infection.

The inflammatory process

When injury, either from trauma or infection occurs, mast cells that are present in the connective tissue release the inflammatory mediators histamine and serotonin. These substances act on the blood vessels causing vasodilatation (increase in the diameter), which increases the blood flow to the affected area providing oxygen and nutrients for the cellular activity that takes place. There also changes within the endothelial cells of the blood vessels where the adhesiveness is increased. This allows the increased number of leukocytes that have been recruited to the area as part of the inflammatory response to enter the inflamed area (Murphy & Weaver, 2016). The increased blood flow causes the heat and redness associated with the inflammatory response.

The inflammatory mediators also make the blood vessels more permeable and, in conjunction with the increased blood flow, allow fluid from the plasma in the blood to leak out of the capillaries into the surrounding tissues. The fluid contains plasma proteins including antibodies and clotting factors. This increases the osmotic pressure within tissues, drawing more fluid out of the blood vessels, which forms swelling within the tissue called oedema.

Other plasma proteins are activated during the inflammatory process; these include the kinins and the complement system as well as the antibodies and clotting factors. Kinins affect the dilation and permeability of the blood vessels and also form bradykinin which, with prostaglandins, stimulate pain nerve fibres. The complement system consists of soluble proteins circulating in blood, becoming activated when in contact with foreign cells such as bacteria and fungi. They also cause vasodilation and attract the phagocytic cells (neutrophils and macrophages) to the affected areas by chemotaxis (release of chemicals to attract them). Another function of the complement is to enhance the process of phagocytosis by opsonisation where the microbes are coated with complement, and are directed to specialised receptors on the phagocytes, which increases their uptake and elimination by the phagocytes. Complement seems to be particularly effective against pyogenic (pus-forming) bacteria such as *Streptococcus pyogenes* and *Staphylococcus aureus*, and children who have a genetic defect in their ability to produce complement are very susceptible to these infections. Complement deficiency may also contribute to autoimmune disease such as systemic lupus erythematosus and other immune deficiencies (Abbas *et al.*, 2016; Helbert, 2017).

The clotting factors are stimulated to arrive at the site of inflammation and migrate through the permeable cell walls of the blood vessels where they start to produce fibrin. This forms an insoluble mesh within the tissue space, which helps to localise the infected area and to trap the invading bacteria and prevent the spread of infection. See Figures 5.5 and 5.6.

Wound healing and abscess formation

Acute inflammation causes tissue damage; an important part of inflammation is to stimulate the process of repair and healing (Macpherson & Austyn, 2012). Where there has been minimal destruction of tissue (e.g., when there has been a cut in a surgical incision)

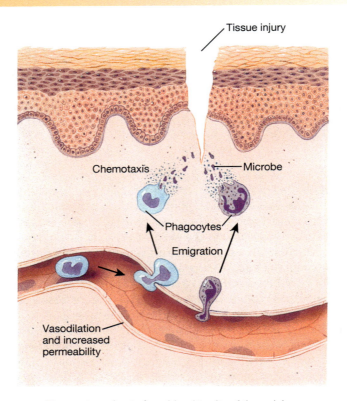

Figure 5.5 Inflammation and the stages that occur. *Source:* Tortora & Derrickson 2009, in: Peate & Gormley-Fleming 2015.

healing takes place by primary healing (also called first intention). Wounds heal by tissue regeneration and repair. Generally, in children, wounds will heal quickly and require minimal intervention (Jonas et al., 2010).

Platelets adhere to the cut surfaces; a blood clot is formed and stabilised by the fibrin laid down with cell debris filling other spaces. Monocytes move into the area and differentiate into inflammatory macrophages and they begin to remove the cell debris by ingesting and digesting the damaged cells (Macpherson & Austyn, 2012). They also stimulate the production of fibroblasts, which form collagen and other connective tissue within the inflamed area bringing wound margins together.

If the inflammation is caused by infection, the tissue damage is more extensive with increased recruitment of neutrophils and macrophages. The healing of the affected area may be delayed with increased formation of collagen and scarring of the tissue, known as healing by second intention. As part of the inflammatory process there may be separation of necrotic (dead) tissue from healthy tissue due to the action of phagocytes within the inflammatory exudate, this is known as slough. Figure 5.7 demonstrates the stages of wound healing.

Acute inflammatory reactions to extracellular bacteria result in the formation of pus. These extracellular bacteria are known as pyogenic (pus-forming) and exist and multiply in extracellular tissues and fluids. Some of these bacteria include: *Staphylococcus aureus,* which can cause skin abscesses; *Streptococcus pyogenes,* which causes throat infections; *Haemophilus influenzae* and *Streptococcus pneumoniae,* which cause respiratory infections.

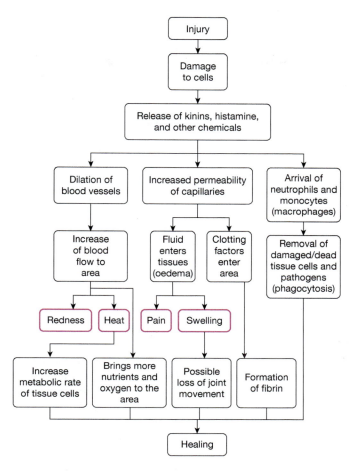

Figure 5.6 Flowchart of inflammatory events. *Source:* Adapted from Marieb 2012, in: Peate & Gormley-Fleming 2015.

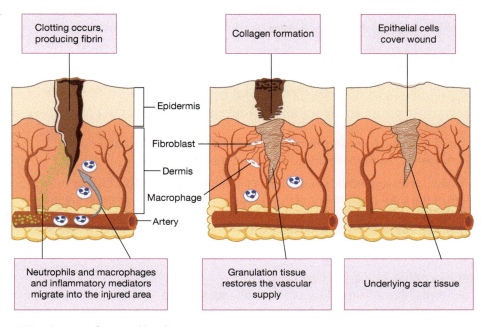

Figure 5.7 Stages of wound healing.

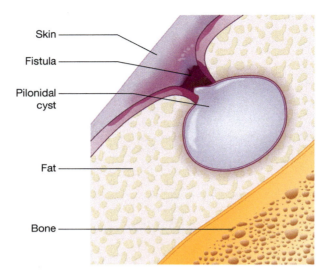

Figure 5.8 Diagram to show pilonidal abscess. *Source:* Google images.

A collection of pus within a cavity is called an abscess, superficial ones often occur under the skin – a boil is a collection of pus within an infected hair follicle. Superficial abscesses often rupture spontaneously on to skin surface discharging pus whereas deeper-rooted abscesses may rupture and only discharge some of the pus to the surface leaving an open infected channel or sinus. Fig. 5.8 demonstrates a pilonidal sinus.

Abscesses can also rupture and discharge into an adjacent organ forming a channel open at both ends called a fistula. In some chronic infections, these abscesses can be surrounded by fibrous tissue forming granuloma but containing live infective organisms as seen in tuberculosis.

Wounds

Jonas *et al.* (2012) describe the types of wounds commonly seen in children:

- cuts from accidental and non-accidental injuries
- animal bites
- burns and scalds
- surgical wounds
- pressure-related, which can be from equipment (e.g., saturation probe) or in relation to a child's immobility
- extravasation following intravenous fluid and drug administration
- congenital abnormalities, e.g., epidermis bullosa.

When assessing a child's wound, the children's nurse needs to consider the size and location of the wound and the underlying cause. Other factors to consider are the progression of the wound healing and any evidence of exudate, infected, sloughy or necrotic tissue. The child will need to be assessed for pain during wound dressing, and analgesia should be administered prior to the procedure as required.

Systemic effects of inflammation

Generally, the inflammatory process will contain the infection within the local area. The effects of this response may also be felt systemically and the child who has an infection can feel unwell with a fever, headache, muscle pains and loss of appetite. This response is

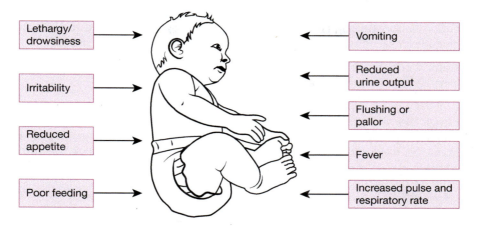

Figure 5.9 Diagram to show systemic signs of infection.

due to the release of cytokines, which are proteins that act as chemical messengers affecting the functions of the immune cells (Murphy & Weaver, 2016). Some of these will stimulate the inflammatory response and affect the endothelial cell changes resulting in increased permeability of the blood vessels and the recruitment of neutrophils and macrophages discussed earlier. Others affect wound healing and tissue repair and some cytokines enter the blood stream and act on distant tissues, such as the bone marrow, the liver and the hypothalamus in the brain.

The main cytokines involved in these systemic effects are interleukin (IL) 1 and IL-6 and tumour necrosis factor (TNF); their effects are summarised in Fig. 5.9. They affect the hypothalamus in the brain, resetting the temperature regulating centre to cause the rise in temperature associated with a fever (Helbert, 2017). These cytokines are sometimes called endogenous pyrogens. The increased temperature inhibits the action of the invading pathogens (Murphy & Weaver, 2016).

Prostaglandins are also released by mast cells as part of the inflammatory process, these affect the sympathetic nervous system, activating the adrenal glands to release adrenaline and noradrenaline. This results in a rise in pulse and respiratory rates causing peripheral vasoconstriction, which conserves heat and decreases the activity of the digestive system (Marieb, 2012). The child presents with characteristic signs of lethargy, fever and anorexia (Ridder et al., 2011).

Feverish illness is very common in young children, particularly in the under 5 age group, and it is the most common reason for parents to seek medical advice. In most cases the fever is due to a self-limiting viral infection but it may also be indicative of a more serious bacterial infection, such as meningitis, pneumonia or a urinary tract infection (National Institute for Health and Care Excellence [NICE], 2013). It is important that children are assessed rapidly and receive the appropriate treatment. Recent guidelines from NICE provide a traffic light system to assist health professionals in this assessment.

🚩 Red Flag

Recording temperature in children
Fever has been defined by the National Institute for Health and Care Excellence (NICE, 2013) as 'an elevation of body temperature above the normal daily variation'.

Recording temperature in children aged 4 weeks to 5 years according to NICE guidance (2013) includes measuring body temperature by one of the following methods:

- electronic thermometer in the axilla
- chemical dot thermometer in the axilla
- infrared tympanic thermometer.

An electronic thermometer under the axilla is recommended for infants under 4 weeks.

It is important to consider reported parental perception of a fever, and health professionals should take this seriously. In addition measurement and recording of heart rate, respiratory rate and capillary refill time should be part of the routine assessment of a child with fever (NICE, 2013; RCN, 2013).

When assessing the child, other considerations include:

- age of the child – the infant less than 3 months old may present with non-specific features, such as poor feeding, drowsiness, and irritability, and may have a bacterial infection that cannot be identified by physical examination;
- identifying illness in other members of the family;
- whether the child is up to date with immunisations;
- recent travel abroad;
- history of any recent infections – this may indicate increased susceptibility to infection associated with immunodeficiency;
- evidence of any rashes – rashes often accompany febrile illness but may also be characteristic of certain conditions in conjunction with other presenting symptoms, e.g., meningococcal meningitis;
- evidence of a focus of infection, e.g., otitis media or abscess.

Investigations for a febrile child with a suspected infection include:

- blood tests – these will include a full blood count (FBC) with a differential white count and inflammatory markers such as C-reactive protein (CRP) and erythrocyte sedimentation rate (ESR);
- blood cultures to determine the presence of the infective organism within the blood;
- urine sample;
- other investigations will depend on the presenting symptoms but may include a chest X-ray, lumbar puncture and wound swabs.

The effect of the cytokines on the bone marrow is the increased production of white blood cells (leukocytosis) to produce neutrophils and macrophages, which migrate to the site of infection.

Sepsis and septic shock

In severe infections, bacterial toxins are released into the blood and the activation of the innate immune system can cause an overwhelming response leading to septic shock. Activation of the cytokines and other inflammatory mediators in high concentrations can cause vasodilation, increased permeability of the capillaries affecting the venous flow to the heart. This results in hypotension and multi-organ failure and is life threatening.

Sepsis leading to septic shock is a medical emergency and is recognised as the leading cause of death in all age groups (NICE, 2016). The importance of rapid assessment of a child with suspected sepsis cannot be over-emphasised. Guidance from NICE (2016) ensures that health professionals use the traffic light system in the assessment of the acutely ill child and have protocols in place for the management of patients with meningitis and meningococcal septicaemia, neonatal infection and neutropaenic sepsis (see also NICE, 2012).

Risk factors contributing to the onset of sepsis and septic shock are:

- age of the child – preterm babies and the infant under 1 year because of their immature immunity;
- the child with impaired immune function, e.g., child with neutropaenia following cytotoxic therapy or child with immunodeficiency;
- the child with a critical illness or injury;
- the presence of indwelling central venous catheters for intravenous fluids and parenteral nutrition;
- invasive procedures such as cannulation;
- surgical incisions and wounds;
- burns;
- long-term antibiotic therapy;
- the child with a chronic illness.

Acquired immunity

The innate immune system provides an immediate response to any invading organism and often is sufficient to eliminate it. However, the immune system is also able to respond to specific organisms and destroy them. This specific immunity involves the B and T lymphocytes and their ability to recognise an antigen. Antigens are foreign molecules found on the surfaces of pathogenic organisms, toxins, cancer cells, transfused blood cells, transplanted tissues, foods and pollens. Receptors on the lymphocytes recognise these antigens and the cells of the adaptive immune system are activated. Specialised antigen-presenting cells (APC) found in the epithelia of the skin (dendritic cell) and gastrointestinal tract capture the antigens, transport them to the lymph tissue and present them to the lymphocytes (Abbas *et al.*, 2016).

B and T lymphocytes are found in the lymphoid organs, which consist of the lymph nodes, the spleen and the specialised mucosal lymphoid tissue found in the gastrointestinal and respiratory tracts. Examples include Peyer's patches, the appendix, and adenoids and tonsils (see Fig. 5.1).

T lymphocytes

Immature T lymphocytes undergo a maturation process within the thymus gland prior to their migration to the lymph tissue. The thymus is situated in the chest area in the upper anterior thorax just above the heart. It is a relatively large organ in babies and grows until puberty when it begins to atrophy; by adulthood there is only a very small amount of tissue left (Helbert, 2017).

During this process, the T lymphocytes learn to recognise the body's own cells and differentiate self from non-self. Non-self cells include cancer cells, transplanted cells and pathogens. Lymphocytes need to be exposed initially to the foreign proteins on the cell membrane to recognise the antigen. Once the T lymphocytes have matured they migrate to the lymph nodes and spleen, and will activate when exposed to that specific antigen by the antigen-presenting cells that have been activated during the innate immune response. This is known as cell-mediated immunity. A summary of the T-cell functions is shown in Table 5.2.

Table 5.2 T-cell functions

Cytotoxic T cells	Destroy and kill abnormal cells, e.g., virus-infected cells, cancer cells, and cells of transplanted tissue. Bind to foreign cells, release enzymes causing the cell to be destroyed by apoptosis.
Helper T cells	When activated act on innate and adaptive immune system. Release cytokines which stimulate the production of B lymphocytes and cytotoxic T cells. Recruit neutrophils and phagocytic cells to the site of the infection.
Regulatory T cells	Suppress activity of B and T lymphocytes, which stops the immune response once the antigen is destroyed. Prevents over-activity of the immune system.
Memory T cells	Antigen-specific memory cells that reactivate rapidly when exposed to the same antigen

Table 5.3 Functions of antibodies

Antibody	Function
IgA	Present in body secretions and mucosal surfaces, e.g., saliva, tears, sweat, nasal secretions, breast milk. Provides localised protection from bacteria and viruses. Provides protection in the neonatal period from gastrointestinal infections.
Ig D	Found on the surface of B cells and activates B cells.
IgE	Found on the surfaces of mast cells and basophils. Activation of mast cells when antigen binds to IgE triggers release of histamine and initiates the inflammatory response. Responsible for allergic reactions when present in excess.
IgG	Most prevalent antibody in serum. Can pass through placenta providing maternal protection to the newborn infant. Neutralises bacterial toxins and prevents attachment of some viruses to body cells. Activates complement system. Opsonisation of antigen for phagocytosis.
IgM	Most predominate immunoglobulin in early phase of the immune response. Causes agglutination of bacteria and activation of complement.

The B lymphocytes, like the T lymphocytes, are initially produced by the bone marrow, but unlike the T cells, they mature in the bone marrow before being released into the blood. The B cells have specialised surface receptors to antigens and when exposed to that antigen with the help of an activated helper T cell they stimulate the B cells to grow and multiply rapidly by a process called cloning. Two types of mature B cells are produced – plasma cells secreting antibodies and memory cells circulating in the blood – and when they meet the antigen again, they can rapidly start to produce plasma cells.

Antibodies are soluble proteins that circulate in the blood and are produced as a response to a specific antigen; using a lock and key analogy, the structure of the antibody matches that of the antigen (Tortora & Derrickson, 2011). The functions of the antibodies are summarised in Table 5.3.

Primary and secondary response to infection

The immune response following the first encounter with an antigen is the *primary response*. This initial exposure results in a delay in the production of antibodies known as the lag phase as the T lymphocytes are activated and stimulate the production of the B lymphocytes. One of the special features of the adaptive immune system is its ability to respond to future encounters with a known antigen, known as immunological memory as a result of the newly formed memory B cells. On subsequent exposure to the antigen the immune

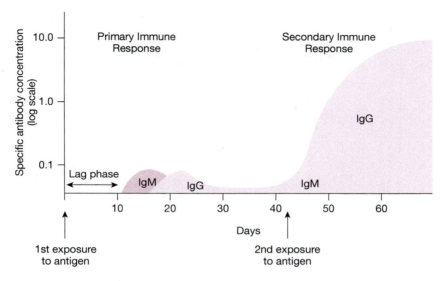

Figure 5.10 Primary and secondary responses to infection. *Source:* Peate & Nair 2011, in: Peate & Gormley-Fleming 2015.

response is much faster and more powerful ensuring that the antigen is destroyed effectively, known as the *secondary response* to infection (see Fig. 5.10).

Immunity can be acquired actively by the individual's response to an antigen and production of antibodies, or passively by the transfer of antibodies to the host. In both types of immunity this can be acquired naturally or artificially.

Natural active immunity is acquired by the body's response to infection. Immunisation with vaccines provides artificially acquired active immunity by allowing immunological memory to develop without a primary infection (Helbert, 2017). Vaccines contain small amounts of the infective organism that are inactivated (killed) or attenuated (weakened) live organisms, this is sufficient to stimulate an immune response without causing disease. Vaccination against communicable diseases is an essential part of public health programmes and children will receive their vaccinations as part of the current vaccination schedule (Public Health England, 2016).

A newborn baby acquires passive immunity naturally by the transfer of maternal IgG through the placenta and IgA in the colostrum of breast milk. A child with immunodeficiency who receives an infusion or injection of antibodies will acquire immunity artificially by passive immunization (see Fig. 5.11).

Alterations in immunity and inflammation

The immune system provides a complex network of mechanisms to protect the individual from foreign antigens, particularly infectious agents. However, at times this ability to protect the individual is compromised and there may be an inappropriate immune response. These can include reactions to environmental antigens such as pollen (allergy), against the body's own cells (autoimmunity), against foreign tissue and cells in transplantation and blood transfusion, and deficiency or abnormal function of the immune system (Rote & McCance, 2014). The result of these reactions can be serious or life threatening.

An excessive immune response is described as a hypersensitivity reaction (Helbert, 2017). This is further categorized by the types of immune response involved (Table 5.4). In each type of hypersensitivity reaction the response is made by the adaptive immune

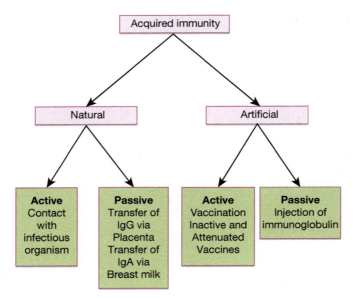

Figure 5.11 Acquired (specific) immunity. *Source:* Adapted from Taylor & Cohen 2013, in: Peate & Gormley-Fleming 2015.

Table 5.4 Types of hypersensitivity reaction

Type of hypersensitivity	Antigen	Onset	Immune response	Characteristics of reaction
Type I Immediate hypersensitivity	Pollen, house dust mite, foods, e.g., cow's milk protein peanut, insect venom	Rapid – can occur within seconds of exposure	IgE-mediated. Degranulation of mast cells and eosinophils resulting in release of immune mediators such as histamine	Allergy Hay fever Eczema Asthma Anaphylaxis (severe reaction)
Type II Tissue-specific hypersensitivity	Cell expressing foreign antigen	Rapid onset	IgG reacts with antigen and interacts with complement and phagocytes	Autoimmunity, e.g., rheumatoid arthritis Haemolytic disease of the newborn Blood transfusion reactions
Type III Immune complex hypersensitivity	Formation of immune complex with antigen and antibody	Onset within hours	Immune complexes deposited at site of production or circulated interacting with complement and neutrophils causing tissue damage	Glomerulonephritis Vasculitis Penicillin allergy
Type IV Delayed hypersensitivity	Pathogen e.g., hepatitis B virus, *Mycobacterium tuberculosis*. Environmental allergen, chemicals, plant extracts e.g., poison ivy	Days	T-cell response to antigen in conjunction with macrophages can also be associated with presentation of HLA	Tuberculin skin testing Contact dermatitis e.g., nickel allergy Graft and transplant rejection

HLA, human leukocyte antigen.

Inflammation, immune response and healing

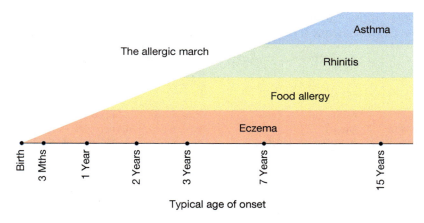

Figure 5.12   Diagram of the allergic march.

system and previous exposure to the antigen (sensitization) is required for the reaction to occur. The reactions can be immediate (minutes or a few hours) as seen in allergies, or delayed (up to several days) depending on the time of re-exposure to the antigen.

Allergy (type I hypersensitivity)

The incidence of allergy is increasing with approximately 1 in 4 individuals affected in the UK; half are children (Allergy UK, 2013). There is a familial association and individuals who are susceptible are said to be atopic. A child can develop an allergy in isolation but there is also evidence that children who are predisposed to allergy can develop allergic disorders at different times, for example, an infant can develop atopic eczema then develop food allergies as a toddler, and rhinitis and asthma may then develop in early childhood. This is referred to as the allergic march (Helbert, 2017) (see Fig. 5.12).

Allergy is defined as immediate hypersensitivity mediated by IgE, and antigens that trigger allergic reactions are known as allergens. They enter the body after being eaten, inhaled, administered as drugs, and by injection into the skin by an insect bite. Exposure to the allergens results in a rapid increase of IgE, which binds to receptors on the mast cells present in the tissues. These are found predominantly in the gastrointestinal tract, respiratory tract and the skin, and the symptoms of allergy will depend on the portal of entry for the allergen. The release of histamine causes constriction of smooth muscle, vasodilation and increased vascular permeability, which can lead to exudation of fluid and proteins into the tissues. See Table 5.5 for allergic diseases that affect children.

Fig. 5.13 describes a range of allergic symptoms.

Care of a child with allergy

Once a child has been diagnosed with an allergy a written individualised care plan must be provided for the child and their family. This outlines the symptoms of mild, moderate and severe reactions, and the appropriate treatment (see British Society for Allergy & Clinical Immunology; www.bsaci.org).

Advice on the avoidance of the allergen can help to minimise the allergic reaction. For a child who has asthma exacerbated by house dust mite, using allergen-proof barriers on mattresses, pillows and duvets, and washing bedding at 60°C can help to control exposure. Families are advised to remove carpeting and vacuum floors with a high-filtration vacuum cleaner.

Table 5.5 Allergic diseases that affect children

Allergic diseases	Allergen	Symptoms
Food allergy	Peanuts, tree nuts, cow's milk, eggs, fish, shellfish, legumes, wheat, seeds and fruits	Increased peristalsis resulting in diarrhoea and vomiting. May also be associated with urticaria and angioedema and anaphylaxis (see below)
Allergic rhinitis and conjunctivitis associated with hay fever	Pollens from trees and grasses Fungal spores and moulds House dust mite	Inflammation of mucous membranes of nasal passages and eyes and production of excessive mucus. Sneezing, discharge and nasal obstruction
Asthma	Tree, grass and weed pollens House dust mite Fungal spores and moulds Animal dander	Constriction of the bronchi with excessive production of mucus, oedema and swelling of the respiratory mucosa causing wheezing, coughing and breathlessness
Urticaria or hives	Food and drug reactions Also associated with exposure to temperature, stress and other systemic diseases	Localised release of histamine and increased vascular permeability result in formation of fluid-filled blisters (wheals) surrounded by areas of redness (flares)
Atopic eczema	Associated with food allergies such as egg, and family history of atopy	Eczema is classified as atopic where there is evidence of IgE antibodies to allergens. A defect in the skin barrier that is thought to be genetic makes it more susceptible to inflammation and allows allergens and bacteria to make contact with the immune system
Insect sting hypersensitivity	Insect venom	Mild to moderate reactions involve swelling and urticaria. Severe reactions can be systemic with wheeze and anaphylaxis

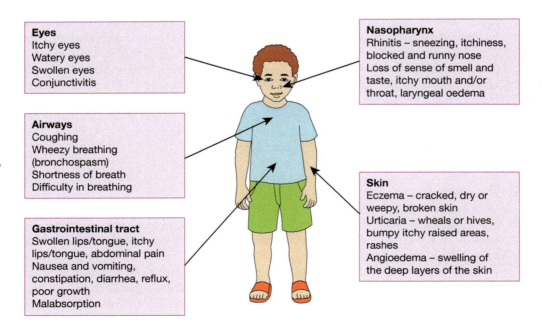

Figure 5.13 Diagram of allergic symptoms.

A child who has a food allergy should avoid the relevant food and be supervised by a paediatric dietician if appropriate. This is difficult to maintain and approximately 50% children with IgE-mediated food allergies report accidental exposure to the allergen (Luyt et al., 2016). Early recognition and treatment of the symptoms can prevent a more severe reaction occurring.

The plan should also include details of any medication, any emergency treatment in the event of a further reaction, together with advice and support for the child's nursery and school. Drugs that are used in the treatment of allergy include antihistamines that block specific histamine receptors. Antihistamines can be sedating or non-sedating (British National Formulary, 2017); non-sedating antihistamines are the treatment of choice. Oral antihistamines are effective in the treatment of nasal allergies and hay fever and for mild to moderate allergic reactions in food allergy. Corticosteroids are effective in allergic reactions and can prevent the immediate hypersensitivity reaction and also help to prevent chronic allergic inflammation (Helbert, 2017). They are used topically, for example, hydrocortisone cream in eczema, and inhaled in the treatment of asthma. Sodium cromoglycate can also be used topically as eye drops and nasal cream in the treatment of allergic rhinitis. For those children who have a severe allergic reaction with respiratory and cardiovascular involvement (anaphylaxis), intramuscular epinephrine (adrenaline) should be administered.

Anaphylaxis

Anaphylaxis is the most severe form of type I hypersensitivity with a systemic reaction resulting in angioedema, affecting the larynx causing airway obstruction, and hypoxia, bronchoconstriction, vasodilation and decrease in blood pressure. This can be life threatening without prompt treatment and is a result of widespread mast cell degranulation due to the systemic presentation of the allergen. The most common allergens to cause anaphylaxis in children are foods, but other triggers include insect stings, drugs, latex, and it can also be exercise-induced. The majority of anaphylaxis in children occurs in those under the age of 5 years and is linked to food allergy. However, there is an increased incidence of anaphylaxis fatality in adolescence associated with nut allergy and asthma (Lissauer & Clayden, 2012). A child who experiences anaphylaxis may present with facial swelling and symptoms of difficulty in swallowing or speaking, severe asthma, abdominal pain, nausea and vomiting, feeling dizzy due to the drop in blood pressure, which can rapidly progress to loss of consciousness (see Anaphylaxis Campaign; www.anaphylaxis.org.uk/).

Care of a child with anaphylaxis

The management of a child with suspected anaphylaxis is an emergency situation. It is likely to occur within the child's home or a community setting such as an immunisation clinic or nursery/school environment. There is a possibility that it may occur during the administration of drugs, for example, intravenous antibiotics, and there should be early recognition of this within the clinical environment. Children's community nurses who are administering medication to children at home should carry an anaphylaxis pack for use in the event of an emergency, and all staff within the clinical areas should be familiar with the location of emergency resuscitation equipment and medication in those areas.

It is important to recognise that the child is seriously unwell and seek emergency medical treatment urgently. Early treatment with the administration of intramuscular epinephrine is the treatment of choice for anyone experiencing anaphylaxis (Resuscitation Council, 2008) and if it is available, parents and carers should use it prior to seeking emergency help (Fig. 5.14). Epinephrine stimulates both α and β adrenergic receptors and

Chapter 5   Inflammation, immune response and healing

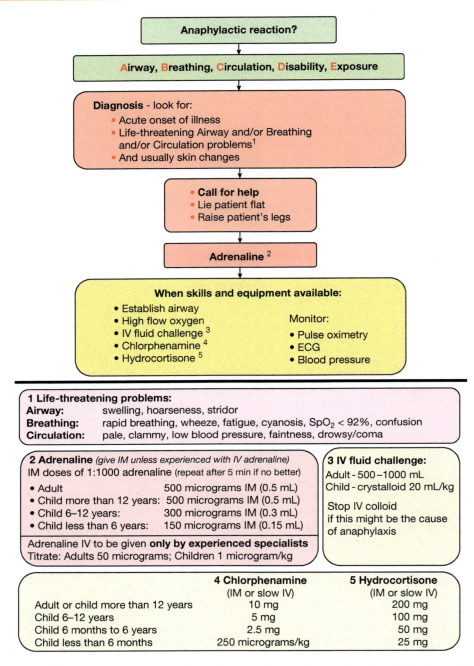

Figure 5.14 Emergency treatment of anaphylaxis. *Source:* Reproduced with kind permission of the Resuscitation Council UK.

this decreases vascular permeability, increases blood pressure, and helps to reverse airway obstruction (Helbert, 2017).

On admission to the emergency unit assessment of the child should follow the **A**irway, **B**reathing, **C**irculation, **D**isability, **E**xposure (ABCDE) approach to recognise potential problems and treat the child. Following administration of the epinephrine, assessment of the child's breathing and circulation should be monitored closely (pulse rate, blood pressure, pulse oximetry) to assess the child's response to the drug. In addition to intramuscular epinephrine the child may require supportive therapy with oxygen and intravenous fluids and also treatment with antihistamine and steroids. These drugs can assist with the treatment of urticaria and also reduce the chance of further reaction. As discussed earlier, children with allergies may also have asthma and this should be treated in line with emergency treatment for asthma with bronchodilator therapy (see British Thoracic Society and Scottish Intercollegiate Guidelines Network (SIGN) Asthma Guidelines, 2016).

A detailed history is taken to establish the allergen that has caused the anaphylactic reaction. Once the child's condition has improved following the emergency treatment, he/she should be observed closely for a minimum of 6 hours until stable. The child may require hospital admission for further observation as there may be a recurrence of the reaction, or if the child has a history of asthma or has had a reaction that has included asthma symptoms. Prior to discharge parents should be given advice about avoidance of the allergen and a written plan detailing an emergency treatment plan. The child may be prescribed an epinephrine autoinjector, and relevant training in administering this should be given to the family. It is essential that these children should have follow-up in an allergy clinic for confirmation of the diagnosis and a personal care plan to support the child and the family. The child and the family should be directed to allergy and anaphylaxis support groups for further support and advice.

Red Flag

An adrenaline autoinjector is a pre-filled disposable syringe and should be carried at all times. Families need to be reminded to check the expiry date as the shelf-life of these devices is 1–2 years. It is important to monitor the child's weight as there are two doses of epinephrine: 0.15 mg (for children who are 15–30 kg) and 0.3 mg (>30 kg). Patients may be prescribed two autoinjectors with advice to administer a second dose after 5 minutes (BNF, 2017).

Autoimmune disease

Autoimmune disease occurs when the adaptive immune system loses its ability to distinguish self from non-self and the immune cells start to attack the body's own cells causing tissue damage through hypersensitivity reactions (type II–IV). Factors that are thought to contribute to the development of autoimmunity are:

- **genetic** – autoimmune conditions are often found in members of the same family, e.g., type 1 diabetes mellitus and coeliac disease;
- **environmental triggers** – the disease may not be evident until it is triggered by something, e.g., ultraviolet light in systemic lupus erythematosus and gluten in the diet in coeliac disease;
- **infection** is thought to also play a significant part and it may be a connection with some or all of these factors that precipitates the inflammatory response associated with these conditions (Helbert, 2017; Abbas et al., 2016);
- **hormones** – there seems to be an increased incidence of autoimmune disease in adolescent girls and young women.

Autoimmune conditions can be either organ-specific affecting one organ or specific type of tissue, or systemic (non-organ-specific) where there is widespread tissue damage.

Diagnosis and management of autoimmune disorders

Autoimmune conditions are rare in children and can be difficult to diagnose. There may be specific symptoms associated with the affected organ, such as the signs and symptoms of diabetes or hyperthyroidism. However, often the symptoms that the child presents with are non-specific and could be associated with other conditions. Symptoms can include recurring fevers, rashes, fatigue, joint pain and weight loss, and further investigation is required. A feature of autoimmune disease can be periods where the child feels well (remission) and periods where the child becomes unwell (remission); this can have a significant impact on the child's ability to attend school and participate in social activities.

Investigations will include blood tests for full blood count and inflammatory markers – CRP and ESR – and further diagnostic tests to include identification of the presence of autoantibodies and rheumatoid factor. CRP and ESR are abnormal proteins which the body can make when attacking itself and are serological markers for autoimmune disease. However, these tests must be interpreted in conjunction with the child's presenting symptoms. Other investigations may include magnetic resonance imaging (MRI) and ultrasound in order to examine the organs and tissues more closely. In some cases biopsy of the affected tissue may assist with diagnosis.

Treatment for autoimmune disease relates to the specific condition the child presents with, the aim is to control and suppress the disease activity.

Transfusion reactions

Red blood cells have antigens expressed on the surface of their cells and form the basis of the ABO blood groups (see Chapter 12 in Peate and Gormley-Fleming, 2015). IgM antibodies against the red cell antigens are produced as natural antibodies and are present in the plasma. This means that an individual with blood group A has anti-B antibodies, group B has anti-A antibodies, group AB has no antibodies, and group O has both anti-A and anti-B antibodies. If a child who is group A receives blood from a group B donor the donor erythrocytes will be destroyed by activation of complement and opsonisation of the donor cell. This occurs extremely rapidly and is a type II hypersensitivity reaction; the resulting cytokine release can cause severe shock and is potentially fatal. Prior to a transfusion, a sample of the child's blood should be cross-matched with the donor blood to ensure compatibility.

The other consideration is the rhesus (Rh) D factor where individuals are classified as Rh positive or negative depending on whether they express the Rh system antigen on the erythrocytes. Unlike the ABO group natural antibodies, Rh antigens are not normally produced, but a Rh-negative mother and Rh-positive father may produce a Rh-positive fetus. This does not cause problems during a first pregnancy but during delivery there may be mixing of fetal and maternal blood so that exposure occurs to a foreign antigen for the mother and IgG anti-Rh antibody is formed. In a subsequent pregnancy with another Rh-positive fetus the IgG antibody will cross the placenta into the fetal circulation causing destruction of the fetal red blood cells. This can cause death in utero or haemolytic disease of the newborn (Macpherson & Austyn, 2012). Treatment for haemolytic disease of the newborn is an exchange transfusion with blood that is cross-matched with that of the mother. This condition can be prevented by giving the mother anti-D antibody which destroys the Rh-positive fetal cells before the mother can make her own before and after delivery (Helbert, 2107).

Immune responses against transplantation

The transplantation of tissue and cells from one person to another to replace damaged or defective cells has significantly improved outcomes for children with cancer, primary immune deficiency where there is a defect in the immune system, and conditions requiring organ transplant. However, the transplantation of foreign tissue and cells can cause an immune response, resulting in the rejection of the transplant. This is a normal reaction when a transplant takes place between genetically non-identical individuals of the same species and is known as allogenic. It occurs when the T lymphocytes of the recipient react against the antigens on the donor cells, which are called transplant antigens. The most significant of these are the major histocompatibility complex molecules (MHC), which are crucial for the presentation of antigen to T cells in the adaptive immune response. The MHC molecules in humans are known as human leukocyte antigen (HLA).

In order to minimise the possibility of rejection during transplantation of tissue, for example, solid organ transplantation such as kidney or cells (stem cell transplant), the donor and recipient should be tissue typed for ABO compatibility and also for HLA as matching the donor and recipient will increase the chances of a successful acceptance of the graft (Rote & McCance, 2014). Ideally a sibling donor will provide the greatest chance of a compatible donor and there is a 1:4 chance that a sibling will be an identical match on tissue typing. One of the major complications of stem cell transplantation is graft-versus-host disease (GVHD), which occurs when the T cells of the donor respond to antigens of the recipient. This can result in effects on the skin (skin rashes), the gastrointestinal tract (diarrhoea and vomiting), the liver (jaundice), and the lungs.

To ensure the greatest possibility of success in organ and stem cell transplantation the child will require immunosuppressive treatment at the time of the transplant. The use of these drugs means that the child is significantly at risk of infection so during hospital admission the child should be nursed in a single room, at home should avoid contact with anyone who has an infection, and avoid crowded places and travelling on public transport. The parents will be advised to seek urgent medical advice if the child becomes unwell with a temperature or has been in contact with measles or chicken pox (varicella) as h/she may require specific immunoglobulin treatment. It is important that during this treatment the child does not have exposure to live vaccines as part of the vaccination programme.

Immune deficiency

Immune deficiencies are caused by a defect in part of the immune system. A defect or deficiency in the immune system can result in an increased susceptibility to infection. Young children have an immature immune system and have not yet developed immunity to common pathogens so it is expected that a young child will have several infections in early childhood. However, children who present with severe, persistent unusual or recurrent infections should be investigated for immune deficiency. These can be:

- Primary immunodeficiency (PID) where one or more components of the immune system are not working due to a genetic abnormality. These are rare conditions that can result in severe life-threatening infections.
- Secondary immunodeficiency where the immune deficiency is acquired as a result of other factors, such as infection, medical treatments, nutritional defects and exposure to environmental toxins. These are much more common than primary immunodeficiency.

Primary immunodeficiency

Primary immunodeficiency conditions are caused by genetic defects and can be inherited as X-linked or autosomal recessive disorders. There may also be a history of parental consanguinity and a family history of unexplained death of children – usually boys (Helbert, 2017) (see Fig. 5.15). However, in many cases the genetic cause may not be inherited but a result of a sporadic genetic mutation. There are over 300 different PID conditions and they can present with a wide range of symptoms that can vary in their severity (PID UK, n.d.).

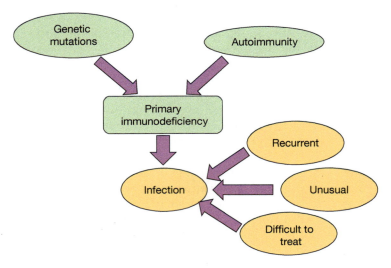

Figure 5.15 Features of primary immunodeficiency. *Source:* Adapted from Helbert 2017.

Care and management of a child with primary immunodeficiency

The diagnosis of PID can take place after admission to hospital with a serious life-threatening infection or following recurrent infections that are persistent, severe or caused by unusual micro-organisms. A full history from the child's parents is important to establish the history of infections, family history and presentation of symptoms. A physical examination is also carried out including a record of the child's weight and height.

Investigations include blood tests that help to identify the immune deficiency. These include:

- full blood count – gives total number of red cells, white blood cells and platelets;
- white cell differentiation – quantifies number of lymphocytes, granulocytes and monocytes;
- lymphocyte subsets – quantifies number of T and B lymphocytes, which can identify whether the defect is B or T lymphocyte;
- serum immunoglobulin levels – quantifies the amount of circulating antibody (IgG, IgA and IgM);
- specific antibody reactions – antibody reactions to vaccines (pneumococcus, *Haemophilus influenzae*, tetanus, measles), which can determine the IgG response by B lymphocytes;
- other blood tests may be carried out for phagocyte function, complement and genetic testing for known mutations in PID, and to exclude secondary immunodeficiency.

The severity and type of antibody deficiency will determine the treatment for children diagnosed with PID. Children who have mild antibody deficiency may receive prophylactic antibiotic therapy; they also receive an early intervention of an alternative antibiotic therapy in the event of an infection. For those children who have more severe antibody deficiency, replacement immunoglobulin treatment is needed. The immunoglobulin provides antibodies against a wide range of pathogens and is obtained from pooled plasma donations (Helbert, 2017). This is known as artificially acquired passive immunity. Replacement immunoglobulin can be administered intravenously or subcutaneously and is normally a lifelong treatment. Diagnosis and treatment may take place in specialist

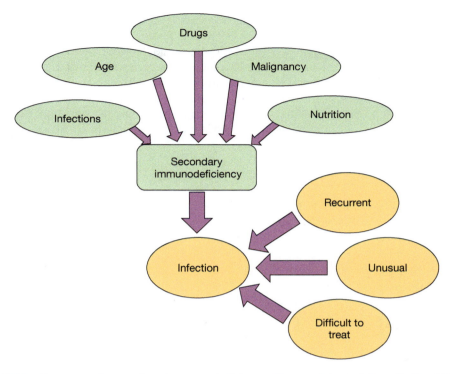

Figure 5.16   Features of secondary immunodeficiency. *Source:* Adapted from Helbert 2017.

centres, which can add to the stress encountered by the families if they have long distances to travel. Once treatment is established, home therapy treatment for the child under supervision of a specialist nurse can be initiated.

Secondary immunodeficiency

Immunodeficiencies that are not caused by a genetic defect are secondary or acquired (Macpherson & Austyn, 2012). Secondary immunodeficiencies can cause the same types of infections as PID depending on which part of the immune system is affected. They are more common than PID and can be related to many factors, such as age of the child, cancer, drugs, nutrition, infection and surgery (see Fig. 5.16).

Acquired immunodeficiency syndrome

Acquired immunodeficiency syndrome (AIDS) is a viral disease caused by human immunodeficiency virus (HIV). It is discussed here briefly as it is a significant cause of severe immunodeficiency having reached epidemic proportions, particularly in Africa and Asia, after first being identified in the 1980s. However, a sustained global approach to combating the disease with a combination of retroviral drugs and support for individual countries has reduced its impact (World Health Organization [WHO], 2016). CHIVA (2014) provide practitioners with guidance for HIV testing for children of HIV-positive parents and/or siblings in the UK and Ireland.

HIV is a virus that affects primarily T helper cells and it is a member of the retrovirus family. It produces an enzyme reverse transcriptase that converts viral RNA to DNA within the host cells of the infected person, and this DNA is incorporated within the host cells where it may lie dormant for some time. If the cell is activated, for example, from an outside stimulus such as another infection, the host cells divide and produce further copies of the infected DNA and the disease will progress. The HIV infects T helper cells that have a protein receptor CD4 within their cell membrane, but will also target dendritic cells and macrophages in the epithelia, lymph tissue and in the circulation. The consequence of this is that the CD4 cells are destroyed and their key function in activating both cell-mediated and antibody-mediated immunity means that the individual has a significant susceptibility to infection, and very often they will be infected by organisms that would not generally affect an individual with a normal functioning immune system. These infections are described as opportunistic infections.

Case Study 1 Child with appendicitis

An 8-year-old girl is admitted to the emergency department with a history of abdominal pain and vomiting for 12 hours. On examination she has pain in the right iliac fossa and her abdomen is tender when palpated. Her vital sign observations on admission were:

Vital sign	Observation	Normal range
Temperature	37.5 °C	36.5–37.2 °C
Pulse	110 beats per minute	70–120
Respiratory rate	36 breaths per minute	20–30 breaths per minute
Blood pressure	85/50 mmHg	80–100 mmHg (systolic)
CRT	2 seconds	<2 seconds
Oxygen saturation	98% in air	98–100%
Level of consciousness	Alert on the AVPU scale	Alert on the AVPU scale
Pain score	4	1 (no pain)

Her PEWS score is 2, her respiratory rate is elevated and her pulse rate is at the upper end of the normal range.
What explanation can you give for this?
Blood test and urinalysis indicate:

Blood test	Result	Normal range
Haemoglobin	12.5 g/dL	11.5–15.5 g/dL
White blood cells	13.2×10^9/L	$4.5–13.5 \times 10^9$/L
Neutrophils	8.5×10^9/L	$1.5–8.0 \times 10^9$/L
Lymphocytes	6.6×10^9/L	$1.5–7.0 \times 10^9$/L
Platelets	420×10^9/L	$150–450 \times 10^9$/L
C-reactive protein	42 mg/L	0–10 mg/L
Urinalysis	+ve Nitrites and leucocytes on testing	

Her white blood cell count is at the upper end of the normal range and she has an elevated neutrophil count and raised C-reactive protein.
What do you think the significance of this might be?
She is admitted to the paediatric ward and following administration of analgesia and starting intravenous fluids the child is monitored closely with hourly recordings of her

vital signs. Six hours later she is still complaining of abdominal pain and her recordings are now as follows:

Vital sign	Observation	Normal range
Temperature	38.5 °C	36.5–37.2 °C
Pulse	125 beats per minute	70–120
Respiratory rate	34 breaths per minute	20–30 breaths per minute
Blood pressure	80/55 mmHg	80–100 mmHg (systolic)
CRT	3 seconds	<2 seconds
Oxygen saturation	98% in air	98–100%
Level of consciousness	Lethargic and responding to voice on the AVPU scale	Alert on the AVPU scale
Pain score	4	1 (no pain)

Her PEWS score is now 4, and the child is reviewed by the paediatric surgeon. On examination her abdomen is tense. Blood tests indicate that the neutrophil count is now 12.2×10^9/L and the C-reactive protein is 110 mg/L.
What explanation can you give for this?
What care and support will the child and family need at this time?
The child is taken to theatre and has her appendix removed. The appendix has perforated and following surgery she requires intravenous antibiotics. Following the surgery she makes a good recovery and is discharged home 4 days later with follow-up from the children's nursing team for wound dressing. She completes her antibiotic treatment orally.

Case Study 2   Child with anaphylaxis

A 2-year-old boy is brought into the emergency department by his parents with a history of swelling of the face and eyes and generalised itching with a rash on his chest. His parents have also noted that he has started to wheeze during the journey to the hospital. His parents report that he had taken a bite of his father's peanut butter sandwich and they noticed the facial swelling within minutes.

The paediatric team urgently reviews the child and a suspected diagnosis of a severe allergic reaction is made. He receives intra-muscular epinephrine 0.15 mg and has oxygen administered via a face mask. He is also prescribed chlorphenamine and hydrocortisone and is monitored closely in the emergency department.

His vital signs on admission are:

Vital sign	Observation	Normal range
Temperature	37.2 °C	36.5–37.2 °C
Pulse	135 beats per minute	90–140
Respiratory rate	42 breaths per minute	20–40 breaths per minute
Blood pressure	75/40 mmHg	80–95 mmHg (systolic)
CRT	2 seconds	<2 seconds
Oxygen saturation	100% in oxygen	98–100%
Level of consciousness	Drowsy and responding to voice on the AVPU scale	Alert on the AVPU scale

His PEWS score is 4, his respiratory rate is above the normal range, he has required oxygen and has an inspiratory wheeze and is drowsy.
What explanation can you give for this?
What is the possible significance of his blood pressure recording and why is this not included within the PEWS score?
Following treatment with the epinephrine his condition stabilises quite quickly but he is monitored closely by the nursing staff and is admitted to the paediatric ward as he has had asthma-type symptoms.
What advice and support should the child and family receive prior to discharge the following day?

Conclusion

This chapter has provided insight into the anatomy and physiology of the immune response and inflammation, and has discussed how the pathophysiology of the altered effects of these can affect a child and his/her family. The focus in this chapter has been to present an overview of the interplay between the innate and adaptive immune systems and to consider how the inflammatory process can manifest locally and systemically within the body. Emphasis has been given on how alterations in immunity can affect the infant and child, and the implications of providing care for the child and the family have been discussed.

References

Abbas, A.K., Lichtman, A.H. & Pillai, S. (2016). *Basic Immunology*, 5th edn. Elsevier, St. Louis.

Allergy UK (2013). *What is an allergy?* [online] Available at: https://www.allergyuk.org/what-is-an-allergy/what-is-an-allergy (accessed 13 March 2017).

British National Formulary (2017). BNF for children. [online] Available at: https://www.medicinescomplete.com/mc/bnfc/2011/ (accessed 27 March 2017).

British Thoracic Society (2016). *BTS/SIGN British guideline on the management of asthma*. [online] Available at: https://www.brit-thoracic.org.uk/standards-of-care/guidelines/btssign-british-guideline-on-the-management-of-asthma/ (accessed 28 February 2017).

Children's HIV Association (CHIVA) (2014). *HIV testing guidelines for children of HIV positive parents and/or siblings in the UK and Ireland*. [online] Available at: http://www.chiva.org.uk/files/2014/2738/8338/testing-guidelines.pdf (accessed 30 March 2017).

Helbert, M. (2017). *Immunology for Medical Students*, 3rd edn. Elsevier, Philadelphia.

Jonas, D., Muldowney, Y., Byrne, I. & Southern, H. (2012). Essential care. In: Coyne, I., Neill, F. & Timmins, F. (eds). *Clinical Skills in Children's Nursing*. Oxford University Press, Oxford, pp. 115–145.

Lissauer, T. & Clayden, G. (2012). *Illustrated Textbook of Paediatrics*, 4th edn. Mosby Elsevier, Edinburgh.

Luyt, D., Ball, H., Kirk, K., & Stiefel, G. (2016). Diagnosis and management of food allergy. *Paediatrics and Child Health* 26(7), 287–291.

Macpherson, G. & Austyn, J.M. (2012). *Exploring Immunology Concepts and Evidence*. Wiley-VCH, Weinheim.

Marieb, E.N. (2012). *Essentials of Human Anatomy and Physiology*, 10th edn. Pearson Benjamin Cummings, San Francisco.

Murphy, K. & Weaver, C. (2016). *Janeway's Immunobiology*, 9th edn. Garland Science, New York.

National Institute for Health and Care Excellence (NICE) (2012). *Neutropaenic sepsis: prevention and management in people with cancer*. Clinical guideline [CG151]. Available at: https://www.nice.org.uk/guidance/cg151 (accessed 28 February 2017).

National Institute for Health and Care Excellence (NICE) (2013). *Fever in under 5 s: assessment and clinical management*. Clinical guideline [CG160]. Available at: https://www.nice.org.uk/guidance/cg160 (accessed 28 February 2017).

National Institute for Health and Care Excellence (NICE) (2016). *Sepsis: recognition diagnosis and early management*. NICE guideline [NG51]. Available at: https://www.nice.org.uk/guidance/NG51 (accessed 30 March 2017).

Peate, I. & Gormley-Fleming, E. (2015). *Fundamentals of Children's Anatomy and Physiology*, 1st edn. Wiley, Oxford.

Peate, I. & Nair, M. (eds) (2011). *Fundamentals of Anatomy and Physiology for Student Nurses*. Wiley, Oxford.

Primary Immunodeficiency (PID) UK 0000 (n.d.). *What are PIDs? The basics*. Available at: http://www.piduk.org/whatarepids/basics (accessed 30 March 2017).

Public Health England (2016). *The complete routine immunisation schedule from summer 2016*. Available at: https://www.gov.uk/government/publications/the-complete-routine-immunisation-schedule (accessed 1 March 2017).

Resuscitation Council (2008). *Emergency treatment of anaphylactic reactions: guidelines for healthcare providers*. Resuscitation Council UK, London.

Ridder, D.A., Lang, M.F., Salinin, S., *et al.* (2011). TAK1 in brain endothelial cells mediates fever and lethargy. *Journal of Experimental Medicine* 208(13), 2615–2623.

Rote, N.S. & McCance, K.L. (2014). Alterations in immunity and inflammation. In: McCance, K.L. & Huether, S.E. (eds). *Pathophysiology: The Biologic Basis for Disease in Adults and Children*, 7th edn. Elsevier, St. Louis, pp. 262–298.

Royal College of Nursing (RCN) (2013). *Caring for children with fever. RCN good practice guidance for nurses working with infants, children and young people*. Royal College of Nursing, London.

Taylor, J.J. & Cohen, B.J. (2013). *Memmler's Structure of the Human Body*, 10th edn. Lippincott Williams & Wilkins, Baltimore.

Tortora, G.J. & Derrickson, B.H. (2009). *Principles of Anatomy and Physiology*, 12th edn. Wiley, Hoboken, NJ.

Tortora, G.J. & Derrickson, B.H. (2011). *Principles of Anatomy and Physiology*, 13th edn. Wiley, Hoboken, NJ.

Weston, D. (2013). *Fundamentals of Infection Prevention and Control*. Wiley, Chichester.

World Health Organization (2016). *Global health sector strategy on HIV, 2016–2021*. WHO, Geneva.

Chapter 6

Shock

Usha Chandran

Aim

The aim of this chapter is to offer an introduction to shock, which can develop into a life-threatening condition. The chapter considers pathophysiological changes and addresses the need for care to be offered in a safe and confident manner.

Learning outcomes

On completion of this chapter, the reader will be able to:

- Have an understanding of basic physiology of shock states in children.
- Know the classification and recognition of clinical shock states in children.
- Understand the pathophysiology of septic shock and be able to explain the changes that occur in a child's vital signs.
- Discuss the pathophysiological changes that occur in anaphylactic shock and articulate the immediate care required for the child.
- Be able to discuss the initial management of shock in children.

Keywords

- cardiac output
- hypovolaemic
- cardiogenic
- stroke volume
- hypotension
- compensatory shock
- anaphylaxis
- hypoperfusion
- distributive
- pre-load
- afterload

Fundamentals of Children's Applied Pathophysiology: An Essential Guide for Nursing and Healthcare Students, First Edition.
Edited by Elizabeth Gormley-Fleming and Ian Peate.
© 2019 John Wiley & Sons Ltd. Published 2019 by John Wiley & Sons Ltd.
Companion website: www.wileyfundamentalseries.com/childpathophysiology

Test your prior knowledge

1. Define cardiac output.
2. Explain compensatory shock and its mechanisms.
3. Hypotension is a pre-terminal sign, explain why this is?
4. List the clinical features of warm shock.
5. List the clinical features of cold shock.
6. Identify four clinical conditions that can lead to left ventricular failure and cardiogenic shock.
7. Identify three causes of distributive shock.
8. Identify the variables that impact on stroke volume.
9. How would you assess a child who has presented with a possible diagnosis of septic shock?
10. Discuss the diagnosis and pathophysiological changes that occur with anaphylactic shock.

Introduction

Shock is a broad term describing a very complex syndrome that affects nearly every organ system of the body. We often describe the child patient as shocked, septic, or even sick looking. Recognizing the child in shock is vitally important as failure to do so has the potential to lead to a life-changing outcome or may even be life threatening. This chapter aims to provide the reader with the information required to give them a good understanding of the pathophysiology of shock and its initial management.

Normal metabolic processes depend on the delivery of oxygen to tissues and removal of toxic waste products to maintain normal function. The cardiac, pulmonary and circulatory systems are integral to these processes. This means good blood flow, sufficient blood (circulating) volume, an efficient cardiac system and the ability of the blood vessel to autoregulate according to need. Shock therefore may be defined as a state of acute circulatory failure.

Shock can be defined at both the cellular level or by its clinical presentation. At the cellular level, it is defined as a state of inadequate substrate for aerobic cellular respiration and the accumulation of cytotoxic waste. In other words, tissues become hypoperfused and there is poor oxygen delivery for normal metabolic processes, and toxic waste products reach dangerous levels. At the clinical level, a constellation of signs and symptoms which you may be familiar with, for example, changes to the normal heart rate, cardiac rhythm changes, deranged capillary refill time, changes to mental state and muscle tone (floppiness), changes to skin colour and warmth, and other complications such as poor kidney perfusion leading to poor urine output, define shock.

Shock is classified according to the cause or abnormality that occurs. Table 6.1 illustrates different types of shock depending on their pathophysiology. Sinniah (2012) found that out of 147 cases of paediatric shock with the highest mortality, 57% were septic shock, 24% hypovolaemic shock, 14% had distributive shock, and 5% cardiogenic shock. Table 6.1 outlines the classification of shock.

Distributive shock

Distributive shock is associated with dysfunctional blood flow and intravascular volume. As blood vessels lose tone and become larger, this causes a relative hypovolaemia and blood does not flow efficiently. For various reasons, for example, toxins and inflammatory

Table 6.1 Classification of shock

- **Hypovolaemic shock.** This is due to a reduction in circulating volume either from intravascular losses (e.g., burns), haemorrhage (e.g., trauma, surgery) or interstitial losses (e.g., burns, ascites, other third spacing or sepsis). Haemorrhage shock and severe dehydration fall into this category.
- **Cardiogenic shock.** This is due to cardiac pump failure or dysfunction. Pump failure can be due to right or left heart or both right and left heart failure. Cardiogenic shock causes impairment of cardiac contractility.
- **Distributive shock.** This is due to a relative hypovolaemia caused by vasodilatation (poor vascular/vasomotor tone) and low total systemic vascular resistance (SVR). Sepsis mediators, anaphylaxis or autonomic dysfunction from head and/or spinal injury can cause this type of shock.
- **Obstructive shock.** This is due to impaired blood flow such as pulmonary embolism (rare in children), cardiac tamponade, tension pneumothorax or pulmonary hypertension. In neonates, coarctation of aorta, interrupted aortic arch and aortic valvular disease can cause obstructive shock. Obstructive shock results in cardiogenic shock and death if left untreated.

proteins (in septic shock) or allergens (in anaphylactic shock), the blood vessels widen to such as extent that they lose their tone and blood pools in the vessels rather than circulating normally. This manifests in symptoms of early shock as the body tries to compensate by increasing the heart rate. Three different types of distributive shock are described in the following sections. These are: sepsis and septic shock, neurogenic shock, and anaphylactic shock.

Septic shock

Sepsis/septic shock is a serious type of distributive shock caused by a dysregulated and overwhelming host response to infection (Singer *et al.*, 2016). In this type of shock, pathogens such as gram negative bacteria and their microbial products, for example lipopolysaccharides (LPS), cause a highly immunogenic and toxic molecule to activate the inflammatory system – the body's natural response to injury (in this case injury to the endothelial system). However, microbial toxins and activated inflammatory cytokines from the inflammatory pathway cause vasodilatation and low systematic vascular resistance (SVR), i.e., poor vessel tone, which increases vessel permeability, causing fluid to leak out of the circulatory system. SVR refers to the resistance offered by all blood vessels to the aortic valve when it opens to eject blood. Low SVR can be caused by the host (child's) own response to inflammation – the systemic inflammatory response syndrome (SIRS). Inflammatory mediators (e.g., cytokines, interleukins) and bacterial toxins (e.g., LPS) cause dilatation of blood vessels and lead to low SVR, also known as warm shock.

In septic shock, 20% of patients will present with this type of warm shock. Other features of warm shock are tachycardia, bounding peripheral pulses, and a warm skin. Warm shock results in high cardiac output and low SVR. These children require proper management as they may decompensate into shock with hypotension secondary to low SVR. Alternatively, they may quickly decompensate into cold shock, which is more difficult to treat. Eighty percent of children in septic shock present with features of cold (or late) shock. In cold shock, the child becomes excessively vasoconstricted, skin is pale, cool or cold to touch with mottling as blood is shunted away and capillary refill time is prolonged. This sympathetically mediated response maintains the child's blood pressure for a while until there is decompensation and the child collapses. By this stage, capillary blood flow becomes sluggish, capillaries become leaky and permeable, there is third-spacing of fluid further exacerbating the hypovolaemic state, and metabolic acidosis. Cold shock is associated with low cardiac output, high SVR and poor outcome. Refractory shock is defined by irreversible shock, multi-organ failure and death.

Initially, as a compensatory mechanism, blood vessels try to maintain tone, which is one of the major differences between adults and children as children will maintain their SVR and blood pressure until the pre-terminal stage. During the compensatory stage, however, you may observe a subtle increase in diastolic blood pressure and a subtle decrease in pulse pressure (difference between systolic and diastolic blood pressure), which results in a normal systolic blood pressure. Monitoring the trends in blood pressure is therefore an important nursing skill and a vital part of nursing practice, and such observations are key to identifying shock at an early stage. This is usually coupled with an early rise in heart rate (tachycardia) to maintain the circulating volume. In almost all types of shock, the body attempts to improve its cardiac output and circulating volume by activating the sympathetic nervous system and it releases endogenous catecholamines, such as adrenaline and noradrenaline, which increase cardiac contractility and heart rate. This is the reason for an early rise in heart rate. Thus a very obvious early sign of any type of shock is tachycardia. Other signs of early shock are warm skin tone, flushed appearance (usually also fever), flash capillary refill time, and bounding pulses. These are signs of a hyperdynamic circulation and fluid resuscitation during this stage may reverse these early symptoms.

Here, the inflammatory response can become so extreme and the vessel tone so excessively dilated that it is not uncommon to volume resuscitate a child to over 100 ml/kg of fluid. This is severe distributive shock caused by sepsis and inflammation, and by this stage the child will have been referred to or transferred to the ICU for intensive care management. This life-threatening emergency presents with features of cold shock: cool or cold peripheries, cyanosed or mottled skin, prolonged capillary refill, oligo-anuria, metabolic acidosis, tachycardia and hypotension. These children are extremely ill and can develop a serious condition known as disseminated intravascular coagulopathy (DIC).

🚩 Red flag

In some types of sepsis, however, for example, neutropenic or neonatal sepsis, the compensatory phase may be too short or even non-existent and patients will decompensate very rapidly.

DIC is an over-activation of the inflammatory and clotting system. Any type of injury, including injury to the endothelial system as in shock, will activate both these systems. The inflammatory system aims to protect the organism while the clotting cascade aims to heal and seal the vessel or injured area. However, in DIC the clotting system also becomes deranged because sepsis is a condition of extensive and ongoing microvascular injury and clotting products become so quickly consumed that it becomes difficult to replace them.

Another complication of DIC is not only the resulting coagulopathy but also the microvascular clotting and fibrin deposits that occur in the small blood vessels, which then occlude tissues from extracting oxygen. As aerobic metabolism requires oxygen, tissue dysoxia initially leads to anaerobic metabolism, metabolic acidosis and a rise in lactate – the by-product of anaerobic metabolism – all of which will eventually lead to cell death. That is why DIC is a marker of poor prognosis and is associated with the mnemonic **D**eath **I**s **C**oming (Moore, Knight & Blann, 2016). Thus DIC is both a clotting and bleeding disorder that is difficult to treat. The underlying condition, i.e., the stimulus for DIC, in this case sepsis, must instead be treated and controlled. Treatment of DIC is therefore only symptomatic and patients will require many blood and blood product transfusions. These patients are usually cared for in the paediatric intensive care unit (PICU). Fortunately, the majority of children with sepsis and septic shock do recover to lead normal lives. International efforts such as the Surviving Sepsis Campaign and Sepsis 6 (NICE, 2016) aim to improve diagnosis and survival rates of children with sepsis through early recognition

Table 6.2 SIRS to septic shock

SIRS is a response to a stimulus (inflammation), which results in two or more of the following:
Temperature >38.5 °C or <36 °C
Heart rate >2SD above normal or bradycardia in children <1 year old (10th centile for age)
Respiratory rate >2SD above normal or pCO_2 < 32 mmHg
Leukocyte count >12 000 cells/mm³, 4000 cells/mm³ or 10% band forms
Hyperglycaemia, altered mental status, hyperlactaemia, increased capillary refill time (CRT)
Sepsis is SIRS with a suspected or confirmed bacterial, viral or fungal cause.
Septic shock is sepsis with cardiovascular dysfunction and signs of organ hypoperfusion.

and timely treatment. Thus, nurses and other healthcare professionals play a vital role in recognising and reporting the signs and symptoms of sepsis early so that children are given the best chance of survival.

See Table 6.2 for an overview of SIRS to septic shock.

Although the early signs of compensated shock may be short-lived, the clinical features of decompensated shock are very obvious. This is due to the vasoconstriction that comes from decompensated shock. Blood vessels will constrict so that the circulating volume is maintained and to shunt blood to vital organs. Such vasoconstriction will manifest as cold, clammy skin, mottling, there may be floppiness and poor muscle tone in infants and young children, and persisting tachycardia.

🚩 Red Flag

If a child with suspected or proven infection has at least two of the criteria set out in Table 6.1, then it should be assumed that sepsis is present and full screening should proceed.

Tachycardia will decompensate further into bradycardia, a pre-terminal sign, if this stage is not adequately or promptly managed. In decompensated shock, capillary refill time is prolonged and there may be low rather than high core temperature. Unlike adults who become hypotensive at an early stage, children will remain normotensive but significantly tachycardic until they become pre-terminal. As blood flow is diverted from the kidneys to more vital organs, there may be oliguria or anuria and poor perfusion to other non-vital organs, for example, gut. Urine output less than 1 ml/kg/h in young children and less than 0.5 ml/kg in older adolescents must be reported in a timely manner as this is a very serious but early feature of poor kidney blood flow and perfusion. Monitoring urine output and maintaining an accurate fluid balance chart is therefore a vital part of the nurse's role.

Cold shock from any cause is a more severe type of shock and is more difficult to treat. It is a life-threatening condition, requires invasive monitoring and intensive care drugs only possible in PICU. Regardless of the type of shock, however, all patients suspected of being septic must have appropriate antibiotics administered without delay as this can be life-saving (Dellinger *et al.*, 2013).

The clinical features of warm and cold shock are highlighted in Fig. 6.1.

Life-threatening complications related to septic shock are outlined in Fig. 6.2.

Neurogenic shock

Another type of distributive shock is neurogenic shock. Neurogenic shock is caused by the sudden loss of autonomic control and impairment of autoregulation resulting from spinal cord injury (SCI) – especially above T6. Here, disruption to the descending pathways of the

Types of shock

Warm: early, compensated, hyperdynamic
- Confusion/agitation or lethargy
- Warm extremities
- Bounding pulses
- Tachycardia
- Tachypnoea
- Wild PP
- Up CO
- ↓ SVR

Cold: late, uncompensated with low CO
- Cyanosis
- Cold
- Clammy
- Rapid, thready pulses
- Shallow respirations
- Thrombocytopenia
- Oliguria
- Myocardial dysfunction
- Capillary leak

GOAL: increase DO_2 AND decrease O_2 demand

Figure 6.1 The clinical features of warm and cold shock.

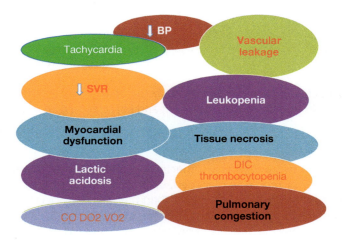

Figure 6.2 Life-threatening complications of septic shock.

sympathetic nervous system results in unopposed vagal (parasympathetic) tone. Loss of tone and dilatation of vascular smooth muscles and an increased venous capacitance results in a decreased SVR. There will be a relative hypovolaemia, meaning that the circulating volume in itself is unchanged but as the blood vessel capacity enlarges, the existing circulating volume becomes inadequate to fill it. The relative hypovolaemia and the disruption to vessel autoregulation result in hypotension.

Neurogenic shock is managed with fluids and drugs that aim to increase the tone of blood vessels. The treatment should support blood pressure until the patient overcomes and the body has time to adapt to the changed system due to the SCI. Bradycardia, another consequence of neurochemical derangement and autonomic dysregulation in SCI, should also be managed with drugs such as atropine or glycopyrrolate. These drugs can be given prophylactically prior to suctioning or turning the patient if they are particularly sensitive to these interventions, which may cause a vagal response. Other dysrhythmias are also possible in severe conditions and should be controlled for as cardiac dysrhythmias can cause poor ejection of blood out of the heart. Bowel and bladder care is important so that constipation or urinary retention, a distended abdomen and pain do not trigger an episode of neurogenic shock in these patients.

Neurogenic shock can occur anytime following injury up to 6 weeks post-injury (Mack, 2013). There is no diagnostic test for this condition so history, the nature of spinal cord injury, and exclusion of other causes for hypotension and bradycardia contribute to the diagnosis of neurogenic shock. Bradycardia in these patients is exacerbated by any condition that increases intra-cranial pressure, such as suctioning, defaecation, coughing, turning the patient, and hypoxia. Initially, the skin can be warm and flushed in this condition but heat loss from profound vasodilatation can cause hypothermia.

Anaphylactic shock

Anaphylaxis is a state of immediate hypersensitivity resulting in distributive shock due to loss of vasomotor tone and massive vasodilatation. The most frequent trigger for anaphylaxis is exposure to food allergens and medications such as antibiotics (e.g., penicillin allergy). The condition is caused by the release of mediators, especially histamine from mast cells and basophils. Histamine has a vasodilatory effect and increases blood vessel permeability. Typical signs of anaphylaxis are stridor, swelling around the mouth and face, wheezing, respiratory distress, vomiting, urticaria.

Red flag

Diagnosis may be difficult due to inconsistent clinical manifestations, so it is essential that a rational approach, ABCDE, is taken.

Stridor, which is a sign of partial airway obstruction, and wheeze, an intrathoracic sound from narrowed airways, can lead to complete airway obstruction and respiratory and cardiac arrest. Poor circulating volume due to vessel dilatation and permeability can lead to cardiac arrest. Intramuscular epinephrine will dampen this inflammatory anaphylactic response and reverse its symptoms. Systemic corticosteroids and antihistamines may be required.

Hypovolaemic shock

Hypovolaemic shock is common worldwide (Hobson & Chima, 2013). Thirty percent of hypovolaemic shock is due to diarrhoeal disease in susceptible nations (Thomas & Carcillo, 1998). At least 8000 children under 5 years old die from untreated dehydration causing hypovolaemic shock (Glass *et al.*, 1991).

Hypovolaemic shock is associated with either a direct loss of fluid, i.e., the water content of the body, or a relative loss of intravascular volume. A direct loss of fluid can be caused by conditions such as gastroenteritis, diarrhoea and vomiting, or diabetes insipidus caused by pituitary dysfunction, which results in excessive urinary loss. Haemorrhage also causes direct loss of fluid, in this case loss of whole blood.

Relative hypovolaemia (e.g., in distributive shock) is caused by increased capillary permeability causing fluid to leak out of the intravascular volume (e.g., sepsis). Other conditions, such as burns, liver failure, pancreatitis, and bowel obstruction, also cause this type of hypovolaemic shock known as 'third-spacing'. For example, ascites in liver failure is a form of third-spacing where large volumes of fluid extravasate out of the circulatory system and accumulate around the abdominal cavity. This fluid is wasted. Without appropriate fluid management and adequate fluid replacement, the patient may become extremely dehydrated and at risk of hypovolaemic shock.

Two types of hypovolaemic shock are discussed in this section: extreme/severe dehydration leading to hypovolaemic shock, and haemorrhagic shock.

Extreme/severe dehydration

In hypovolaemic shock, there is actual loss of fluid (e.g., diarrhoea and vomiting) or inadequate intake leading to dehydration and shock. When dehydration is so severe that it degenerates to shock, the usual clinical features of shock (e.g., vasoconstriction) will be observed. These features are related to compensatory mechanisms that activate the renin-angiotensin-aldosterone system. This is an important feedback system as the system strives to conserve the circulating volume and maintain blood pressure. Another related mechanism, the release of anti-diuretic hormone (ADH) from the posterior pituitary gland also conserves fluid and urine output to improve circulating volume. The consequence of these feedback systems is poor urine output, which is an important nursing observation to report and manage.

Other consequences of vasopressin (ADH) release are vasoconstriction and shunting of blood to vital organs. Thus another feature of hypovolaemic shock is weak, thready peripheral pulses and prolonged capillary refill. However, in certain conditions, such as diabetic ketoacidosis (DKA), these signs can be misleading. The hyperosmolar, hyperglycaemic circulation of DKA draws fluid out of cells into the vascular compartment as the blood is more viscous than the fluid surrounding the cell. Thus in DKA, despite significant cellular dehydration, capillary refill time can remain normal and there is polyuria rather than oliguria (which occurs much later in the presentation). Monitoring capillary refill time in DKA can be unreliable and must be interpreted cautiously. This demonstrates the importance of understanding the pathophysiology of different types of shock.

Hypovolaemic shock can also be classified according to serum sodium levels. In hyponatraemic hypovolaemia, serum sodium is less than 130 mmol/L. Serum sodium is within 130–150 mmol/L in isonatraemic hypovolaemia while in hypernatraemic hypovolaemia, serum sodium is over 150 mmol/L. The rapid correction of sodium levels with aggressive fluid resuscitation is dangerous and will risk cerebral oedema, brain herniation and brain-stem death.

Haemorrhagic shock

Haemorrhagic shock is the second most important cause of hypovolaemic shock. Common causes are post-operative bleeding and trauma (Hobson & Chima, 2013). In this type of shock, there is loss of red blood cells (RBC). RBC are essential for the delivery of oxygen to tissues and enhance the oxygen-carrying capacity of the blood. Any injured or post-operative child with tachycardia and a poor peripheral pulses warrants an expert examination to exclude bleeding as a source. The definitive treatment for haemorrhagic shock is haemostasis and replacement of RBC via blood transfusions (Wheeler, Wong & Shanley, 2014).

As with all types of shock in children, tachycardia is a very early symptom of hypovolaemic shock which should be reported promptly. Other features of hypovolaemic shock are cyanotic extremities, very dry mucus membranes, weak thready pulses, dark sunken eyes, absence of tears, poor skin turgor, lethargy or coma in the terminal stages, and deep, rapid respirations (Hazinski, 2013).

As children compensate very well in the early stages of haemorrhagic shock, tachycardia is the most common early sign of impending shock. With a class I haemorrhage i.e., 10–15% blood loss, the child will compensate with a 10–20% increase in heart rate while blood pressure and capillary refill time remain unchanged. Even with 15–30% blood loss (class II haemorrhage), there is little change apart from tachycardia, tachypnoea and perhaps a prolonged capillary refill. However, there may be diminished pulse pressure (difference between systolic and diastolic blood pressure) and an anxious demeanour. Tachycardia, tachypnoea, hypotension, oliguria and mental state changes become very evident at class III haemorrhage (30–40% blood loss). Class IV haemorrhage results in over 40% blood loss and the child becomes hypotensive, anuric and loses consciousness. In the United Kingdom, a CODE RED protocol is activated wherever there is significant bleeding. In cases where bleeding persists, a surgical review is mandatory. If an injured child continues to deteriorate despite achieving haemostasis, other causes of shock must be investigated, for example, tension pneumothorax (a type of obstructive shock) or spinal shock (a type of distributive shock).

In haemorrhagic shock, the actual loss of RBC results in the delivery of poorly oxygenated blood. Thus, in haemorrhagic shock, both supplementary oxygen and the transfusion of red blood cells to increase the oxygen-carrying capacity of the blood are important. The administration of supplemental oxygen (where appropriate) and monitoring of oxygen saturation levels (SpO_2) is a fundamental requirement for any child in shock, which nurses must appreciate. See Fig. 6.3 for paediatric code red.

Cardiogenic shock

Whilst all other types of shock are defined by poor intravascular volume, cardiogenic shock is defined as a decreased cardiac output with tissue hypoxia in the presence of adequate intravascular volume (O'Laughlin, 1999). In other words, there is adequate circulating volume but the heart is unable to pump this out efficiently or effectively. Thus, Sachdev *et al.* (2012) define cardiogenic shock as: sustained hypotension for a minimum of 30 min (systolic blood pressure for less than 2SD for age, a reduced cardiac index <2.2 L/min in the presence of elevated pulmonary occlusion pressure (pressure measured in the left heart during cardiac catheterisation in the cardiac lab or during cardiac surgery).

Cardiogenic shock can have both a cardiac and non-cardiac cause. For instance, in aortic stenosis there is adequate circulating volume but the narrowed aorta obstructs blood flow out of the left ventricle to the rest of the systemic circulation and causes cardiogenic shock and poor tissue perfusion. In the newborn with aortic stenosis, where the ductus arteriosus continues to remain, patent blood is diverted via this fetal circulation to maintain perfusion. Once the ductus arteriosus begins to close soon after birth, the baby will develop 'critical' life-threatening obstruction to blood flow and the ductus arteriosus must be kept open with drugs (prostaglandin E_1) to support the baby until definitive treatment is undertaken as an emergency. This is an example of both cardiogenic and obstructive shock in the infant. Another example of cardiogenic shock is cardiac tamponade where excess fluid around the heart causes an obstruction to the pumping action of the heart – another life-threatening condition. Septic shock can cause cardiogenic shock if the contractility of the heart is affected by sepsis. In this type of cardiogenic shock, there is no element of obstruction.

Cardiac conditions that cause cardiogenic shock can be both congenital and/or acquired. Table 6.3 outlines the causes of cardiogenic shock in children. Specialist children's cardiac ICU with specially trained personnel and equipment are required to care for children with congenital or acquired cardiac conditions because they are at high risk of developing cardiogenic shock.

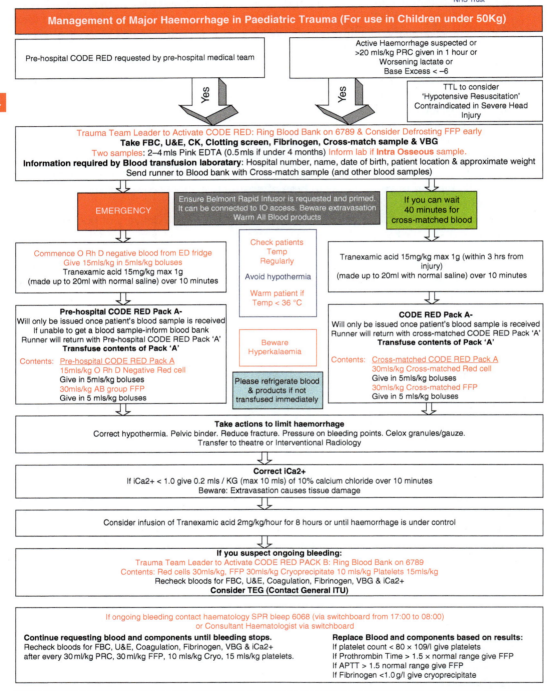

Figure 6.3 Paediatric code red. *Source:* R. Beynon, St George's University Hospitals Foundation NHS Trust. Reproduced with permission.

Table 6.3 Causes of cardiogenic shock in children

Congenital heart disease	Dysrhythmias	Metabolic	Ischaemia	Trauma
HLHS	SVT	Acidosis	Myocarditis	Tension pneumothorax
CoA	VT	Hyperkalaemia	Chemotherapy toxicity	Haemo-pericardium
Interrupted aorta	AV block	Hypercalcaemia	Anaemia	Myocardial contusion
TGA		Inborn errors of metabolism	Myocardial infarction	Cardiac aneurysm
AS		Drug toxicity	Kawasaki disease	
Tricuspid/mitral atresia			Calcium-channel blockers	
MS				
ASD				
VSD				
ASVD				

Table 6.4 Cardiogenic shock related to right ventricular failure

- **Systolic dysfunction (decreased contractility)**
  - RV infarction
  - Ischaemia
  - Hypoxia
  - Acidosis
- **Increased afterload**
  - Pulmonary embolism
  - Pulmonary vascular disease
  - Hypoxic pulmonary vasoconstriction
  - Positive pressure ventilation with PEEP
  - High alveolar pressures
  - Acute respiratory distress syndrome
  - Pulmonary fibrosis
  - Sleep-disordered breathing
  - Chronic obstructive pulmonary disease
- **Arrhythmias**

Source: Adapted from Sachdev *et al.* 2012.

Cardiogenic shock can be differentiated into right and left ventricular failure. Table 6.4 shows causes of right ventricular failure (RVF). Table 6.5 highlights causes of left ventricular failure (LVF). It is important to appreciate these differences as treatment strategies can differ.

Table 6.6 provides an overview of the pathophysiology of the signs and symptoms of cardiogenic shock.

Early markers of compensation are tachycardia and tachypnoea. Assessment of urine output, signs of cyanosis, cold extremities, observation of the patient's mental status or behaviour, and hypotension will all point to the child who is beginning to decompensate. Persisting hypotension in children despite correction for hypovolaemia, arrhythmias, hypoxia and acidosis requires prompt attention and treatment. Table 6.7 outlines the goals of treatment of children with cardiogenic shock.

Treatment strategies aim to increase stroke volume and cardiac contractility, and reduce afterload. These may include cautious fluid resuscitation to minimise overload, drugs to support offload and/or support the heart (diuretics, inotropes, chronotropes, inodilators), and in extreme cases, mechanical support such as ECMO.

Table 6.5 Cardiogenic shock related to left ventricular failure

- **Systolic dysfunction (decreased contractility)**
  - Ischaemia/infarction
  - Global hypoxaemia
  - Valvular disease
  - Myocardial depressant drugs (beta-blockers, calcium-channel blockers, anti-arrhythmics)
  - Myocardial contusion
  - Respiratory acidosis
  - Metabolic derangements
- **Diastolic dysfunction**
  - Ischaemia
  - Ventricular hypertrophy
  - Restrictive cardiomyopathy
  - Prolonged hypovolaemic or septic shock
  - Ventricular interdependence
  - Pericardial tamponade
- **Increased afterload**
  - Aortic stenosis
  - Hypertrophic cardiomyopathy
  - Dynamic aortic outflow tract obstruction
  - Coarctation of aorta
  - Malignant hypertension
- **Valvular or structural anomaly**
  - Mitral stenosis
  - Endocarditis
  - Mitral aortic regurgitation
  - Obstruction
  - Papillary muscle dysfunction or rupture
  - Ruptured septum
- **Arrhythmias**

Source: Adapted from Sachdev *et al.* 2012.

Table 6.6 Pathophysiology of the signs and symptoms of cardiogenic shock

Sign/symptom	Pathophysiology
Tachypnoea	Reflex response to rise in pulmonary venous pressure, LV volume and pressure
Dyspnoea	Pulmonary congestion, compression of bronchi by dilated pulmonary arteries or atria and pulmonary oedema
Feeding difficulty	Lack of energy to suck and tire quickly
Faltering weight	Inadequate calories due to feeding difficulty and extra work of breathing causes increased metabolic demand
Irritability	Reduced oxygen transport to the brain
Oliguria	Impaired renal perfusion
Diaphoresis	Increased sympathetic activity
Increased precordial activity	Chamber dilatation
Tachycardia	Increased sympathetic activity as a compensatory mechanism to increase oxygen delivery to tissues
Gallop sounds	Increased afterload, decreased compliance
Hepatomegaly, oedema	Systemic venous congestion
Reduced capillary filling	Reduced tissue perfusion
Lung crackles	Alveolar oedema

Source: Adapted from Sachdev *et al.* 2012.

Table 6.7 The goals of treatment of children with cardiogenic shock

- General supportive care to maintain systemic perfusion
- Relieve systemic and pulmonary congestion
- Improve myocardial performance
- Optimise afterload
- Treat and manage the underlying cause

Source: Adapted from Sachdev *et al.* 2012.

A common pathway to the pathophysiology of shock

As discussed earlier, the hallmarks of shock are poor circulating volume, hypoperfusion, organ dysfunction and organ failure. When there is poor circulating or blood volume, the normal and more efficient aerobic metabolic pathway using oxygen as the main substrate utilises another pathway, i.e., an anaerobic metabolism. Anaerobic metabolism is inefficient and produces the toxic by-product lactic acid. Lactic acid creates an acidic environment and disrupts enzyme processes, causing enzymes to become denatured. Lactate, which is normally cleared by the liver, can be measured at the bedside and is a common procedure undertaken by emergency department and critical care unit nurses. It is a very useful marker of organ perfusion and a determinant of whether the patient requires more filling to improve cardiac output and blood pressure, or drugs to improve vascular tone and cardiac function. A rise of more than 2 mmol/L of lactate in the blood gas increases the risk of morbidity and mortality (Wheeler *et al.*, 2014).

Ultimately, the treatment goal in shock is to improve cardiac function and circulating volume so that oxygen increases. This is the key principle of fluid resuscitation in the initial stages of shock, which adopts the principle of the Frank–Starling law of the heart. Thus, strategies for fluid resuscitation are to bolus 5–20 ml/kg of fluid rapidly to restore circulating volume in hyperdynamic states. In cardiogenic shock or renal failure, fluid resuscitation is undertaken cautiously to prevent overload as an overloaded heart cannot contract efficiently. The aim of fluid resuscitation is to manipulate pre-load and end-diastolic pressures because cardiac contractility is enhanced if the cardiac muscle fibres are stretched to an optimal level (not over- or under-stretched) in order to eject the stroke volume more forcefully.

Fluid overload is undesirable and detrimental. Fluid overload can lead to respiratory congestion, increasing ventilation/perfusion mismatch and poor gas exchange in the lungs. In such cases, special drugs to 'offload' the patient's heart and diuretics to remove excess fluids may be required. Non-invasive ventilation is sometimes used to manage respiratory congestion leading to pulmonary oedema. However, positive pressure ventilation can also exacerbate poor venous return and cause cardiac or haemodynamic instability.

Fluid overload can be assessed by observing for signs of peripheral and pulmonary oedema, hepatomegaly, fine basal crackles on lung auscultation, pink, frothy sputum and jugular venous distension in the older child. A chest X-ray will reveal fluid that has accumulated in the lungs: pulmonary oedema, and pleural effusions. Echocardiogram can be useful.

An adequate circulatory system is required to deliver oxygenated blood to tissues for maintaining their integrity. This requires a good venous return, adequate pre-load and end-diastolic pressure. Without good venous return, there will be poor ejection of systemic blood, which will cause poor flow and organ perfusion. Additionally, there must be a clear and patent pathway for blood to flow to the lungs so that haemoglobin can be oxygenated. Any obstruction to blood flow, inefficient or failing pulmonary function, low haemoglobin levels or structurally poor haemoglobin (e.g., in sickle cell disease), and poor oxygen saturation will all affect the oxygen content of arterial blood (CaO_2) and in turn oxygen delivery to the tissues. Heart and pulmonary diseases, such as asthma or bronchiolitis, which lead to excessive gas-trapping and increased transpulmonary pressure plus positive pressure ventilation for respiratory failure, can impede venous return and thus pre-load.

It can be seen from the afore-mentioned that the ultimate aim in managing shock is to restore the circulating volume and oxygen delivery to tissues. A number of key variables are fundamental to this aim. These variables are:

1. cardiac output (to deliver oxygen to tissues)
2. oxygen content in the blood
3. haemoglobin to bind oxygen.

Cardiac output is dependent on two variables as shown in Fig. 6.4.
Stroke volume (Fig. 6.5) is the volume of blood ejected by the heart in one beat. Stroke volume depends on pre-load, afterload and cardiac contractility.

For more information on cardiac output and stroke volume, read Chapter 9 in Peate and Gormley-Fleming (2015). It is essential for you to understand these principles to appreciate the pathophysiology of shock and its management.

The variables for oxygen delivery (DO_2) are highlighted in Fig. 6.6. Management focuses on the manipulation of one or more of these variables to reinstate oxygen delivery to tissues (see Fig. 6.3).

As identified in Fig. 6.6, cardiac output (CO) is one of the variables associated with oxygen delivery but CO is dependent on stroke volume (SV) and heart rate (HR). Older children can augment their cardiac output by increasing both SV and HR but SV is relatively fixed in young children who cannot increase their SV to any great extent. This is because young hearts are less compliant and cannot stretch easily enough to accommodate an increasing stroke volume Thus, in young children, sympathetic stimulation leads to tachycardia very quickly and is one of the early signs of compensatory shock. Changes in HR are therefore very significant in unwell or sick children and must be closely monitored.

Extreme or prolonged fast HR (tachycardia), however, is dysfunctional. Extreme tachycardia shortens the diastolic phase of the cardiac cycle. As perfusion to cardiac muscle occurs during diastole, a shortened diastolic phase will affect cardiac perfusion. A very

Cardiac output = heart rate × stroke volume

Figure 6.4 Cardiac output and its variables.

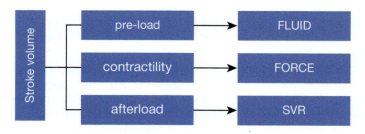

Figure 6.5 Stroke volume and its variables.

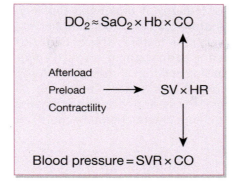

Figure 6.6 Oxygen delivery, blood pressure and its variables. Reproduced with permission.

rapid heart rate will also increase myocardial oxygen consumption. This can cause the heart to become ischaemic. Children who are monitored on an electrocardiogram (ECG) will show an S-T depression on their ECG complex if the heart is ischaemic or under strain. Observing for this sign is an important duty for nurses who monitor children's ECG. Bradycardia is a pre-terminal event.

In older children, extreme or prolonged tachycardia can also cause another complication known as loss of 'atrial kick'. Atrial kick is the last few volumes of blood that the heart ejects from atria to ventricles just before atrial diastole (relaxation). Atrial kick contributes to end-diastolic volume and pressure, which influences the contractility of the heart. Cardiac contractility is associated with stroke volume and cardiac output. Thus, atrial kick is an important haemodynamic in shock. The last few millilitres of blood contributing to atrial kick are very important as it not only prevents cardiac and pulmonary congestion but it also influences how efficiently the heart contracts in systole. This is to do with the Frank–Starling principle of the heart. Fluids and/or drugs can be given to normalise heart rate and must be closely monitored.

Strategies for caring for and managing the child in shock

It cannot be stressed strongly enough that the fundamental principle for managing shock is to recognise the signs and symptoms and to treat it early. The aim is to improve the circulating volume, improve cardiac output and blood pressure, and prevent or minimise the risk for organ failure. Although different protocols exist for managing this in different shock states, the aim is to restore circulating volume and perfusion pressure. Perfusion pressure is related to blood pressure and stroke volume, and is the pressure at which organs are perfused. Strategies for achieving adequate perfusion pressures are fluid/volume resuscitation, afterload manipulation and vasopressor drugs plus surgical management where indicated. In extreme cases, mechanical support, for example, extra-corporeal membrane oxygenation (ECMO) or extra-corporeal life support (ECLS) may be warranted.

Monitoring end-organ perfusion

Monitoring end-organ perfusion is one of the most important and fundamental functions of the nurse and healthcare team. Poor end-organ perfusion is an early sign of shock. Poor end-organ perfusion includes changes to mental state and behaviour like confusion, agitation or lethargy. A prolonged capillary refill time of longer than 2 seconds, a skin temperature gradient, cool peripheries, pale, mottled skin and poor urine output are also very clear features of poor perfusion, which nurses should monitor closely. The paediatric early warning scores (PEWS), a track and trigger tool for identifying and recognising children at risk, is a useful tool for monitoring end-organ perfusion for children in shock states. Recovering patients show improvements in behaviour and mental status, and recover a normalised capillary refill of less than 2 seconds, normal skin colour and temperature, moist, mucus membranes and a good urine output.

A systematic approach to assessing the patient in shock

The ABCDE approach is a systematic approach to assessing the patient in shock.

Airway (A): The patient's airway may be at risk for a number of reasons. The moribund, obtunded patient, floppy and with a low coma score or unconsciousness will be unable to protect their own airway. Patients requiring large volumes of fluid boluses (>60 ml/kg) will also be at risk. Patients undergoing invasive procedures require sedation, which may compromise their airway. A good GCS, cough and gag reflex is a part of the airway assessment.

Breathing (B): Patients who are shocked require oxygen therapy but this must be balanced against oxygen toxicity in neonates in particular, and in cardiac patients with cyanotic conditions and duct dependency. Central and peripheral cyanosis must be reported. Oxygen must be prescribed and titrated to condition, need, saturations and blood gases. Respiratory rate and effort, work of breathing and use of accessory muscles, chest wall expansion, the efficiency and effect of breathing are important parameters. Sputum must be analysed for appearance, volume, consistency, colour and smell. Fine crackles on auscultation may indicate pulmonary oedema. Coarse crackles may suggest sputum/secretions from infection or aspiration. Wheezing and stridor may be due to anaphylaxis. A chest X-ray may be required.

Circulation (C): Colour, skin temperature and central and peripheral capillary refill time are assessed to determine perfusion status. Core temperature, heart rate and rhythm, pulse rate, volume, character and rhythm are assessed. Central and peripheral pulses are palpated and compared. ECG monitoring may be in situ. Blood pressure trends are monitored and reported. Central venous pressure may be monitored and a central venous gas may be required to determine volume status. Septic screens, full blood count, clotting and coagulation profiles and urea and electrolytes will be monitored. An echocardiogram may be performed.

Disability (D): Glasgow coma score is assessed and managed. A floppy patient is seriously unwell. Blood glucose level is monitored.

Exposure (E): The patient must be fully exposed and assessed. There may be obvious bleeding. A distended abdomen may suggest internal bleeding. Bruises may indicate low platelets or clotting disorder. Rashes must be carefully assessed. A petechial rash may point to meningococcal septicaemia. An urticarial rash may be a sign of anaphylaxis. Other discolouration or anomalies give clues to the reason for the shocked state and response to treatment.

Family (F): The family will also require support during this time.

As the patient begins to recover, a more holistic approach, such as the Roper's activities of living model, can be taken. In the unfortunate state that the patient is in irretractable shock, then a dignified approach to end-of-life care is required.

Summary and conclusion

In summary, shock is a serious life-threatening condition. This chapter has described the different types of shock syndrome and their management. It has provided an overview of the important concepts associated with shock and circulatory dysfunction and its management. The importance of oxygen delivery, fluid resuscitation, perfusion and end-organ assessment, monitoring and a systematic approach to the assessment of the shocked patient has been stressed. It is important for nurses to appreciate the application of these concepts and the underlying pathophysiology of shock if they are to be active partners in care. Fortunately, with proper care and treatment, the majority of patients recover from shock and go on to lead normal lives.

References

Dellinger, R.P., Levy, M.M., Rhodes, A. & Annane, D. (2013). Surviving sepsis campaign: international guidelines for management of severe sepsis. *Intensive Care Medicine* 39(2), 165–228.

Glass, R.I., Lew, J.F., Gangarosa, R.E., LeBaron, C.W. & Ho, M.S. (1991). Estimates of morbidity and mortality rates for diarrheal diseases in American children. *J Pediatr* 118(4 pt 2), S27–S33.

Hazinski, M.F. (2013). *Nursing Care of the Critically Ill Child*, 3rd edn. Elsevier Mosby, St. Louis.

Hobson, J.H. & Chima, S.R. (2013). Pediatric hypovolemic shock. *The Open Pediatric Medicine Journal* 7, 10–15.

Mack, E.H. (2013). Neurogenic shock. *The Open Pediatric Medicine Journal* 7(Suppl 1: M4), 16–18.

Moore, G., Knight, G. & Blann, A. (2016). *Haematology*, 2nd edn. Oxford University Press, Oxford.

National Institute for Health and Care Excellence (NICE) (2016). Sepsis: recognition, diagnosis and early management. NICE guideline [NG51]. NICE, UK.

O'Laughlin, M.P. (1999). Congestive heart failure in children. *Pediatric Clinics of North America* 46, 263–273.

Sachdev, M.S., Aggarwal, N., Joshi, R.K. & Joshi, R. (2012). Cardiogenic shock in children. [Review article.] [online] Available at: https://www.researchgate.net/publication/278021324 (accessed 15 March 2016).

Singer, M., Deutschman, C.S., Seymour, C.W., *et al.* (2016). The Third International Consensus Definitions for Sepsis and Septic Shock (Sepsis-3). *JAMA* 315(8), 801–810.

Sinniah, D. (2012). Shock in children. *IeJSME* 6(Suppl 1), S129–S136. https://pdfs.semanticscholar.org/8485/636ffb90f8816b31f2061538a1481484770e.pdf (last accessed April 2018).

Thomas, N.J. & Carcillo, J.A. (1998). Hypovolemic shock in pediatric patients. *New Horizons* 6(2), 120–129.

Wheeler, D.S., Wong, H.R. & Shanley, T.P. (eds) (2014). *Pediatric Critical Care Medicine, Volume 2: Respiratory, Cardiovascular and Central Nervous Systems*. Springer-Verlag, London.

Chapter 7

Pain and pain management

Helen Monks, Kate Heaton-Morley and Sarah McDonald

Aim

This chapter provides an overview of mechanisms of pain and pain management. There is an emphasis on an individual approach to care provision along with the role others, including family, can play in relieving or alleviating pain.

Learning outcomes

On completion of this chapter, the reader will be able to:

- Outline the anatomy and physiology of children's pain.
- Discuss common myths relating to pain in infants, children and young people.
- Describe common approaches to pain assessment for infants, children and young people.
- Describe common pharmacological and non-pharmacological pain management interventions for infants, children and young people.

Keywords

- nociceptive pain
- ascending/descending pain pathway
- reflex arc
- gate control theory
- neuropathic pain
- cognitive development
- pain perception
- behavioural cues
- pharmacological/non-pharmacological
- opioids/non-opioids
- distraction

Fundamentals of Children's Applied Pathophysiology: An Essential Guide for Nursing and Healthcare Students, First Edition.
Edited by Elizabeth Gormley-Fleming and Ian Peate.
© 2019 John Wiley & Sons Ltd. Published 2019 by John Wiley & Sons Ltd.
Companion website: www.wileyfundamentalseries.com/childpathophysiology

Test your prior knowledge

1. Identify the body system and any anatomy and physiology involved in transmission, sensation and perception of pain.
2. What do you understand by the terms acute and chronic pain?
3. How would you assess a child's pain?
4. Identify a pain assessment tool for school-age children.
5. What common behaviours do children display when in pain?
6. How can the family be involved in the assessment and management of their child's pain?
7. Name five non-pharmacological techniques used for controlling pain in children.
8. Discuss one of the pharmacological methods used to control acute pain.

Introduction

Many definitions of pain exist. The following definition is perhaps one of the most well known.

> Pain is an unpleasant sensory and emotional experience associated with actual or potential tissue damage or described in terms of such damage. Pain is always subjective. Each individual learns the application of the word through experiences related to injury in early life.
>
> (International Association for the Study of Pain [IASP], 1979, p. 250)

This definition has since been revised but the original still has great relevance today.

It is important to note that pain does not always arise from tissue damage. Pain can arise from relatively 'normal' activities such as touch, or even from tissue that does not exist (phantom limb pain). Therefore pain is a complex phenomenon.

The definition from IASP (1979) is especially important for children's nurses because:

- it relates to the physiology of pain
- it relates to how pain is perceived by a child
- it relates to the experience of pain during childhood and the affect this has on the way that pain is experienced in adulthood.

Therefore, whilst it is possible to generalise and offer some explanations about the way in which children experience pain from an anatomical and physiological perspective, it seems from the definition that much about the way in which pain is experienced is individual and dependant on biopsychosocial factors (Table 7.1).

In view of these biopsychosocial factors it is easy to see why the pain experience is considered unique to the individual. This experience relates to the perception as well as the response to pain. Some people are thought of as having a high or low pain threshold – it seems likely that, while some humans have largely equitable physiological factors, other factors such as psychological state can vary enormously and therefore significantly affect the pain experience.

For children some of these factors have heightened significance. According to the child's age and stage of development the cognitive experience of pain may be very different, for example, small children may perceive pain as a punishment and older children may relate pain to more sinister reasons like death and dying (Twycross, Dowden & Stinson, 2013).

For children, the experiences and responses formed in early life can have a dramatic impact not just in the present but also for the future. Not least, pain can be an important

Table 7.1 The experience of individual and biopsychosocial factors

Characteristics of host	
Biological	genetics, sex, endogenous pain control
Psychological	anxiety, depression, coping, behaviour
Cognitive	
Disease	
History	
Present disease	
Environment	
Socialisation	
Lifestyle	
Traumas	
Cultural	expectations, upbringing, roles

Source: Holdcroft & Power 2003.

developmental learning tool; children learn to avoid certain actions because they have discovered that pain is a consequence, in other words warning of danger (Franck, Greenberg & Stevens, 2000). Pain also has an important protective function in terms of warning and diagnosis of illness or disease, as many have painful symptoms (Tortora & Derrickson, 2009). For these reasons this type of pain is often referred to as protective pain.

🚩 Red Flag

Some children cannot feel pain because of altered physiology such as nerve damage and therefore pain does not serve as a warning of danger. However, some children may feel pain but cannot react to the danger, such as immobile children unable to withdraw from a painful stimulus.

Pain perception, assessment and management in children is a complex subjective issue. A significant factor influencing a child's pain experience is their developmental stage. This is not limited to age-related expectations – it includes previous experience, context and the child's perceptions of the pain experience.

Anatomy and physiology of pain in children

In order to offer effective and safe care to those in pain, the nurse is required to describe the anatomy and physiology of pain transmission and sensation, and to understand the key features of nociceptive and neuropathic pain. There are several common myths that are related to the physiology of children's pain; being aware of these can help provide care that is child- and family-centred.

The nervous system is divided into two parts:

1. the peripheral nervous system (PNS) comprising the cranial nerves, spinal nerves and autonomic nervous system;
2. the central nervous system (CNS) comprising the brain and spinal cord.

Pain is a complicated phenomenon. Although much is known about how we feel pain, scientists are still discovering information about the anatomy and physiology of pain.
Pain can be broadly divided into two groups: nociceptive pain and neuropathic pain.

Nociceptive pain

Essentially there are four stages to the process:

1. Pain receptors (nociceptors) in the skin are stimulated.
2. A message travels to the spinal cord.
3. Neurotransmitters within the dorsal horn of the spinal cord communicate with nerves and pass the message to the brain.
4. The thalamus 'unravels' the message and sends it to various parts of the brain to be analysed and interpreted.

Stages 1 and 2 are within the PNS.
Stages 3 and 4 are within the CNS.
See Fig. 7.1.
McCaffery and Pasero (1999) describe the processes involved for nociceptive pain as:

- transduction
- transmission
- perception
- modulation.

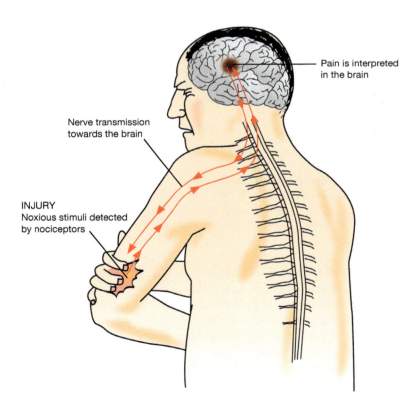

Figure 7.1 Pathway of pain transmission and interpretation. *Source:* Nair & Peate 2013. Reproduced with permission of Wiley.

Transduction

A noxious (harmful, from the Latin *noxa* meaning 'harm') stimulus to the nerve cell is detected by nociceptors (detectors of harm) and transformed into an electrical signal. Noxious stimuli are usually divided into three main types (Nair & Peate, 2013):

1. mechanical, e.g., laceration
2. thermal, e.g., burn
3. chemical, e.g., inflammation caused by release of histamines.

Nociceptors are free nerve endings of nerve fibres found in almost every tissue in the body (Tortora & Derrickson, 2011).

Transmission

During this phase the information is sent via nerve fibres (A and C, see later) to the dorsal horn in the spinal cord and ultimately to the thalamus in the brain. This is known as the ascending pain pathway. Transmission occurs by way of synapses where information is passed on by complex electrical and chemical processes (Marieb, 2015).

Perception

This is when pain is felt. The thalamus sends the information to various parts of the brain to be analysed and interpreted. The somatosensory cortex enables pain to be described and located, the limbic system enables emotional response and the reticular system enables action to be taken in response to pain (Melzack & Wall, 1996). It is thought that the limbic system is important in the memory of pain which serves as a protective measure for the future (avoidance of experiences that have previously been found to be painful) (Godfrey, 2005).

Modulation

This is the body's response to pain, in that there are various factors that increase or reduce the feeling of pain. It is the descending pain pathways that are responsible for the increase or decrease in the pain signals.

Neuropeptides are released, which are also known as endogenous opioids (the body's own analgesia). There are three major groups: endorphins, encephalins, and dynorphins (Nair & Peate, 2013). Differences in an individual's production of these properties could explain why, for the same painful procedure, some people feel levels of pain that are different from those felt by others (Briggs, 2010). Activities such as distraction can inhibit the pain signals (Melzack & Wall, 1965). In this way distraction has long been used as a technique to help children cope with painful procedures (Twycross *et al.*, 2013) and children are sometimes observed to self-distract by playing fervently when in discomfort, which helps them to cope with their pain (McCaffery & Beebe, 1989). This concept is widely regarded to be explained by the gate control theory (Melzack & Wall, 1965), which is described later in this section.

Ascending pain pathways

The ascending pain pathways (Fig. 7.2) originate from the spinal cord and are primarily responsible for sending information to the brain. This pathway is divided into three tracts. Two are specifically involved in transmission of pain impulses to the brain: the spinothalamic tract and the spinoreticular tract (Twycross, Dowden & Bruce, 2009).

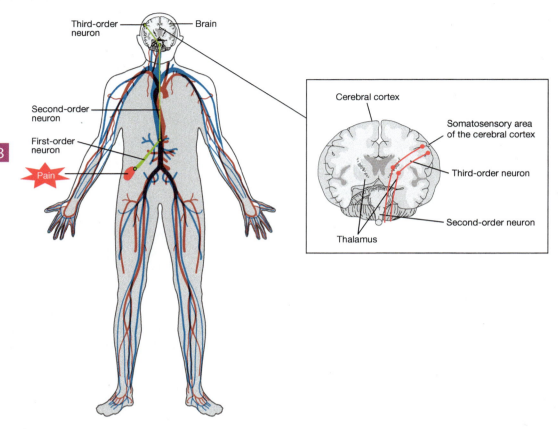

Figure 7.2 The ascending pain pathway. *Source:* Nair & Peate 2013. Reproduced with permission of Wiley.

Once the nociceptors are stimulated and a pain message (impulse) is generated, it travels by way of the ascending pain pathway toward the thalamus in the brain, where it is subsequently analysed and interpreted. The pathway consists of first-, second-, and third-order neurones that pass the message on consequentially:

- First-order neurones travel from the nociceptors to the spine.
- Second-order neurones travel from the spine to the thalamus in the brain.
- Third-order neurones travel between various parts of the brain.

Neurotransmitters convey the message between the neurones. A-delta fibres and C fibres are first-order sensory fibres (the first wave of communication). The speed at which the message travels depends on the diameter of the fibre and whether the fibre is myelinated or not (Table 7.2). Myelinated nerve fibres have an axon which is encased in a lipid covering that

Table 7.2 Size and speed of first-order sensory fibres

Sensory fibre	Diameter (μm)	Myelinated	Speed of conduction (m/s)
A-beta (Aβ) fibres	6–12	Yes	35–75
A-delta (Aδ) fibres	1–5	Yes	5–35
C fibres	0.2–1.5	No	0.5–2

Source: Nair & Peate 2013.

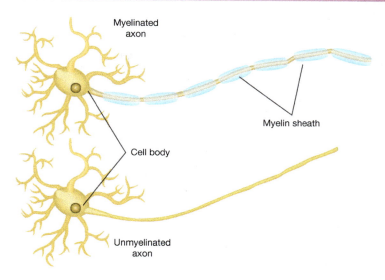

Figure 7.3 Basic structure of myelinated and unmyelinated nerve fibres. *Source:* Nair & Peate 2013. Reproduced with permission of Wiley.

acts as an insulation, helping to increase the speed of travel. This is where the terms white and grey matter originate: in preserved brains myelinated parts (axons) appear white and unmyelinated parts (cell bodies and dendrites) appear grey (Colbert *et al.*, 2012) (Fig. 7.3). A-delta fibres are larger in diameter and are myelinated whereas C fibres are smaller in diameter and not myelinated. Hence the capability of C fibres to conduct messages is slower than A-delta fibres (Nair & Peate, 2013). This is thought to provide the basis for the theory that pain is felt in two waves, for example, when you stub your toe – the first being the initial sharp pain and the second being the dull pain that follows (Tortora & Derrickson, 2011).

Reflex arc

This is where the messages about noxious stimuli are processed quickly and in a particular way in order to produce a rapid protective motor response, such as lifting a foot up quickly if a sharp object is stepped upon. As the term suggests, a reflex is elicited to force the body away from the harmful stimulus. Two neurones are involved in this process: a sensory (afferent) neurone and a motor (efferent) neurone. The noxious stimulus triggers a sensory impulse which travels to the spinal cord in the usual way but here two synaptic transmissions occur at the same time: one travels as normal to the brain to be analysed and interpreted; the other is transmitted to an interneurone which transmits to a motor neurone, which in turn, produces a motor response (Marieb, 2015).

Descending pain pathways

Descending pain pathways originate within the brain and can inhibit ascending nerve signals. Therefore it is within the descending nerve pathway that modulations occur and it is here that Melzack and Wall's gate control theory (1965) can be illustrated.

Gate control theory

A number of theories exist to explain how pain is experienced but the one that continues to hold widespread support is the gate control theory (Fig. 7.4) proposed by Melzack and Wall in 1965.

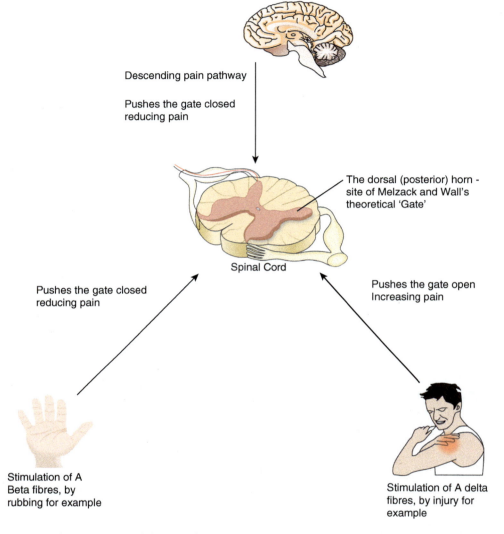

Figure 7.4 The gate control theory of pain. *Source:* Nair & Peate 2013. Reproduced with permission of Wiley.

Simply speaking, the theory is that the pain impulse has to pass through a theoretical gate to enable the brain to receive, perceive and interpret the impulse as painful. Broadly the theory works on the basis that stimulation of A-delta fibres and C fibres pushes the gate open and the stimulation of A-beta fibres pushes the gate closed, but that also the presence (or absence) of other factors like fear or distraction may open or close the gate (McCaffery & Beebe, 1989).

As certain constituents of the message push the gate open, the impulse is allowed to travel to the brain, and pain is felt. In the same way, other factors may be present which inhibit the opening of the gate (or close it after it has been opened) leading to a lack of perception of pain or having the effect of relieving the pain. The actual mechanisms involved are very complex and comprise a complicated interplay involving chemical and electrical reactions between all the connections involved (Marieb, 2015).

Effects of pain on vital signs

The nature of pain is more than a chain of anatomical and physiological processes; likewise the effects of pain are more complex than just physical reactions.

Nevertheless it is important to note that pain can significantly affect the vital signs of children. Common deviations in vital signs as a result of pain can be:

- increased heart rate (tachycardia)
- increased rate of breathing (tachypnoea)
- high blood pressure (hypertension)

(Twycross, Dowden & Bruce, 2009)

Common myths about anatomy and physiology of children's pain

It is clear that the perception of pain is a complex phenomenon. Children's pain has additional complexities particularly concerning anatomical structures, which in some cases are not fully developed, along with developing emotional and cognitive states.

Unfortunately this can give rise to some unfounded and incorrect assumptions about children's pain, which can lead to significant mismanagement.

Some myths relating to the assessment and management of children's pain will be addressed later in this chapter but two common myths related to the anatomy and physiology of children's pain are noted here.

Myth: Infants cannot feel pain because of an immature nervous system
The work of Anand, Sippell and Aynsley-Green (1987) established that infants feel pain. Since that time other studies have supported this notion. It is, however, accepted that some differences are present, for example, nociceptive pain messages travel to the spinal cord through unmyelinated rather than myelinated fibres (Mathew & Mathew, 2003).

Myth: Infants do not feel as much pain as adults
Mathew and Mathew (2003) note that several factors suggest that infants are actually likely to feel pain more intensely than older persons.

Neuropathic pain

The pathophysiology of neuropathic pain is not as clearly understood as nociceptive pain and consequently is often more difficult to assess and manage (Twycross et al., 2009). Neuropathic pain is the abnormal processing of sensory input, perhaps due to damage to the peripheral or central nervous system (McCaffery & Pasero, 1999). In this way a stimulus that is normally felt as a non-painful sensation, for example, the light stroking of a hand, can be felt as extremely painful (McCaffery & Pasero, 1999).

Acute and chronic pain

There are many types of pain documented but acute and chronic are two of the types most commonly referred to.

Acute pain

Melzack and Wall (1996) describe the characteristics of acute pain as the combination of pain, tissue damage and anxiety, but there is (at some point) recovery. Modern definitions of acute pain build on this further:

> Acute pain may be defined as pain that subsides as healing takes place, that is to say, is of a limited duration and has a predictable end.
>
> (Royal College of Nursing [RCN], 2009, p. 8)

Chronic pain

By contrast Melzack and Wall (1996) note that chronic pain persists after healing has occurred, is no longer a symptom of injury or disease, and has no useful function. Although much more is known about chronic pain these days, the definition remains rather more nebulous than that of acute pain, but there is a general view that pain is considered chronic when it has persisted for longer than 3 months (IASP, 2011).

Common approaches to assessing pain in infants, children and young people

There are a number of common approaches to pain assessment. The nurse needs to understand the context of the pain experience for children and young people, and be able to identify appropriate validated pain assessment tools for infants, children and young people.

The pain experience for children

It is widely acknowledged that pain is a biopsychosocial experience that is made more complex by the subjective nature of the experience of pain through the life span. It is therefore difficult to truly relate to what another individual is experiencing – a headache will be interpreted differently by different people. This phenomenon is made more complex when attempting to assess pain in infants, children and young people due to their age, development, communication abilities, previous experience (or lack of), gender, ethnicity, cultural and family influences.

Acute pain occurs from noxious stimuli and may be experienced by children in the form of accidents and injury, surgical interventions, and some procedural events, such as dressing changes and phlebotomy. Chronic, persistent or recurrent pain derives from numerous complex stimuli and can be linked to long-term conditions such as sickle cell disease or juvenile idiopathic arthritis. Common types of recurrent pain in children and young people are headaches, abdominal pain, back pain and musculoskeletal pain (King *et al.*, 2011). Children have exposure to different painful experiences at different stages of their development. They adapt to these experiences and consequently alter their perceptions, responses and coping strategies to the pain experience.

⚑ Red flag

It is imperative that healthcare professionals appreciate the individual nature of pain and its meaning to infants, children and young people and their families.

Factors affecting children and young people's perceptions of pain

- previous experiences, good or bad
- inability to communicate
- peer pressure
- ethnicity and gender (stereotyping)
- coping mechanisms
- anxiety
- lack of control
- support from parents/family
- age
- fatigue
- professional attitudes/ward culture
- type and amount of information given
- understanding of the meaning of pain
- fear

Cognitive development and the perception of pain

An understanding of the phenomenon of pain and its assessment developed first from an adult perspective (Kortesluoma & Nikkonen, 2006). More is being understood about the child's perception of pain, but it should be acknowledged that each child and family are individual and may not exhibit or report their pain in the same way as another. Exploring this phenomenon through a biopsychosocial perspective is essential and becomes a more valid assessment when this is supplemented by incorporating knowledge of the cognitive development of the child.

Neonates and infants

Neonates and infants respond to pain in a physiological and behavioural manner. This may result in bradycardia and/or apnoea, and the cry may be intense and high pitched with stiffening of the body and a grimacing expression on the face. Repeated painful stimuli may have consequences on growth, development and susceptibility to infection (Boxwell, 2010). It is imperative that the physical dimension of pain is anticipated and treated prophylactically.

Pre-school child

For the pre-school child the physical pain and context of events are important – pain during rough play while children are enjoying themselves may be brushed off and attention to it dismissed. However, the same level of pain inflicted while the child is frightened or fatigued may have a different response. The expression of pain here is predominantly behavioural: anger, aggression, crying, and physical withdrawal or over-activity (Twycross & Smith, 2006). Pre-school children may be incapable of understanding cause and effect and have little concept of time, and the significance of associated events often takes precedence over physical pain. Indeed, the child may find separation from loved ones more 'psychologically' painful than physical pain or illness (Carter & Simons, 2014).

Therefore minimising the psychological distress becomes of equal importance to the relief of physical pain. Often the presence of a well-loved cuddly toy or a sticking plaster with a favourite character on it will be the child's pain relief of choice as psychological comfort is as important as physical comfort.

School-age child

As children develop and progress through school their cognitive development becomes more reasoned and the development of logical thinking is evident. The school-age child has increased language and verbal skills although age is not a reliable indicator of cognitive ability. Indeed, the child may suffer psychological stress alongside illness and the pain experience and, as a result, may regress developmentally. In addition, some children are predisposed to immaturity and may fantasise about internal body processes and disease, which can result in increased anxiety levels and enhanced perceptual awareness (Twycross & Smith, 2006). For example, children may exhibit surprise once a plaster is removed from a broken leg to see that their leg is actually still there and the magic plaster made it better.

Carter and Simons (2014) warn that a child's imagination can summon up dramatic and frightening scenarios due to pain and fear being intertwined. Children's version of logic can inadvertently encourage frightening misconceptions which may be enhanced by their peer group or family members – such as the 6-year-old boy who was helpfully told by another boy that his tonsils would be removed by slitting this throat open! As a consequence of misconceptions, post-operative pain may be challenging to manage.

Adolescents

Adolescents are more able to think in abstract terms and understand the nature of the pain experience, and are more able to communicate their feelings. However, great care should again be taken with assumptions based on age, as young people may be emotionally immature and lack the necessary coping skills. Forgeron and Stinson (2014) suggest that anxiety, depression, self-esteem and emotional states can affect how the young person perceives pain. Although often independent, the adolescent may be in need of great compassion and understanding.

Cognitively impaired child

Cognitively impaired children present a challenge for parents and carers alike because of their altered processing and communication abilities. It is sometimes difficult to know if they perceive pain and sensation in the same manner as a child without impairment. McDonald and Cooper (2001) suggest that children with physical and learning disabilities may show higher pain thresholds and their autonomic, motor and sensory systems may have an effect on the pain experience meaning. This may indicate that they have reduced sensitivity to pain. Because of the communication difficulties with this group of children, it is imperative that accurate pain assessments are performed regularly in collaboration with carers who know them and their behaviours well.

Gender and cultural aspects of pain in children, young people and their families

It is generally accepted that alongside cognitive and psychological factors, such as fear, anxiety, emotion and fatigue, the attitudes of the child and family toward pain and illness are of significant consequence (Schechter, Berde & Yaster, 2003). The meaning and behavioural norms in response to pain may be learned from parents, family members and experiences in the social environment. Glasper and Richardson (2006) define this as culture, meaning that it is dynamic, helps to identify life habits and customs, and gives the child and family a group identity and a pattern for living. Culture is important and thoroughly internalised.

Almost three decades ago, McGrath (1990) identified that when reporting pain, boys were expected to 'play it away' while girls were advised to rest, given medication and afforded sympathy. This may have given credence to the assumption that giving attention may lead to the child developing sophisticated somatic complaints, and that an excessive sustained reliance on others or on medication may result in an inability to use natural capacity to suppress pain. Research by Perquin *et al.* (2000) established that girls aged 12–14 experienced the most pain and reported it more than boys. The relationship of reporting pain with age and gender must be borne in mind when performing pain assessment.

East (1992) considers cultural aspects to be of significance when children and families deal with and report pain. British children tend to be stoical about their pain, but prefer to have company while in pain, whereas Australian children often prefer to be alone. The Irish are said to be stoical also, but may be more concerned about the future consequences of their pain. Edwards *et al.* (2001) report that African Americans use more distraction and praying/hoping to cope with pain. The Muslim view is that one is purged of one's sins through pain and illness (Sheikh & Gatrad, 2001).

Carter (1994) claims that nurses' culture affects their perception of a child's pain and it should also be acknowledged that there may be a difference in the level of educational background between families and the healthcare team. It is clear that assessing pain in infants, children and young people and their families is a complex issue and demands a holistic, non-judgemental approach. Care should be taken to be mindful of the psychosocial aspects mentioned earlier before moving on to specific assessment techniques outlined in the following sections.

Methods of pain assessment (see Table 7.3)

QUESTT approach (Baker & Wong, 1987)

Question the child
Use pain rating scales
Evaluate behaviour and physiological changes
Secure parental involvement
Take cause of pain into account
Take action and evaluate results

Self-report

The RCN (2009) recommend that despite the subjective complexity of pain, children's self-report of their pain is the preferred approach where possible. Forgeron and Stinson (2014) advise that the use of pain diaries and tracking a child's pain over time may be useful. Also, it is necessary to assess quality of sleep, social functioning, and physical and emotional health as these can give an overview of the effect of pain on the child and family. Often, it is appropriate for a carer to report and assess pain on a child's behalf, using appropriate and validated tools (RCN, 2009).

Chapter 7 — Pain and pain management

Table 7.3 Validated, age-appropriate pain assessment tool suggestions

Age	Tool
Infants and neonates	Comfort **C**rying, **R**equires O$_2$ for saturation above 95, **I**ncreased vital signs, **E**xpression and **S**leeplessness (CRIES) Premature Infant Pain Profile (PIPP) Neonatal Infant Pain Scale (NIPS)
Toddlers and young children	**F**aces, **L**egs, **A**ctivity, **C**ry, **C**onsolability (FLACC) Children's Hospital of Eastern Ontario Pain Scale (CHEOPS) COMFORT Visual analogue scales (such as faces scale)
Older children and young people	Visual analogue scales (such as faces, numbers) Poker chip Colour analogue scale Word descriptor scale
Children with cognitive impairment	**F**aces, **L**egs, **A**ctivity, **C**ry, **C**onsolability (FLACC) Paediatric pain profile (PPP) Non-communicating children's pain checklist revised (NCCPC-R)

Source: Adapted from www.rcn.org.uk/childrenspainguideline. A more comprehensive and detailed algorithm appears within the guidelines with evidence for the validated tools cited.

Behavioural cues

Twycross *et al.* (2013) found that nurses considered behavioural cues important when assessing pain but that difficulty is encountered when the child does not behave in a manner that makes it explicit that they are in pain. In addition, Dickin and Green (2010) propose that as children develop, their behaviour may become more withdrawn and they may conceal pain as a means of protection, so behavioural cues should be used in combination with physiological and self-report techniques. Panjganj and Bevan (2016) reinforce this message as their literature review reveals that children's behavioural cues were misinterpreted by nurses. It is important to monitor these behavioural cues and interpret them, together with the child's family.

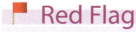
Red Flag

The common behaviours indicated in Table 7.4 may not be limited to a particular age race, gender or culture.

Table 7.4 Pain and behavioural cues

Age of child	Common behaviours exhibited
Infants	Grimacing, high-pitched crying, changes in breathing pattern, difficulty in calming, quivering chin, difficulty sucking, hiccupping, avoiding eye contact, wanting to be still
Toddlers and young children	Increase in crying, irritability or restlessness, loss of interest in play, difficulty sleeping, reduction in eating or drinking, quiet or curled, need to be held, pulling at affected body part, saying something hurts, difficulty sleeping
School-age child	Difficulty sleeping, moaning/crying, holding or protecting area of discomfort, loss of interest in play, decrease in activity level, complaining of pain, reduction in eating or drinking
Adolescent	Increasingly quiet, loss of interest in friends and family, decrease in activity level, increase in anger or irritability, changes in eating habits

Source: Adapted from Turner-Cobb 2014.

Involving parents and family members

A previously mentioned, children may absorb some pain perception from their families and therefore also coping styles and an ability to communicate their pain experience. Forgeron and Stinson (2014) acknowledge that behaviours exhibited by parents have been shown to affect how the child copes with pain. So if parents often talk about their pain symptoms, the child mirrors this with more symptom complaints. Parents assess their children's pain through a range of different cues identified earlier and take into account how different their behaviour is from their usual selves. Carter and Simons (2014) comment that while nurses and other professionals have pain assessment tools, parents use a mental checklist and intuition based on their intimate, subjective knowledge of their child. Parents may be assessing their child's pain in addition to being concerned about the cause of the pain or illness, and managing their own and their child's distress. Forgeron and Stinson (2014) advise that nurses should work with the parents to help them support their child, but recognise that their excessive worry can sometimes negatively affect their child's ability to cope.

Common myths about the assessment of children's pain

Myth: A playing/sleeping child cannot be in pain

It is well recognised that a child can engage in self-distraction and may use play as a coping mechanism. Indeed increased activity is often a sign of pain. Conversely, if a child is sleeping – this may be as a result of exhaustion from dealing with the pain (Eland, 1985 in Twycross & Smith, 2006).

Myth: Children cannot tell you where the pain is

Young children are able to demonstrate on a body chart where they hurt despite not knowing the body-part names (Van Cleve & Svedra, 1993 in Twycross & Smith, 2006), and by the age of 3–4 years they can also tell adults how much it hurts (Harbeck & Peterson, 1992 in Twycross & Smith, 2006).

Pain management

It is essential for the nurse to understand the importance of effective pain management for children and young people, and to be able to explain the management of acute, chronic and procedural pain in children and young people.

It is suggested by Twycross *et al.* (2013) that the management of pain in children is still substandard despite the availability of clinical guidelines for management. This part of the chapter will discuss the factors that influence pain management, effective strategies and pain management practices in the care of the child.

Children with unrelieved pain can experience both physical and psychological effects that are undesirable. These physical effects include rapid, shallow breathing, increased oxygen requirements and increased stress hormones (WHO, 1997). The psychological effects include anxiety, distress, decreased appetite and sleeplessness (WHO, 1997). Untreated pain can have profound effects on the future attitudes and behaviour of the child (Wilson-Smith, 2011).

The importance of the family in the management of pain cannot be underestimated, as parents may know which analgesia works best for their child. Parents have an important role in the non-pharmacological management of pain as they can provide essential distraction.

The management of pain is not solely the responsibility of the nurse. A multidisciplinary approach to pain management can lessen the side effects of treatment and potential complications (Williams & Rose, 2015). Acute pain management teams within paediatrics were developed in the 1990s and have foundations on a solid and established evidence base (RCoA, 1990). The multidisciplinary team may involve a number of professionals with the overall responsibility lying with the consultant and specialist nurses (RCoA, 2014).

Current guidance emphasises the need for individual children to have in place appropriate, flexible and safe plans that cater for their development, age and clinical condition. This of course requires the use of a validated pain assessment tool (APAGBI, 2012). Pain management is the involvement of an appropriate and individualised approach that uses both non-pharmacological and pharmacological approaches (AHRQ, 2008).

For effective pain management strategies to be adopted, it is important to understand the type of pain that the child is experiencing. Acute, chronic and procedural pain are common types of pain experiences that children encounter.

Acute pain

This type of pain is usually short-lived and can last from days to weeks. There are a number of causes of acute pain including injury, medical procedures and surgery (Schechter, 2006).

Chronic pain

This is classified as pain that persists over 3 months. Chronic pain persists beyond the time of expected tissue healing. It can be idiopathic, as a consequence of disease or injury. Macintyre *et al.* (2010) suggest that the two types of pain are placed on a continuum.

Procedural pain

This type of pain has been described as the most distressing and feared aspect of medical care (Howard *et al.*, 2012; Duff & Bliss, 2005). Of all children admitted to hospital, within 24 hours at least three-quarters of these children will experience at least one painful procedure (Stevens *et al.*, 2012). Examples of these procedures include venepuncture, cannulation, insertion and removal of tubes (e.g., catheters), and lumbar punctures.

Pain management

The first step in the effective management of any type of pain is accurate assessment to identify the appropriate treatment. Effective treatment includes encompassing the biological, psychological and social aspects of the child. The overarching aim in the management of pain in children is (APA, 2012):

- early identification
- prevention
- administration of appropriate analgesia
- reduction of stress response
- multimodal approach
- prevention of adverse reactions
- consideration of emotional aspects
- continued control post discharge.

Interventions
Psychological:

- relaxation
- hypnosis
- biofeedback
- CBT
- acceptance and commitment therapy
- music therapy
- distraction

Physical:

- TENS
- massage
- desensitisation
- acupuncture
- physiotherapy

Pharmacological:

- non-opioid
- opioid
- adjuvants
- PCA/NCA
- local/regional anaesthesia

Myth: Children are more sensitive to pain-relieving drugs than adults

If the prescription is based on the child's weight and is age appropriate then children are no more sensitive to analgesia than adults (Charlton, 2005).

The WHO (2012) 3-step management of pain

STEP 1 (For mild pain)
Non-opioid +/− adjuvant
STEP 2 (For moderate pain)
Weak opioid +/− adjuvant
STEP 3 (For severe pain)
Strong opioid +/− non-opioid =/− adjuvant

Pharmacological management

There are four components to the successful management of pain in children using the pharmacological approach. McGrath (1996) describes them as: by the child, by the ladder, by the clock, and by the mouth. The WHO analgesic ladder guides the nurse in the selection of analgesics that become progressively stronger based on the patient's level of pain (McGrath, 1996).

The pharmacodynamics of a drug are the mechanism of the drug and how the drug affects the body (Kanneh, 2002; Begg, 2008). There are two types of analgesia that have varying modes of mechanism. These are centrally acting drugs and peripherally acting drugs (Reaney & Trower, 2010). Centrally acting drugs act on the opioid receptors in the spinal cord and brain, whereas peripherally acting drugs inhibit the production of prostaglandins.

The administration of analgesia in children often relies on informal evidence and experience. The reasoning for this is the lack of indicative data to support the administration of pain-relieving drugs to children. A significant number of 'off-label' medications are therefore administered (WHO, 2007).

Non-opioid analgesia

This group of analgesics is given for mild pain and is the cornerstone of effective pain management. When used in conjunction with opioids, a multimodal approach can treat moderate to severe pain. The American Association of Anaesthesiologists (ASA) (2012), define the multimodal approach as a combination of two or more drugs, either from the same route or different routes, that have a different mechanism of action.

By combining a non-opioid with an opioid, a greater pain relief effect is experienced in comparison with administration of either drug alone. It is important for optimum effect that the correct dosages be used (BNFC, 2016) (Table 7.5).

Opioid analgesia (Table 7.6)

Opioid medication is used in conjunction with non-opioid analgesics for the treatment of moderate to severe pain. There are varying routes of administration and the choice of route may depend on the severity and duration of pain with consideration of the condition of the child.

Opioid drugs work by binding to opioid receptors in the spinal cord, central nervous system and peripheral nervous system (Twycross et al., 2013). There are three main receptors and these are: mu (μ), delta (δ), and kappa (κ). Whichever receptor the opiate binds to will determine the systemic effect.

Table 7.5 Non-opioid drugs

Drug	Trade name	Action	Route/s	Dose	Considerations
Paracetamol	Calpol® (oral suspension) Panadol® (capsule, tablet) Perfalgan® (intravenous)	Inhibits cyclooxygenase, selective to COX-2	Oral, IV, PR	Loading dose 2–3 mg/kg then 15–20 mg/kg 4–6 hours, max. 75 mg/kg/day	Not licensed for children under 2 months by mouth and 3 months rectally
Ibuprofen	Brufen® (oral suspension) Anadin® (tablet)	Cyclooxygenase inhibitor, reduction of prostaglandins	Oral	30 mg/kg/day 3–4 doses	Not licensed under 3 months or body weight under 5 kg
Diclofenac	Voltarol®	See above for NSAIDs	Oral, PR, IV, deep IM	6 months–17 yrs 0.3–1 mg/kg/day in 3 doses	Not licensed for children under 1 yr by mouth and 6 yrs by rectum. IV not licensed for children.

Source: BNFC 2016.

Pain and pain management Chapter 7

Table 7.6 Examples of opioid drugs

Drug	Trade name	Action	Route	Dose	Considerations
Codeine phosphate	Codeine	Metabolised in the liver and converted to morphine	Oral, PR	0.5–1 mg/kg/4-hourly; max. 60 mg/dose	Not licensed for children under 12 years and those with obstructive sleep apnoea
Morphine	Oramorph® (oral solution) Sevredol® (tablet) Morphine sulfate (IV)	Morphine is an opioid receptor agonist. Its main effect is binding to and activating the μ-opioid receptors in the central nervous system	PO, IV, SC	0.2–0.4 mg/kg/3–4-hourly (oral) 0.05–0.1 mg/kg/2–4-hourly (intravenous)	With oral use: Oramorph solution and MXL® capsules not licensed for use in children under 1 year. Sevredol tablets not licensed for use in children under 3 years. Oramorph unit dose vials and Filnarine® SR tablets not licensed for use in children under 6 years. MST Continus® preparations licensed to treat children with cancer pain (age-range not specified by manufacturer).
Tramadol hydrochloride	Zydol® Tramadol®	Binds to the μ-opioid receptors and inhibits the reuptake of serotonin and norepinephrine	PO, IV	1–2 mg/kg/4–6-hourly. Max. dose 100 mg/dose	Tramadol is licensed for children over the age of 12

Source: BNFC 2016.

Routes of opioid administration

Opioids can be administered via a large variety of routes. The choice of route is dependent on the specific needs of the child and the effect required.

- Oral
- Intranasal
- Intramuscular
- Intravenous
- Subcutaneous
- Inhaled
- Transdermal
- Epidural
- intrathaecal
- transmucosal

Notes:
Intranasal – diamorphine can be used intranasally for acute and procedural pain (Mudd, 2011).

Medication Alert

IM injections are best avoided in children as there are other more effective routes (Macintyre et al., 2010).

Intravenous – morphine can be given via IV route in intermittent doses.
Subcutaneous – SC morphine can be given via SC cannula.
Bolus administration – bolus administration usually is used in the short term.
Continuous morphine infusion – CMI is considered if pain is prolonged and intermittent and bolus administration is not appropriate. It is used for children who are cognitively unable to use the PCA method of control.
Patient-controlled analgesia – PCA is considered for children, typically over the age of 5 years, who are able to understand the process of self-administration of analgesia via a programmable pump (Maxwell & Yaster, 2000).

PCA administration

This is a method of intravenous analgesia, typically for use with morphine. The child is able to control the administration by means of a hand-held button attached to a computerised pump (Reaney & Trower, 2010). The pump is programmed to deliver an appropriate dose of analgesia based on the child's weight.

The use of patient-controlled analgesia in children experiencing moderate to severe pain is said to be the gold standard of pain management (Grass, 2005). The use of a PCA can allow for three methods of administration that can not only be used in isolation, but can also be used in combination. The following are examples of the different modes of PCA administration:

- Patient-administered bolus – This is infused at a set amount and the device has a 'lockout' facility to ensure that the child cannot overdose.
- Nurse administered (NCA) – This is a PCA that is controlled by the nurse. This method is chosen if the child is unable, for various reasons, to effectively use the PCA function. This can include end of life, cognitive impairment or physical disability (Franson, 2010).
- Continuous opioid infusion – Typically morphine is used and this method is for when PCA or NCA are not appropriate. This method allows constant pain relief to be administered to the child. There is function to administer bolus medication in breakthrough pain (Macintyre et al., 2010).

Individual assessment will determine the choice of method. It may be decided that continuously infused morphine is used in combination with PCA doses. The nursing care of a child who has a morphine PCA is detailed in Table 7.7.

Medication Alert

The use of codeine as an analgesic for children and adolescents is now restricted (EMA, 2013). The EMA have advised that it should only be used to relieve acute moderate pain in children older than 12 years in the event of paracetamol or ibuprofen being ineffective.

Regional analgesia

- Central blocks
- Peripheral blocks

Central blocks

Neuraxial analgesia (regional analgesia) is administration of local anaesthetic into the epidural or intrathecal space to prevent the transmission of pain messages sent by the

Table 7.7 Patient observations during PCA administration and for 4 hours following discontinuation

Observation	Frequency	Rationale
Heart rate	Hourly	Opioids can cause bradycardia
Respiratory rate	Hourly	Opioids can cause respiratory depression
Sedation score	Hourly	Opioids can cause sedation
Pain score	Hourly	To assess effectiveness of analgesia
Nausea and vomiting	Hourly	Opioids can cause nausea and vomiting, particularly in the initial stages
Pruritus	At least 4-hourly	Opioids can cause itching and urticaria
Urinary retention	Regular output monitoring	Opioids can induce urinary retention

Source: BNFC 2016.

nerves to the brain. This type of pain management can provide a more targeted delivery. This in turn can reduce the adverse effects of systemic opioids (ASA, 2004).

Epidural analgesia is effective in the management of some types of postoperative pain; for example, major abdominal, urologic, or lower extremity orthopaedic surgical procedures (Aram et al., 2001; Jylli, Lundeberg & Olsson, 2002). The caudal space is used as a single dose in the neonate and younger child (Patel, 2006).

Peripheral blocks

Peripheral nerve blocks are useful for specific site pain relief. They can be continuous via an infusion or single dose via a catheter (Dadure & Capdevila, 2012). Local anaesthetic of bupivacaine or levobupivacaine (see Table 7.8) is often used and opioids can be added (APA, 2012).

Table 7.8 Observations required for a child with a continuous epidural with levobupivacaine with/without fentanyl

Observation	Frequency	Rationale
Pain score (validated and appropriate)	Hourly	To monitor effectiveness of the analgesia
Sedation score	Hourly	Fentanyl can cause sedation
Heart rate	Hourly	Levobupivacaine can cause a decrease in heart rate
Respiratory rate	Hourly	To monitor for high motor block
Oxygen saturation	Continuous	To detect respiratory problems
Blood pressure	Hourly	Levobupivacaine can decrease blood pressure
Bromage score	4-hourly	Levobupivicaine can affect motor nerves
Sensory block	4-hourly	Monitor the spread of the block
Catheter site	6-hourly	To observe for leakage/redness
Pressure areas	At least 4-hourly	Local anaesthetic blocks can lead to loss of sensation
Agitation	Regularly	Levobupivacaine can cause agitation
Pruritus	Regularly	Fentanyl can cause itching
Nausea and vomiting	Hourly	Fentanyl is an emetic. Hypotension can lead to nausea
Temperature	4-hourly	Indication of catheter infection

Source: Based on Sheffield Children's Hospital Guidelines (2015). This guidance is for the Sheffield Children's Hospital NHS Foundation Trust and following local policies and procedures is advised.

Management of procedural pain

There are considerations that need to be addressed prior to and during the procedure that will aid the child and limit the distress encountered. Psychological preparation and parental presence is an important aspect in the management of painful procedures (Polkki, Pietila & Vehvilamen-Julkunen, 2003). There are a number of pharmacological strategies that may be considered, such as topical anaesthetics, Entonox®, pre-analgesia and sedation, which may assist in the management of such procedures. Assessment of pain, anxiety and fear should be considered in preparation.

Non-pharmacological management

The non-pharmacological approach to pain management in children can be used in conjunction with pharmacological management. Acute pain in children is usually accompanied by psychological distress and anxiety, which requires an integrated treatment approach (Duff, 2003; Young, 2005; Medrick, 2010). These approaches can be broadly defined as distracting measures and physical comfort measures (Konner, 2010).

Children are able to channel their imagination and are able to distract themselves from their surroundings in a way that adults find difficult. Children are able to allow themselves to be more open in the use of activities that may enable them to focus less on their pain (Twycross et al., 2009).

It is the healthcare practitioner who may decide on the appropriate intervention. The decision on that intervention needs, among other factors, to account for the child's age, cognition, behaviour and type of pain (Oakes, 2011).

Infants

It is well documented that the use of small amounts of oral sucrose in infants reduces the pain response during painful procedures (Harrison et al., 2010). Infants have a positive physiological response to oral stimulation which, together with physical comfort, can minimise pain during venepuncture and heel lancing (Krauss et al., 2016). Appropriate interventions in this age group include using mobiles, music and familiar objects.

Preschool

Preschool children benefit from physical comfort along with distraction. Interactive and passive distraction is valuable in the management of procedural pain. Cannulation and other procedural interventions can induce high levels of anxiety and can impair co-operation in this age group as they find it difficult to control their apprehension (Kagan & Herschkowitz, 2005). Appropriate interventions in this age group include reassurance and praise, reading books, blowing bubbles, simple stories and giving simple choices.

The younger child

Until the age of 5–7 years, a child may not have comprehension of verbal reasoning. School-age children develop the comprehension of reassurance and reasoning, and by now are able to recall past experiences (Kagan & Herschkowitz, 2005; White, 1996; Cohen, 2001). This age group enjoy hand-held games as well as relaxation, role-play with medical equipment, and the appropriate involvement of choice.

Adolescents

This age group are becoming more independent, prefer to listen to their favourite music and have an interest in technology. They are able to understand how muscle relaxation and controlled breathing can assist in pain management, and can be involved in decision making.

Case Study 1

Sophie is 11 and is admitted to hospital for the first time in her life with abdominal pain. Her Mum is with her and is understandably anxious to find out what is causing Sophie's pain. She cannot stay long as she has to get back to nursery to collect Sophie's younger brother, Danny. She will come back later after taking Danny to her estranged husband's flat.

1. What pain tools are appropriate to help to assess Sophie's pain?
2. What other factors would need to be considered?
3. What non-pharmacological methods could used to help Sophie?

Case Study 2

Alfie is a 10-year-old boy who has severely injured his right ankle playing football at school. He arrives in the emergency department via ambulance and accompanied by his teacher. His ankle is swollen and he is unable to move his leg. He is usually fit and well and is a keen footballer. His parents have been contacted and are on their way.

1. What type of pain is Alfie experiencing and how can you assess the amount/type of pain?
2. What drugs do you think Alfie should be given?
3. How do these drugs work and what are their main side effects?
4. Are there any other considerations to be taken when administering analgesia to Alfie?

Conclusion

While it is a fact that there are anatomical and physiological processes involved in the sensation and perception of pain, for children and young people there are also many other factors which influence the sensation and perception of pain. This means that pain is a unique experience for each child, and is affected by gender, age and development, culture, and previous experiences within the context of the family. It is essential that the assessment is performed in partnership with the child and family where possible. In view of this there can be no single approach for assessment and management of pain – it is bespoke for each child. Consequently, for the effective management of children's pain a biopsychosocial and multimodal approach is required, which remains a challenge for children's nurses.

References

Agency for Healthcare Research and Quality (AHRQ) (2008). *Patient safety and quality: An evidence-based handbook for nurses.* [online] Available at: http://www.ahrq.gov/qual/nurseshdbk/ (accessed October 2016).

American Society of Anesthesiologists (ASA) (2004). Practice guidelines for acute pain management in the perioperative setting. An updated report by the American Society of Anesthesiologists Task Force on Acute Pain Management. *Anesthesiology* 100(6), 1573–1581.

American Society of Anesthesiologists (ASA) (2012). Practice guidelines for acute pain management in the perioperative setting. An updated report by the American Society of Anesthesiologists Task Force on Acute Pain Management. *Anaesthesiology* 116(2), 248–273.

Anand, K.J. Sippell, W.G. & Aynsley-Green, A. (1987). Randomised trial of fentanyl anaesthesia in preterm babies undergoing surgery: effects on the stress response. *Lancet* 329(8524), 62–66.

Aram, L., Krane, E.J., Kozloski, L.J. & Yaster, M. (2001). Tunneled epidural catheters for prolonged analgesia in pediatric patients. *Anesthesia and Analgesia* 92(6), 1432–1438.

Association of Paediatric Anaesthetists of Great Britain and Ireland (APA) (2012). Good practice in postoperative and procedural pain management, 2nd Edition, 2012. In: *Pediatric Anesthesia*, Vol. 22, Suppl. 1, pp. 1–79. Wiley; https://onlinelibrary.wiley.com/doi/pdf/10.1111/j.1460-9592.2012.03838.x (last accessed 11 April 2018).

Baker, C. & Wong, D. (1987). Q.U.E.S.S.T.: a process of pain assessment in children. *Orthopaedic Nursing* 6(1), 11–21.

Begg, E.J. (2008). *Instant Clinical Pharmacology*, 2nd edn. Wiley, Chichester.

Boxwell, G. (2010). *Neonatal Intensive Care Nursing*, 2nd edn. Routledge, London.

Briggs, E. (2010). Understanding the experience and physiology of pain. *Nursing Standard* 25(3), 35–39.

British National Formulary for Children (BNFC) (2016). [online]. Available at: https://www.medicinescomplete.com/mc/bnfc/current/PHP78520-analgesics.htm?q=analgesics&t=search&ss=text&tot=47&p=1#_hit (accessed November 2016).

Carter, B. (1994). *Pain in Infants and Children*. Chapman & Hall, London.

Carter, B. & Simons, J. (2014). *Stories of Children's Pain: Linking Evidence to Practice*. Sage, London.

Charlton, J.E. (ed.) (2005). *Core Curriculum for Professional Education in Pain*, 3rd edn. IASP Task Force on Professional Education. IASP Publications, Seattle.

Cohen, L.L., Blount R.L., Cohen, R.J., et al. (2001). Children's expectations and memories of acute distress: short- and long-term efficacy of pain management interventions. *Journal of Pediatric Psychology* 26, 367–374.

Colbert, B., Ankney, J., Lee, K. Stegall, M. & Dingle, M. (2012). *Anatomy and Physiology for Nursing and Healthcare Professionals*, 2nd edn. Pearson, London.

Dadure, C. & Capdevila, X. (2012). Peripheral catheter techniques. *Paediatric Anaesthesia* 22(1), 93–101.

Dickin, L. & Green, H. (2010). Pain assessment and management. In: Glasper, A., Aylott, M. & Battrick, C. (eds). *Developing Practical Skills for Nursing Children and Young People*. Hodder Arnold, London, Chap. 17.

Duff, A. (2003). Incorporating psychological approaches into routine paediatric venepuncture. *Archives for Diseases in Childhood* 88, 931–937.

Duff, A. & Bliss, A.K. (2005). Reducing stress during venepuncture. In: David, T.J. (ed.). *Recent Advances in Paediatrics 22*. Royal Society of Medicine Press, London, pp. 149–157.

Edwards, C.L., Fillingham, R.B. & Keefe, F. (2001). Race, ethnicity and pain. *Pain* 94, 133–137.

East, E. (1992). How much does it hurt? *Nursing Times* 88(40), 48–49.

European Medicines Agency (EMA) (2013). *Restricting the use of codeine when used for pain relief in children*. Available at: http://www.ema.europa.eu/ema/index.jsp?curl=pages/news_and_events/news/2013/06/news_detail_001829.jsp&mid=WC0b01ac058004d5c1 (accessed April 2017).

Forgeron, P.A. & Stinson, J. (2014). Fundamentals of chronic pain in children and young people. Part 1. *Nursing Children and Young People* 26(6), 29–34.

Franck, L., Greenberg, C. & Stevens, B. (2000). Pain assessment in infants and children. *Pediatric Clinics of North America* 47(3), 487–512.

Franson, H. (2010). Postoperative patient-controlled analgesia in the pediatric population: a literature review. *American Association of Nurse Anesthetists Journal* 78(5), 374–378.

Glasper, A. & Richardson, J. (2006). *A Textbook of Children's and Young People's Nursing*. Churchill Livingstone, London, Chap 4.

Godfrey, H. (2005). Understanding pain, part 1: physiology of pain. *British Journal of Nursing* 14(16), 846–852.

Grass, J.A. (2005). Patient-controlled analgesia. *Anesthesia and Analgesia* 101(5 Suppl), S44–S61.

Harrison, D., Bueno, M., Yamada, J., et al. (2010). Analgesic effects of sweet-tasting solutions for infants: current state of equipoise. *Pediatrics* 126(5), 894–902.

Holdcroft, A. & Power, I. (2003). Management of pain. *British Journal of Medicine* 326(7390), 635–639.

Howard, R.E., Lloyd-Thomas, A., Thomas, M., et al. (2010). Nurse-controlled analgesia (NCA) following major surgery in 10,000 patients in a children's hospital. *Paediatric Anaesthesia* 20(2), 126–134.

International Association for the Study of Pain (IASP) (1979). Pain terms; a list with definitions and usage. *Pain* 6, 249–252.

International Association for the Study of Pain (IASP) (2011). *Classification of Chronic Pain*, 2nd edn (Rev.). Available at: https://www.iasp-pain.org/PublicationsNews/Content.aspx?ItemNumber=1673 (last accessed April 2018).

Jylli, L., Lundeberg, S. & Olsson, G. L. (2002). Retrospective evaluation of continuous epidural infusion for postoperative pain in children. *Acta Anaesthesiologica Scandinavica* 46(6), 654–659.

Kagan, J. & Herschkowitz, N. (2005). *A Young Mind in a Growing Brain*. Lawrence Erlbaum Associates, Mahwah, NJ.

Kanneh, A. (2002). Paediatric pharmacological principles: an update, part 1. Drug development and paediatric pharmacodynamics. *Paediatric Nursing* 14(8), 36–42.

King, S., Chambers C.T., Huguet A., *et al.* (2011). The epidemiology of chronic pain in children and adolescents revisited: systematic review. *Pain* 152(12), 2729–2738.

Konner, M. (2010). *The Evolution of Childhood: Relationships, Emotion*, Mind. Belknap Press, Cambridge, MA.

Kortesluoma R.L. & Nikkonen, M. (2006). 'The most disgusting ever': children's pain description and views of the purpose of pain. *Journal of Child Health Care* 10(3), 213–227.

Krauss, B.S., Calligaris, L., Green, S.M. & Barbi, E. (2016). Current concepts in management of pain in children in the emergency department. *Lancet* 387(10013), 83–92.

Macintyre, P.E., Schug, S.A., Scott, D.A., Visser, E.J. & Walker, S.M.; APM:SE Working Group of the Australian and New Zealand College of Anaesthetists and Faculty of Pain Medicine (2010). *Acute Pain Management: Scientific Evidence*, 3rd edn. ANZCA & FPM, Melbourne.

Marieb, E. (2015). *Essentials of Human Anatomy and Physiology*, 11th edn. Pearson, London.

Mathew, P.J. & Mathew, J.L. (2003). Assessment and management of pain in infants. *Postgraduate Medical Journal* 79(934), 438–443.

Maxwell, L. & Yaster, M. (2000). Perioperative management issues in pediatric patients. *Anaesthesiology Clinics of North America* 18(3), 601–632.

McCaffery, M. & Beebe, A. (1989). *Pain: Clinical Manual for Nursing Practice*. Mosby, St. Louis.

McCaffery, M. & Pasero, C. (1999). *Pain: Clinical Manual*, 2nd edn. Mosby, St. Louis.

McDonald, A.J. & Cooper, M.G. (2001). Patient-controlled analgesia: an appropriate method of pain control in children. *Pediatric Drugs* 3(4), 273–284.

McGrath, P. (1990). *Pain in Children: Nature, Assessment and Treatment*. Guilford Press, New York.

McGrath, P. (1996). Development of the World Health Organization guidelines on cancer pain relief and palliative care in children. *Journal of Pain Symptom Management* 12, 87–92.

Mednick, L. (2010). Preparation for procedures. In: Shaw, R. & Demaso, D. (eds). *Textbook of Pediatric Psychosomatic Medicine*, 1st edn. APA Publishing, Washington, DC.

Melzack, R. & Wall, P. (1965). Pain mechanisms: a new theory. *Science*, 150(3699), 971–979.

Melzack, R. & Wall, P. (1996). *The Challenge of Pain*, 2nd edn. Penguin, London.

Mudd, S. (2011). Intranasal fentanyl for pain management in children: a systematic review of the literature. *Journal of Pediatric Healthcare* 25(5), 316–322.

Nair, M. & Peate, I. (2013). *Fundamentals of Applied Pathophysiology*, 2nd edn. Wiley, Oxford.

Oakes, L.L. (2011). *Compact Clinical Guide to Infant and Child Pain Management*. Springer Publishing, New York.

Panjganj, D. & Bevan, A. (2016). Children's nurses' post-operative pain assessment practices. *Nursing Children and Young People* 28(5), 29–33.

Patel, D. (2006). Epidural analgesia for children. *Continuing Education in Anaesthesia, Critical Care and Pain* 6(2), 63–66.

Perquin, C.W., Hazebroek-Kampschreur, A., Hunfield, J., *et al.* (2000). Pain in children and adolescents: a common experience. *Pain* 87(1), 51–58.

Polkki, T., Pietila, A.M. & Vehvilamen-Julkunen, K. (2003). Hospitalized children's descriptions of their experiences with post-surgical pain relieving methods. *International Journal of Nursing Studies* 40, 33–44.

Reaney, R. & Trower, C. (2010). In: Trigg, E. & Mohammed, T. (eds). *Practices in Children's Nursing. Guidelines for Hospital and Community*, 3rd edn. Churchill Livingstone Elsevier, Edinburgh.

Royal College of Anaesthetists (RCoA) (1990). *Commission on the Provision of Surgical Services: Report of a Working Party on Pain after Surgery*. RCoA, London.

Royal College of Anaesthetists (RCoA) (2014). *Guidelines for the provision of anaesthetic services for acute pain management*. RCoA, London.

Royal College of Nursing (RCN) (2009). *The recognition and assessment of acute pain in children. Update of full guideline*. RCN, London.

Schechter, N. (2006). Treatment of acute and chronic pain in the outpatient setting. In: Finley, G.A., McGrath, B.J. & Chambers, C.T. (eds). *Bringing Pain Relief to Children: Treatment Approaches*. Humana Press, Totowa, pp. 31–58.

Schechter, N., Berde, C. & Yaster, M. (eds) (2003). *Pain in Infants, Children and Adolescents*. Lippincott, Philadelphia.

Sheikh, A. & Gatrad, A. (2001). *Caring for Muslim Patients*. Radcliffe Press, Oxford.

Stevens, B.J., Harrison, D., Rashotte, J., et al.; CIHR Team in Children's Pain (2012). Pain assessment and intensity in hospitalized children in Canada. *Journal of Pain* 13(9), 857–865.

Tortora, G. & Derrickson, B. (2009). *Principles of Anatomy and Physiology*, 12th edn. Wiley, Hoboken, NJ.

Tortora, G. & Derrickson, B. (2011). *Principles of Anatomy and Physiology*, 13th edn. Wiley: Hoboken, NJ.

Turner-Cobb, J. (2014). *Child Health Psychology: A Biopsychosocial Perspective*. Sage, London.

Twycross, A. & Smith, J. (2006). The management of acute pain in children. In: Glasper, A. & Richardson, J. (eds). *A Textbook of Children's and Young People's Nursing*. Churchill Livingstone, London, Chap. 7.

Twycross, A., Dowden, S. & Bruce, E. (eds) (2009). *Managing Pain in Children: A Clinical Guide*. Wiley

Twycross, A., Dowden, S. & Stinson, J. (eds) (2013a). *Managing Pain in Children: A Clinical Guide for Nurses and Healthcare Professionals*, 2nd edn. Wiley, Oxford.

Twycross, A., Finley, G. & Latimer, M. (2013b). Pediatric nurses' post operative pain management practices: an observational study. *Journal for Specialists in Pediatric Nursing* 18(3), 189–201.

White, S. (1996). The child's entry into the age of reason. In: Sameroff, A. & Haith, M. (eds). *The Five to Seven Year Shift: The Age of Reason and Responsibility*. University of Chicago Press, Chicago.

Williams, G. & Rose, M. (2015). Managing acute pain in children and young people. In: *Core Standards for Pain Management Services in the UK*. Faculty of Pain Medicine of the Royal College of Anaesthetists. RCoA, London.

Wilson-Smith, E. (2011). Procedural pain management in neonates, infants and children. *Reviews in Pain* 5(3), 4–12.

World Health Organization (WHO) (1997). How to examine the impact of unrelieved pain. *Cancer Pain Release* 10(3).

World Health Organization (WHO) (2007). *Promoting Safety of Medicines for Children*. WHO, Geneva.

Young, K. (2005). Pediatric procedural pain. *American Emergency Medicine* 45, 160–171.

Chapter 8

Disorders of the nervous system

Petra Brown

Aim

The aim of this chapter is to provide the reader with an overview of the nervous system, and an understanding of the pathophysiological changes that are associated with disorders of this system.

Learning outcomes

On completion of this chapter, the reader will be able to:

- Outline the organisation, structure and function of the nervous system.
- Understand the pathophysiology of common childhood neurological disorders.
- Consider the priorities of a neurological nursing assessment of the young patient.
- Examine some key red flags in the assessment of neurological conditions.
- Discuss the management and nursing care of young patients with neurological disorders.

Keywords

- central and peripheral nervous system
- autonomic and somatic nervous system
- brain and spinal cord
- meninges
- cerebrospinal fluid (CSF)
- intracranial pressure (ICP)
- seizure
- haemorrhage
- tumour

Fundamentals of Children's Applied Pathophysiology: An Essential Guide for Nursing and Healthcare Students, First Edition.
Edited by Elizabeth Gormley-Fleming and Ian Peate.
© 2019 John Wiley & Sons Ltd. Published 2019 by John Wiley & Sons Ltd.
Companion website: www.wileyfundamentalseries.com/childpathophysiology

Chapter 8 — Disorders of the nervous system

Test your prior knowledge

1. List the two anatomical areas of the central (CNS) nervous system.
2. Describe the functions of the central (CNS) nervous system.
3. Name the four main anatomical areas of the brain.
4. Describe the four main functions of cerebrospinal fluid.
5. Review the role of neurotransmitters in the central (CNS) nervous system.
6. Outline the structure of the peripheral (PNS) nervous system.
7. Compare the structure and function of the autonomic and sympathetic nervous system.
8. Draw a diagram of a motor neurone cell.
9. Review fetal and childhood development of the nervous system.

Introduction

In conjunction with the endocrine system, the nervous system interacts with all body systems to maintain homeostasis. It is a complex system which co-ordinates and controls voluntary and involuntary action. It orientates us to the internal and external environment through sensory mechanisms. The nervous system assimilates experiences and information through memory, intelligence, learning and dreaming. It provides us with instinctual information and reflexes, at birth and beyond.

Structure of the nervous system

While the nervous system functions as a whole, it is useful to subdivide its anatomical structure and physiological components (Table 8.1, Fig. 8.1), to assist in understanding its complexity.

Central and peripheral nervous system

The nervous system may be divided into the central nervous system (CNS) and peripheral nervous system (PNS).

Physiologically, the nervous system is subdivided and organised as shown in Fig. 8.1.

Cellular structure of the nervous system

Highly specialised neurone (nerve) and neuroglia (nerve fibre) cells provide the cellular building blocks of the nervous system. Neurones are nerve cells primarily involved with the transmission of information, while neuroglial cells provide a variety of supportive functions.

Table 8.1 Anatomical structure of the nervous system

Central nervous system (CNS)	Peripheral nervous system (PNS)

• Brain
• Spinal cord
	• Cranial nerves
	• Spinal nerves
	• Sensory (afferent) neurones
	• Motor (efferent) neurones
	• Somatic nervous system (voluntary)
	• Autonomic nervous system (involuntary)
	   • sympathetic
	   • parasympathetic

Disorders of the nervous system Chapter 8

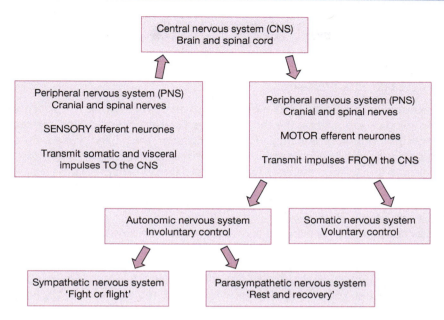

Figure 8.1 Organisation of the nervous system.

Transmission of nerve impulses

There are three types of nerve impulse transmission in the nervous system. Simple linear transmission passes electrical action potentials along neurones, through the exchange of sodium and potassium across cell membranes. This causes polarisation and depolarisation along the neurone. Saltatory conduction passes electrical action potentials along myelinated neurones. The action potential jumps between the nodes of Ranvier, thus travelling much faster than by simple linear transmission. The third type of transmission occurs via chemical neurotransmitters at synaptic endings. These include acetylcholine in the CNS and at neuromuscular junctions. Dopamine and norepinephrine (noradrenaline) are found within the CNS and autonomic nervous system. Other common synaptic neurotransmitters include serotonin and GABA (gamma-aminobutyric acid).

Disorders of the nervous system
Introduction

This section will outline some of the common neurological disorders encountered in childhood. The term applies to any condition that is caused by a dysfunction in the brain or nervous system, resulting in physical, behavioural and cognitive symptoms. The nervous system is a highly complex and integrated system and disorders are categorised by their causative nature. These include neurological dysfunction, cerebral dysfunction, head and spinal trauma, motor dysfunction, neurological tumours, infection and seizures.

Causes of neurological dysfunction
Prenatal causes

These occur in the womb during pregnancy. To recap, the nervous system develops early in the third week of embryonic development to form a neural tube, in a process called neurulation. During the fourth and eleventh week, distinct areas of the brain are formed.

The peripheral nervous system develops from the neural crest at around 4 weeks, alongside the spinal, cranial and autonomic nervous system. Growth continues until at birth, all the major structures of the nervous system are present. Exposure to factors, which may hinder neural development in pregnancy, may cause intellectual, behavioural and developmental problems.

- Neurotoxins can enter and damage a fetus's nervous system, via the placenta leading to neurological problems as the child develops. Fetal alcohol syndrome is linked to alcohol ingestion during pregnancy. Tobacco ingestion has been linked to challenging behaviours and developmental impairment. Lead and mercury ingestion have been linked to intelligence, memory, learning and development problems.
- Nutritional deficiencies in the last 3 months of pregnancy can decrease the number of brain cells. Spina bifida is linked to a maternal deficiency of folic acid before or during the early stages of pregnancy.
- Infections can be transmitted across the placenta from the mother. They can cause developmental problems and cerebral palsy in the case of chorioamnionitis. The Zika virus causes microcephaly, wherein the baby's head is smaller than normal and the brain may not be fully developed. Other infections, which cause prenatal dysfunction, include toxoplasmosis, rubella, cytomegalovirus, HIV, herpes simplex, hepatitis B and syphilis.
- Birth complications such as hypoxic brain damage can occur if the umbilical cord blood supply is interrupted or compromised during birth. The resultant lack of oxygen and nutrients can cause brain damage.

Congenital causes

Genetic abnormalities can lead to a variety of neurological disorders. In the main, genetic disorders are inherited rather than mutations of normal DNA. Inheritance is through an equal combination of parental chromosomes that create the fetal DNA. Human cells have 22 pairs of autosomes and 1 pair of sex chromosomes making a total of 46 chromosomes. This DNA contains the 'code', which makes us who we are and a number of factors can interact, in complex ways, to cause neurological and other disorders.

- Genetic mutations cause abnormalities that lead to alteration in development and can therefore cause neurological damage. Phenylketonuria is such an example, where the child inherits a faulty gene from each parent.
- Chromosome disorders have widespread effects because each chromosome contains approximately 20 000 genes. Down syndrome is caused by the presence of an extra copy of chromosome 21. Turner syndrome is caused by the loss of a chromosome. Microdeletions and microduplications of gene fragments can lead to conditions such as Cri-du-chat, 5p– and Prader-Willi syndromes.
- Metabolic disorders can cause neurological damage and need to be detected early. Babies with the inherited condition phenylketonuria (PKU) are unable to metabolise phenylalanine, which is present in food. High blood concentrations cause brain cell damage and affect intellectual ability. Many countries now routinely test babies at birth for the presence of phenylketonuria.

Acquired causes

These develop after birth and may be caused by trauma, infection, exposure to toxins, autoimmune disorders, epilepsy and neurological tumours.

Cerebral dysfunction

Cerebral dysfunction may be focal or global and alters the function of the brain and cerebral processes. Focal or localised dysfunction is caused by structural abnormalities such as tumours, local haemorrhage, congenital and acquired malformations. Global cerebral dysfunction affects the whole brain and is caused by metabolic, hypoxic, toxic, infective, haemorrhagic or traumatic events

Pathophysiology of raised intracranial pressure (ICP)

There are four interconnected cerebral ventricles in the brain. They are filled with cerebrospinal fluid (CSF) which continuously circulates through the ventricles and in the subarachnoid space around the brain and spinal cord.

ICP is one of the main sequela of cerebral dysfunction (Fig. 8.2). It may be caused by an increase in the volume within the cranium such as tumour growth, oedema, inflammation (meningitis), developmental abnormalities, excessive cerebrospinal fluid (hydrocephalus) or bleeding (haemorrhage).

The CSF has four main functions, which include mechanical protection of the delicate brain tissue against sudden contact with the hard bones of the skull. CSF supports the mass of the brain, preventing ischaemia in the lower parts. Chemical protection against fluctuations in pH and ionic composition and circulation of oxygen, nutrients and removal of waste products from cerebral metabolic processes, such as carbon dioxide.

Abnormal changes in ICP will influence cerebral blood flow. A raised ICP will lead to reduced blood flow, preventing adequate delivery of oxygen (O_2) and nutrients such as glucose to the brain cells. This lack of oxygen rapidly leads to brain tissue hypoxia. Concurrently carbon dioxide (CO_2) removal is impaired by a reduced blood flow and its accumulation will result in acidosis and a fall in pH.

Autoregulation and chemoregulation become impaired, leading to vasodilation of the cerebral blood vessels. This is initially the brain's attempt to increase blood, O_2 and nutrient flow to cerebral cells. In the confined space of the skull, there is nowhere for this increase in blood volume to go, causing fluid to 'leak' out of the cerebral arteries. This oedema formation leads to a further increase in ICP, causing blood flow to become more impaired. The brain is extremely sensitive and a lack of oxygen for more than 3 minutes will result in cerebral cell death.

As the ICP rises, CSF is prevented from draining from the ventricles into the subarachnoid space, leading to a further increase in ICP. If this pressure persists, the fluid build-up

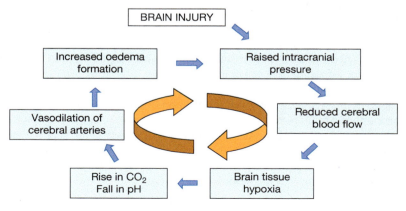

Figure 8.2 Raised intracranial pressure (ICP).

compresses and damages brain tissue. Raised ICP ultimately causes herniation of brain tissue through the foramen magnum at the base of the skull. This compression and herniation of the brain stem, through the space where the spinal cord enters, is also referred to as coning and inevitably results in death.

Initially, clinical signs of raised ICP include:

- decreasing levels of consciousness
- headache that increases in intensity with coughing and straining
- slow pupil constriction when exposed to bright light
- visual disturbances such as blurred vision due to papilloedema, which is swelling of the optic disc
- convulsion and seizure activity
- abnormal breathing patterns
- impaired motor or sensory function and responses
- speech and swallowing difficulties
- altered mood and challenging behaviour.

In later stages, if condition worsens and ICP continues to rise:

- decerebrate or decorticate posturing
- bulging anterior fontanelle (babies only)
- head enlargement when cranial sutures have not fused (babies only)
- vomiting
- high temperature without a clear indication of infection
- Cushing's reflex, also known as the vasopressor response, will result in the clinical signs known as Cushing's triad:
  - raised systolic blood pressure with widening pulse pressures
  - bradycardia, reduction in the heart rate
  - irregular, shallow or slow respirations.

Treatment of a raised ICP will vary depending on the causative condition. The overall aim is to decrease ICP and this may be achieved in several ways, such as reducing the cerebral volume caused by a tumour or inflammation. Draining excess CSF and decreasing the cerebral blood volume, will reduce a raised ICP. Lowering the brain's metabolic rate will reduce cerebral demand of oxygen and nutrients and can be achieved through administration of prescribed sedation, anti-emetics and pharmacological seizure management.

Hydrocephalus

Hydrocephalus causes global cerebral dysfunction, due to increased levels of cerebrospinal fluid (CSF) in the brain and spinal cord. It can be congenital or acquired after birth.

Congenital hydrocephalus is present at birth and can be caused by conditions such as spina bifida, inflammation or tumours. Maternal infections during pregnancy such as mumps or rubella can also be a cause.

Acquired hydrocephalus occurs after birth and usually develops after an injury, illness or development of a brain tumour.

In both, the CSF volume increases, leading to an increase in intracranial pressure (ICP). If this increased pressure persists, the fluid build-up compresses and damages brain tissue. Specific clinical signs of hydrocephalus are caused by the increasing CSF volume and pressure inside the cranium that result in:

- head enlargement in babies and children with congenital hydrocephalus
- bulging anterior fontanelle (babies only)

- dilated scalp veins and separation of skull sutures (later sign)
- downward eye gaze (also known as the 'setting-sun' sign)
- convulsions
- other signs of raised ICP.

Hydrocephalus is an acute life-threatening emergency, which must be treated promptly. Early diagnosis is critical in the older child, whose skull bones have fused, leaving little room for swelling and which will rapidly lead to raised ICP.

Treatment involves implanting a thin tube, called a shunt, in the brain. The excess CSF in the brain runs through the shunt to another part of the body, usually the peritoneal cavity. From here, the CSF is absorbed into the blood stream. The shunt has a valve inside it to control the flow of CSF and to ensure it does not drain too quickly (Corns & Martin, 2012).

Red Flag

Clinical signs of Cushing's triad: Altered respiratory pattern, fluctuating or high blood pressure with widening pulse pressures and bradycardia indicate raised ICP with potential brainstem involvement. This constitutes a medical emergency and immediate action must be taken to avoid herniation of the brainstem and subsequent death (Corns & Martin, 2012).

Cerebral trauma
Fractured skull

Skull fractures can be linear, depressed or open. Linear fractures show no signs of skull depression and are treated conservatively. Depressed skull fractures with a depression of more than 1 cm and open skull fractures may need surgical intervention and repair of the damaged structure. Evidence of a meningeal tear, CSF leakage, cranial nerve damage, seizure activity or a risk of infection make this more likely.

Table 8.2 illustrates specific signs and symptoms that may be present in a child with a fractured skull.

Table 8.2 Vital signs and symptoms of a fractured skull

Symptoms can include:
- Bruising around the eyes ('panda/raccoon eyes'), which is caused by a basal skull fracture. A rupture of the meninges causes blood to pool in the peri-orbital area via the cranial sinuses.
- Bruising over the mastoid bone ('Battle's sign'), behind the ear, is usually caused by a fracture of the posterior cranial fossa. This is a later sign and often does not appear for 24 hours post injury.
- Blood in the ear canal.
- Cerebrospinal fluid (CSF) leakage from the nose or ears, due to a basal skull fracture.
- A palpable dent or spongy area of the head, indicating a depressed skull fracture.

Signs depend on the area of injury and can include:
- Evidence of raised ICP.
- Visual disturbance, due to optical nerve compression/damage or rising ICP.
- Facial muscle weakness, altered facial sensation and loss of smell due to cranial nerve damage.
- Speech impairment.
- Loss of hearing due to inner ear haemorrhage or ruptured eardrum.
- Dizziness, vertigo and other balance problems.
- Impaired motor or sensory function and responses.

Consider a C-spine injury in all head injuries.

Source: Glasper *et al.*, 2011.

Urgent assessment using an ABCDE approach and a full neurological assessment, including Paediatric Early Warning System (PEWS), AVPU (alert, voice, pain, unresponsive) and Glasgow Coma Scale (GCS), is imperative to assess the level of consciousness and awareness (Table 8.3).

Emergency nursing care includes assisting with intubation and ventilation if the airway and breathing are compromised by damage to the respiratory centre in the brain. Immobilise the cervical spine if a fracture is suspected. Continuously monitor vital signs for indications of rising ICP, using the GCS and PEWS chart (Table 8.3). A full neurological assessment should include level of consciousness, cranial nerves, motor and sensory function and cerebellar function. Assess for other injuries and open wounds, including a fractured skull. Only treat/suture if this will not delay further investigations/transfers. Assess pain levels, using an age-appropriate pain tool and administer analgesia. Administer an anti-emetic as prescribed because vomiting can raise ICP further. Assess the efficacy of analgesia and anti-emetic. Ensure family-centred care is implemented, through effective communication and liaison with the child, family and carers. Offer reassurance and support if the child needs to be prepared for transfer to an intensive care or neurological unit (Glasper, McEwing & Richardson, 2011).

Table 8.3 Investigations to assess level of consciousness

1. The AVPU response scale can be used quickly to assess the level of consciousness. A score lower than V is a cause for concern and requires urgent medical referral
   A the patient is awake
   V the patient responds to verbal stimulation
   P the patient responds to painful stimulation
   U the patient is completely unresponsive.

2. The Glasgow Coma Scale (GCS) is used to provide a practical method for the assessment of conscious level in response to defined stimuli. The GCS can be used without modification for children over 5 years old. Under 5 years old, it will be difficult for children to 'obey commands' or give a verbal response that indicates that they are 'orientated'. Thus, the Paediatric Glasgow Coma Scale (PGCS) may be more appropriate. (Amended PGCS stimuli are shown below in brackets.)

GCS stimuli include:
- Eye opening
  4. Eyes opening spontaneously
  3. Eye opening to speech
  2. Eye opening to pressure
  1. No eye opening or response
- Verbal response
  5. Orientated (smiles, oriented to sounds, follows objects, interacts)
  4. Confused (cries but consolable, inappropriate interactions)
  3. Words (inconsistently inconsolable, moaning)
  2. Sounds (inconsolable, agitated)
  1. No verbal response
- Motor response
  6. Obeys commands (infant moves spontaneously or purposefully)
  5. Localises (infant withdraws from touch)
  4. Normal flexion (infant withdraws from pressure)
  3. Abnormal flexion to pain (decorticate response)
  2. Extension to pain (decerebrate response)
  1. No motor response

Each response has a value and these should be considered individually and as a combined score. A combined score of less than eight represents a significant risk of mortality. The GCS should be recorded regularly on a GCS chart. This will allow the nurse to observe trends that can indicate improvement or deterioration of the patient's condition.

Source: Glasgow Coma Scale 2014.

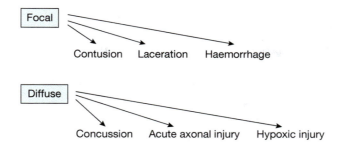

Figure 8.3 Focal and diffuse brain injury types.

Head injury

This occurs when trauma to the head results in damage to the brain. There are three main types of traumatic brain injury (TBI).

- Closed head injuries – where no damage is visible. These are common in car accidents where the moving head suddenly stops or the child experiences a blow to the head.
- Open wounds – such as occur in conjunction with a fractured skull. The brain is exposed and may have been damaged by an object or a blow to the head.
- Crushing injuries – where the head is crushed and brain damage occurs.

Brain injuries may be classified as either focal or diffuse (see Fig. 8.3). Focal injuries are localised to one area, whereas diffuse injuries occur throughout the brain and CNS.

Focal head injuries include contusions, lacerations and haemorrhage

Contusions or bruising, occur as the brain comes into contact with the hard inner skull. The most common areas of injury are the frontal and temporal lobes. The cerebral trauma results in the leakage of blood from microscopic vessels and the possibility of a tear in the delicate meninges, causing a haemorrhage.

Lacerations are tears in the brain tissue. A fractured skull or the entrance of a foreign object, such as a bullet into the skull, usually causes a laceration. This will result in the rupture of large blood vessels causing bleeding into the brain leading to haemorrhage, haematoma formation, cerebral oedema and raised ICP.

Haemorrhage occurs when large or small blood vessels are damaged causing bleeding into the brain. Blood is supplied to the brain from the aorta via the internal carotid and vertebral arteries. Venous blood returns to the heart via the jugular veins and superior vena cava. The brain is very susceptible to interruption in blood supply, which leads to rapid O_2 and glucose deprivation of the delicate neural tissues.

A haemorrhage is classified according to the space it occurs in (Fig. 8.4).

- Intracerebral haemorrhage occurs deep within the brain tissue.
- Subdural haemorrhage occurs in the subdural space between the dura mater and arachnoid mater. It commonly occurs in abusive head trauma or shaken baby syndrome, although other symptoms would also need to be taken into consideration to make a full diagnosis (New Scientist, 2016).
- Subarachnoid haemorrhage occurs in the subarachnoid space between the arachnoid mater and pia mater. It can result from a tear in the pia mater allowing blood to enter the subarachnoid space. It can also result from the rupture of aneurysms or arteriovenous malformations, often present in the circle of Willis. The circle of Willis connects cerebral arteries, allowing for rapid redistribution of arterial blood to be diverted to dependant areas of the brain.

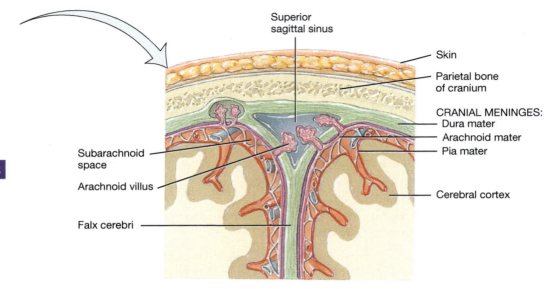

Figure 8.4 Anterior view of frontal section through the skull showing the cranial meninges. *Source:* Tortora & Nielsen 2009.

Diffuse head injuries include concussion, acute axonal and hypoxic injury. Concussion is usually a mild diffuse injury and is the most common brain injury. It may cause temporary loss of consciousness (lasting minutes to hours), confusion, amnesia, visual disturbances, vestibular imbalance, headaches and nausea and vomiting.

Axonal injury is usually caused by high-speed acceleration/deceleration injuries. It causes diffuse haemorrhages throughout the brain and may cause the patient to become deeply unconscious.

Hypoxic injury is caused by oxygen deprivation such as a cardiac arrest or near drowning and may not be associated with a head injury. However, it must be noted that hypoxic injury may compound the effects of a brain injury.

Red Flag

Sudden loss of the Moro reflex, tonic neck reflex and withdrawal reflexes in young infants indicates a neurological emergency.

Spinal trauma
Spinal cord injury

The spinal cord extends from the medulla oblongata to the second lumbar vertebrae. The spinal cord has three main functions.

- Transmission of efferent motor information from the brain to skeletal muscles and other muscles, primarily in the white matter of the spinal cord.
- Transmission of afferent sensory information to the brain, which is also primarily via the white matter.
- Coordination of autonomic and somatic reflex arcs is mediated by the central grey matter.

The main cause of spinal cord injuries are car accidents, falls, and sports-related activities. Benign and cancerous spinal tumours can compress the spinal cord and nerves, leading to similar damage and loss of function.

There are many types of injury to the spine and spinal cord, which can cause varying levels of dysfunction. Spinal cord bruising and concussion cause temporary disruption to motor and sensory function.

Spinal cord compression must be relieved quickly to prevent ischaemia and permanent damage. Crush and penetration injuries of the lower spine can lead to cauda equina, in which the nerve roots at the bottom of the spinal cord become compressed. It is a rare syndrome and represents a medical emergency.

Red Flag

The following symptoms could be a sign of Cauda equina syndrome, which needs urgent medical treatment to prevent permanent damage to the spinal cord.
S: Saddle anaesthesia – loss of feeling around the buttocks and genital area
P: Pain – severe nerve pain in the back or legs
I: Incontinence – bladder and bowel incontinence/retention/constipation
N: Numbness – weakness and loss of sensation in the legs
E: Emergency treatment needed (Cauda Equina UK, 2013).

Full transection of the spinal cord will cause total paralysis and lack of sensation below the level of the spinal injury.

Spinal shock occurs rapidly following spinal cord injury and leads to a loss in reflex function, flaccid paralysis, loss of sensation and loss of bowel and bladder control below the level of the injury. Disruption of sympathetic spinal nerve communication also causes hypotension, poor venous circulation, sweating and peripheral vasodilation. The inability to control body temperature through vasoconstriction and increasing metabolic rate causes the child's temperature to assume the environmental temperature. Spinal shock has a duration of a few days to weeks. The re-appearance of reflex activity, hyperreflexia and spasticity indicate that spinal shock has resolved.

Motor dysfunction
Cerebral palsy

Cerebral palsy is a non-progressive disorder of movement, muscle tone and posture that is caused by injury or the abnormal development of the immature brain during fetal development and in the first year of life. Damage to an area of the brain will cause corresponding motor dysfunction. Other parts of the brain may be damaged and therefore cerebral palsy can be associated with epileptic seizures, learning difficulties, incontinence, dysarthria, scoliosis, and vision and hearing impairment.

Causal factors include impaired embryonic implantation, genetic abnormalities, infection, trauma and exposure to radiation and toxic substances, in the womb. Maternal diabetes mellitus, toxaemia and nutritional deficiencies can also cause fetal neurological damage. Anoxia, trauma and infections are the most common factors that cause perinatal neurological injury. Low birth weight and birth asphyxia are commonly identified risk factors for cerebral palsy. Physical trauma can occur to the central nervous system during birth. Vascular abnormalities, blood stasis and thrombus formation may lead to cerebral infarction, intraventricular or subarachnoid haemorrhage.

Cerebral palsy is classified according to the area of the brain that is damaged and its effects on the body.

- Spastic or pyramidal cerebral palsy accounts for 80% of cases (NICE, 2011a). Increased muscle tone (hypertonia), stiff and weak muscles, abnormal tendon, and primitive reflexes are present and caused by damage to the corticospinal pathways in the brain.
- In dyskinetic cerebral palsy muscle tone varies between stiffness (hypertonia) and floppiness (hypotonia). This causes random and uncontrolled body movements and jerky involuntary spasms and postures. It is associated with severe difficulty in performing purposeful movements that require fine motor coordination. It is caused by injury to the basal ganglia or thalamus.
- Ataxic cerebral palsy presents with balance, gait and coordination problems, resulting in jerky and clumsy movements. Children may also experience involuntary tremors or shaking in their hands. This is caused by injury to the cerebellum.
- In mixed cerebral palsy features of more than one of the types mentioned will be present.

Management varies with age, type, severity and associated disorders. An ongoing multidisciplinary medical, social and educational team approach should be adopted that is patient-centred and takes into account the wishes of the child and family (NICE, 2012).

Spina bifida

Spina bifida is a defect of neural tube closure during fetal development. It leads to failure of the posterior vertebral laminae to fuse causing an incomplete closure of the spine and membranes around the spinal cord. There is no causal factor although folic acid deficiency during early pregnancy increases the risk. The two commonly seen types of malformation include meningocele and myelomeningocele.

Spina bifida meningocele

A meningocele defect results in herniation of the meninges through the vertebral defect but does not involve the spinal cord or nerve roots. This cystic dilation does contain CSF but often causes no neurological deficit. It can occur anywhere along the spine and is dependent on the location of the vertebral defect. A small lump may be seen on the baby's back at birth. This can be corrected with surgery.

A lack of herniation in the presence of a vertebral defect is termed spina bifida occulta. It is the mildest form of posterior neural tube defect and usually causes no neurological dysfunction. Most people are unaware they have the condition.

Spina bifida myelomeningocele

A myelomeningocele defect results in herniation of the meninges, CSF, spinal cord and nerves, through the posterior arch of a vertebra. Most are located in the lumbar and sacrolumbar regions of the spine, which are the last part of the neural tube to close. A transparent membrane usually covers a meningocele defect, which may be intact or easily leak CSF. Thus, surgical repair must be carried out urgently at birth to prevent infection and further nerve damage. Most cases are diagnosed during pregnancy by a blood test or ultrasound and the fetus is usually delivered by Caesarean section to minimise damage during labour.

It is one of the most common developmental abnormalities of the nervous system. It causes damage to the spinal cord, which leads to a loss of motor, sensory, reflex and autonomic functions below the level of the herniation. Muscle weakness, paralysis, a lack of sensation, and bowel and urinary incontinence may be present. The severity of the symptoms can vary depending on the location of the defect and whether the child develops hydrocephalus.

Neurological tumours

Neurological tumours can occur anywhere in the nervous system but are most common in the brain, spinal cord and sympathetic nervous system. Their cause is unknown.

Central nervous system tumours

Neurological tumours in the brain and spinal cord, which are in the CNS, form the second most common group of cancers in children, accounting for a more than a quarter (26%) of all childhood cancers (Childhood Cancer Research Group, 2010).

Brain tumours can be benign (non-cancerous) or malignant (cancerous). Benign tumours remain in situ and do not spread into other areas. However, they can cause pressure and cause neurological damage to the areas around them in a similar way to malignant tumours.

A tumour in the intracranial space causes cerebral tissue compression as its size increases. This affects the ventricular system, causing ventricular dilatation and obstruction to the flow of CSF. Increasing tumour size elevates the CSF pressure, preventing it from draining from the ventricles into the subarachnoid space. This in turn will lead to an increase in ICP, which must be relieved to avoid permanent cerebral damage or death (Fig. 8.2).

Malignant brain tumours are cancerous and can spread into the normal tissue around them. They are high risk and early diagnosis is essential. In childhood, there are two common types, glial and embryonal, named after the type of cell from which they originate.

Glial tumours or gliomas

They arise from the supportive neuroglial cells in the nervous system. Astrocytoma is the largest subgroup (Cancer Research UK, 2014a) of childhood malignant brain and neural tumours and arises from astrocyte cells that form part of the blood–brain barrier. Normal astrocyte cells wrap around synaptic endings of neurones and blood capillaries, mediating the permeability of endothelial cells in the blood capillaries of the CNS.

Embryonal tumours

These are the second most common malignant subgroup (Cancer Research UK, 2014a), arising from nerve cells that are immature. Of these, the most common and fast-growing tumour is the medulloblastoma. It usually develops in the cerebellum, at the back of the brain and may spread to other parts of the brain or into the spinal cord.

Both can occur anywhere within the brain or spinal cord and are unlikely to spread. Subject to their position and rate of growth, they can be difficult to treat and remove.

Initial investigations are concerned with gaining a full medical history, carrying out a full medical examination and a CT/MRI scan (Table 8.4).

Treatment may involve surgery to obtain diagnostic biopsy samples, tumour resection and a reduction in ICP. Tumours found in the brainstem, thalamus and deep grey matter areas are inoperable. Adjunct treatment includes chemotherapy, radiotherapy and dexamethasone to reduce cerebral oedema (NICE, 2006).

Nursing management after surgery will require paediatric intensive care unit (PICU) support initially, followed by a period of post-operative recovery during which neurological, endocrine and wound assessments are key in recognising signs of deterioration. Rehabilitation, parental education and a multidisciplinary approach should be taken to support the child and parents (NICE, 2006).

Sympathetic nervous system tumours

These can be malignant or benign, akin to tumours found in the brain and CNS. Neuroblastoma is a common malignant tumour and neurofibromatosis type 1 is classed as a benign tumour.

Table 8.4 Vital signs and symptoms of paediatric brain tumours

Can be difficult to ascertain in young children who are unable to verbalise. Symptoms can mimic common childhood ailments and can include: • seizures • limb weakness • difficulty walking • speech impairments • swallowing difficulties • strange sensations • learning impairments • challenging behaviours • vision/hearing impairments	Signs and symptoms can be predicted by the location of the tumours. • ataxia – posterior fossa • visual disturbances – optic nerve of posterior fossa • seizures – temporal lobe • behavioural changes – frontal lobe • hormone imbalance – pituitary gland

Neuroblastoma

Nearly all the malignant tumours of the sympathetic nervous system are neuroblastoma, accounting for 5% of all childhood cancers. Neuroblastoma is a cancer of the neural crest cells in the nervous system and it is the most frequently occurring cancer in children under the age of one (22%) (Childhood Cancer Research Group, 2010).

Forty-six percent of neuroblastomas develop in the adrenal gland, 26% in other abdominal sites and 13% in thoracic sites (Cancer Research UK, 2014b). Hence, initial symptoms can vary depending on the site of the primary tumour. The most common sign is an abdominal mass, which can cause pain, lack of appetite, weight loss and constipation. A tumour in the neck or chest can cause difficulties swallowing and breathing if it becomes enlarged. Difficulty walking and passing urine may be signs of a tumour pressing on the peripheral spinal nerves. Bone metastasis can cause joint and bone pain and bone marrow abnormalities such as anaemia, bleeding, pallor and blood cell production.

Specific investigations include X-ray, ultrasound, CT, MRI and an mIBG bone scan to ascertain the location and potential spread of the tumours. Neuroblastoma cells excrete vanillylmandelic acid (VMA), which can be detected in urine and 90% of children with neuroblastoma will have excess levels of VMA (Labtestsonline, 2013).

Treatment of neuroblastoma depends on the location and spread of the tumour. If a tumour is localised, surgery only is the treatment of choice. In high-risk, aggressive neuroblastoma, multi-agent chemotherapy, resection of the primary tumour followed by an autologous stem cell transplant is the treatment of choice (NICE, 2015).

Neurofibromatosis type 1 (NF1)

This is the most common type of benign nervous system tumour. It is caused by a spontaneous mutation, or via autosomal dominant inheritance, of the 17th chromosome. It affects 1 in 3000 live births per year in the UK and there are approximately 25 000 people in the UK diagnosed with NF1. Children with this disease are at increased risk of developing malignant brain tumours (Walker *et al.*, 2006). Of these, 5% will develop brain tumours and there is a 10% lifetime chance of developing a malignant nerve sheath tumour, and 15% will develop an optic pathway glioma (NHS Choices, 2015).

Children develop coffee-coloured patches and freckles in the armpits, groin or under the breast. Neurofibromas are benign tumours that form under the skin, on nerve sheaths. The numbers of these vary from small lumps to large swellings.

Sixty percent of children will have some degree of cognitive defect or learning difficulty, which is usually mild. Fifty percent of children with NF1 have attention deficit hyperactivity disorder (ADHD). Fifteen percent of children develop an optic pathway glioma or tumour and may have vision problems. Physical development problems can include scoliosis in 10% of children, macrocephaly in 50% of children and epilepsy in about 7% of children (NHS Choices, 2015).

Treatment is focused on regular annual monitoring and a multidisciplinary team approach when complications arise. Monitoring should include a detailed skin assessment for the appearance of new neurofibromas or changes in existing ones. Blood pressure, vision checks and a bone assessment for scoliosis and other bone disorders. Assessment of progress at school with a view to eliciting any learning difficulties or physical development should also be undertaken.

Intracranial infection

The most commonly seen infection includes meningitis, which is an infection of the meninges lining the brain and cranium. Encephalitis is an infection of the brain that causes acute and rapid swelling.

Meningitis

The meninges consist of three protective layers surrounding the brain and they are continuous with the spinal cord meninges (Fig. 8.4). The three cranial meninges are the dura mater, arachnoid mater, and pia mater. Cerebrospinal fluid (CSF) circulates between the latter two in the space called the subarachnoid space.

Meningitis is an acute inflammation of these membrane layers and the cause is usually bacterial or viral rather than the rarer fungal meningitis.

It can be difficult to diagnose in babies and young children, which is a concern as the peak age is in children under 5 years of age. A second peak occurs in 15–19 year olds, which is unique to meningitis and not seen in other infectious diseases (Oxford Vaccine Group, 2016).

The two main bacterial pathogens are meningococcal infection (*Neisseria meningitidis*), which is a gram-negative bacteria, and pneumococcal infection (*Streptococcus pneumoniae*), which is a gram-positive bacteria. Group B streptococcus (GBS) is the main cause of neonatal and newborn meningitis.

Bacterial meningitis may result in brain damage, hearing loss or a learning disability in 10–20% of survivors (WHO, 2015).

Mumps, enteroviruses and the Epstein–Barr virus can cause viral meningitis. It is less life threatening than bacterial meningitis and does not require the administration of antibiotics.

Diagnosis is by a lumbar puncture, in the absence of signs of raised ICP, to determine the presence of bacteria in the CSF. Blood cultures are taken to identify the causative organism.

Treatment of viral meningitis is supportive as there are no effective antiviral drugs for most viruses that cause meningitis. Most children recover from viral meningitis without any medical treatment within 7–14 days. Nursing care is aimed at easing the presenting symptoms such as a headache, vomiting and photophobia.

Treatment for bacterial meningitis is often started, by administering IV antibiotics, before a firm diagnosis is made. If the causative organism is viral following tests, then these will be discontinued. In cases of meningococcal meningitis, prophylactic antibiotics are given to immediate family members and close contacts.

If the child is critically ill then care on a PICU is indicated to support their airway, breathing and circulation (ABCs).

If the child is conscious then they should be closely monitored and assessed for changes in their neurological and cardiovascular function (see Table 8.5. In particular, nurses should

Table 8.5 Vital signs and symptoms of meningitis and meningococcal disease

Meningitis	Meningococcal disease/septicaemia

Early symptoms are non-specific and may include:
• fever
• vomiting
• irritability
• drowsiness
 	
In infants under 18 months
• a tense or bulging anterior fontanelle is a sign of raised ICP
• a distinctive high-pitched or moaning cry may be present
 	
In older children
• headache
• neck stiffness
• photophobia
 	
At any age
• seizures
• positive Kernig's sign (inability to extend the knee when the leg is flexed at the hip when lying down)
• positive Brudzinski's sign (severe neck stiffness causes a patient's hips and knees to flex when the neck is flexed)
• confusion
• sleepy and difficult to wake
	Early symptoms are non-specific but the child becomes rapidly unwell.
	• a rash will be present in more than 50% of cases. This can be:
	  • sparse or profuse
	  • tiny petechial spots to large non-blanching purpuric lesions
	• pale or mottled skin
	• fever
	• cold hands and feet
	• shivering
	• high respiratory rate
	• cardiovascular instability
	• neurological instability:
	  • raised ICP
	  • altered GCS
	• GI symptoms, including abdominal pain, vomiting and diarrhoea
	• myalgia (muscle pain) in the legs
	• joint pain
	• weakness
	• restlessness
	• confusion
	• sleepy and difficult to wake

be vigilant for signs of deteriorating consciousness level, increased ICP and shock. The GCS and PEWS can be used for this purpose (Table 8.3). Measure and record fluid balance to ensure adequate hydration and diuresis. Ensure a quiet environment with reduced light and stimulation. Provide support for parents and communicate effectively on progress, treatment and procedures.

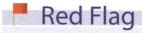

Red Flag

An unwell child who develops a purpuric, non-blanching petechial rash may have overwhelming meningococcal disease and sepsis. This constitutes a medical emergency (Meningitis Research Foundation, 2015).

Meningococcal disease

Meningococcal meningitis and meningococcal septicaemia can on their own, or collectively, cause meningococcal disease, which is a life-threatening systemic infection. It continues to have a high mortality rate of 10% and early diagnosis and aggressive treatment improves outcomes. Several different bacteria can cause meningitis. *Neisseria meningitidis* has the potential to cause large epidemics. There are 12 serogroups of *N. meningitidis* that have been identified, 6 of which (A, B, C, W, X and Y) can cause epidemics (WHO, 2015).

Nursing management includes the assessment of airway patency, breathing and circulation. Record these on a PEWS chart and refer to the early management of meningococcal disease/bacterial meningitis in children and young people algorithm (Meningitis Research Foundation, 2015). Commence resuscitation as indicated and continue to assess cardiovascular function, including blood pressure, ECG, peripheral capillary refill and core body temperature. Treatment is aimed at restoring circulatory volume and may require fluid administration and the use of inotropes. Neurological assessment, using a GCS, is aimed at monitoring for early signs of raised ICP (Table 8.3). Assist with the rapid collection of blood samples for FBCs, U&Es, blood cultures, clotting screen, blood sugar and meningococcal serology. Assist and prepare the child for a lumbar puncture and send CSF promptly to the laboratory for analysis. Administer antibiotics, analgesia and anti-emetics as prescribed and monitor efficacy.

Psychological support of the parents and carers is imperative during this critical period in the child's care and the nurse can play a key role in facilitating effective communication. Information about progress and procedures that are being carried out can be reassuring.

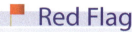
Red Flag

A capillary refill time of 3 seconds or more should be considered abnormal in children (Fleming et al., 2015).

Encephalitis

Encephalitis is an acute inflammation of the brain and when combined with meningitis is known as meningoencephalitis. The very young are at higher risk because of their immature immune system.

Infective encephalitis is usually caused by a viral infection such as rabies, polio and measles. Bacterial infections can also cause encephalitis and include syphilis, toxoplasmosis, Lyme disease and malaria. Chronic encephalitis occurs slowly and can be due to conditions such as HIV. Autoimmune encephalitis also occurs slowly and can be initially difficult to diagnose with no obvious cause. It can cause abnormal body movements and seizures.

Young children may present with symptoms that are initially non-specific and similar to meningitis. Diagnosis is by CT/MRI scan, lumbar puncture and electroencephalogram (EEG). Treatment depends on the cause and may include antibiotic, antiviral, and steroid drugs. Encephalitis can be life threatening and most children will require PICU admission, close monitoring and intensive care.

Some children may develop neurologic long-term consequences following encephalitis, including memory problems, behavioural changes, speech impairments, and epilepsy.

Seizure disorders
Pathophysiology of a seizure

Seizure activity is another main sequela of cerebral dysfunction. A seizure is a transient occurrence of signs and/or symptoms due to abnormal, excessive or synchronous nerve activity in the brain. A seizure does not necessarily mean that a person has epilepsy. Seizures fall broadly into two main groups: focal, which are localised to one hemisphere, or generalised, which spread to other parts of the brain and involve both hemispheres. Uncontrolled electrical activity that leads to an abnormal electrical discharge in the brain in either the sensory, motor or the autonomic nervous regions, can cause many different forms of seizure. Levels of consciousness can vary too and aware, impaired, and unknown awareness are used to describe the level of consciousness during a seizure.

The International League Against Epilepsy (ILAE, 2016) has proposed a new operational classification of seizure types which allows clinicians greater flexibility in naming seizures.

Epilepsy

Epilepsy is the term used to describe a group of neurological conditions of the brain characterised by an enduring predisposition to generate epileptic seizures. The ILAE (Fisher et al., 2014) task force proposed that epilepsy is considered a disease of the brain defined by any of the following conditions:

- At least two unprovoked (or reflex) seizures occurring >24 hours apart.
- One unprovoked (or reflex) seizure and a probability of further seizures similar to the general recurrence risk (at least 60%) after two unprovoked seizures, occurring over the next 10 years.
- Diagnosis of an epilepsy syndrome.

Epilepsy is considered resolved for individuals who had an age-dependent epilepsy syndrome but are now past the applicable age. This also includes those who have remained seizure-free for the last 10 years, with no anti-seizure medicines for the last 5 years.

Diagnostic tests include CT and MRI scans to detect scarring, tumours or damaged areas that could cause epilepsy. An EEG (electroencephalogram) measures the present electrical activity in the brain at the time of the test. It cannot detect past or future epileptic activity and it may be necessary to have an ambulatory EEG test, which is designed to record the activity over a longer period of time. An EEG test is useful for determining the location of a seizure during abnormal electrical activity.

Immediate first aid management involves ensuring the safety of the child without restraining them or trying to move them unless they are in immediate danger. Cushion the child's head. Do not put anything in the child's mouth. Time the length of the seizure and stay with them until fully recovered. Do not attempt to wake them up or give them anything to drink. Gently place in the recovery position once the seizure has finished. Act in a calm and reassuring way. Look for an epilepsy identity card/jewellery or an individual healthcare plan (Epilepsy Action, 2016).

Emergency help should be called if:

- the seizure lasts for more than 5 minutes
- one tonic–clonic seizure follows another one without the child regaining consciousness
- it is the child's first seizure
- an injury has occurred during the seizure (Epilepsy Action, 2016).

The child should be treated immediately to prevent status epilepticus developing. If in the community, call an emergency ambulance. In the hospital setting call for immediate assistance, secure the airway, give oxygen and assess cardiac and respiratory function and a blood glucose measurement. Secure intravenous access and follow the status epilepticus algorithm as appropriate. Note that these are age-dependent and may not apply to infants, those born prematurely or less than 28 days of age (NICE, 2011b). Initial treatment for status epilepticus usually involves the administration of anti-convulsant medication, oxygen and if required, anaesthesia to allow intubation and ventilation. Ensure that support is provided for the family throughout this time.

Ongoing treatment is aimed at controlling the seizures to prevent further occurrences. Children experiencing seizures are more at risk of accidents and seizures may put them at an academic and social disadvantage.

Febrile convulsion

Febrile convulsions, fits or seizures are associated with a high temperature in the absence of CNS infection; they are not the same as epilepsy. The pathophysiology of febrile convulsions is not fully understood, although there appears to be a genetic predisposition to the condition. They occur in children between 6 months and 5 years of age. One in 50 children will develop a febrile convulsion by the age of 5 (Great Ormond Street Hospital, 2014). Most children will outgrow this common illness.

Febrile convulsions can occur when children develop a temperature above 38 °C. Viral, ear, throat, gastrointestinal or post immunisation infections are the most common. Signs and symptoms mimic those of a tonic–clonic epileptic seizure. Loss of consciousness is accompanied by jerking limb movements and loss of continence. It can be distressing for the parent/carers who can be reassured that they do not cause any lasting effects or brain damage (Clinical Knowledge Summaries (CKS), 2013). The fit is usually very brief, lasting less than 5 minutes in a simple febrile seizure. First aid and emergency help guidance is similar to the child having an epileptic seizure (CKS, 2013; Epilepsy Action, 2016) and detailed earlier in this chapter. Admission is not always required after the first febrile seizure unless it lasts longer than 15 minutes, recurs within 24 hours and/or has focal characteristics, which indicate that it is a complex febrile seizure.

The cause of infection and the risk of serious illness should be assessed even in a short duration, simple febrile seizure to exclude the presence of central nervous infection such as meningitis, meningococcal disease or encephalitis (CKS, 2013).

Antipyretics such as paracetamol and ibuprofen should be used to reducing a child's fever; however, this does not prevent recurrence. Dehydration should also be prevented. Evidence suggests that immunisation-related febrile seizures are not likely to recur with future immunisations and parents should be advised to continue with future childhood immunisation (CKS, 2013).

Conclusion

Although we are born with the majority of our nervous system intact, there continues to be rapid development and growth throughout childhood. Our brain continues to grow and we develop cognitive ability as the neural pathways are made permanent within the brain. Neurone myelination continues, allowing us to develop fine motor control. Any trauma or disease of the nervous system can affect this trajectory of growth and development. We are able to compensate to a certain degree owing to the plasticity of the nervous system, which allows us to relearn or re-pattern areas of damage in the brain by creating new neural pathways.

References

Cancer Research UK (2014a). Children's cancers incidence statistics. Children's brain, other CNS and intracranial tumour incidence. Available at: http://www.cancerresearchuk.org/health-professional/cancer-statistics/childrens-cancers/incidence#heading-Five (last accessed 15 April 2018).

Cancer Research UK (2014b). Children's cancers incidence statistics. Children's sympathetic nervous system (SNS) tumour incidence. Available at: http://www.cancerresearchuk.org/health-professional/cancer-statistics/childrens-cancers/incidence#heading-Eleven (last accessed 15 April 2018).

Cauda Equina UK (2013). SPINE. Red Flag Signs and Symptoms. Available at: http://caudaequinauk.org.uk/cauda-equina-syndrome/ (last accessed 17 April 2018).

Childhood Cancer Research Group (2010). Childhood Cancer Registrations, Great Britain, 2006–2007 dataset. Available at: http://www.ccrg.ox.ac.uk/datasets/registrations.shtml (accessed 1 June 2016).

Clinical Knowledge Summaries (CKS) (2013). Febrile seizures. Available at: https://cks.nice.org.uk/febrile-seizure (accessed 1 June 2016).

Corns, R. & Martin, A. (2012). Neurosurgery: hydrocephalus. *Surgery (Oxford)* 30, 142–148.

Epilepsy Action (2016). What to do when someone has a seizure. Available at: https://www.epilepsy.org.uk/info/firstaid (accessed 1 June 2016).

Fisher, R.S., Acevedo, C., Arzimanoglou, A., *et al.* (2014). ILAE official report: a practical clinical definition of epilepsy. *Epilepsia* 55(4), 475–482.

Fleming, S., Gill, P., Jone, C., *et al.* (2015). The diagnostic value of capillary refill time for detecting serious illness in children: a systematic review and meta-analysis. *PLoS ONE* 10(9), e0138155. Available at: http://journals.plos.org/plosone/article?id=10.1371/journal.pone.0138155 (accessed 11 November 2016).

Glasgow Coma Scale (2014). The Glasgow structured approach to assessment of the Glasgow Coma Scale. Available at: http://www.glasgowcomascale.org (accessed 11 November 2016).

Glasper, E.A., McEwing, G. & Richardson, J. (2011). *Emergencies in Children's and Young People's Nursing*. Oxford University Press, Oxford.

Great Ormond Street Hospital (2014). Febrile convulsions. Available at: https://www.gosh.nhs.uk/file/1716/download?token=1LZnVj67 (last accessed 16 April 2018).

International League Against Epilepsy (ILAE) (2016). Operational classification of seizure types by the International League Against Epilepsy: Position Paper of the ILAE Commission for Classification and Terminology. Available at: https://onlinelibrary.wiley.com/doi/full/10.1111/epi.13670 (last accessed 16 April 2018).

Labtestsonline (2013). VMA. Available at: http://labtestsonline.org.uk/understanding/analytes/vma/tab/test (accessed 1 June 2016).

Meningitis Research Foundation (2015). Management of bacterial meningitis in children and young people. Available at: https://www.meningitis.org/getmedia/21891bb1-198a-451a-bc1f-768189e7ecf1/Bacterial-Meningitis-Algorithm-Oct-2017 (last accessed 17 April 2018).

National Institute for Health and Care Excellence (NICE) (2006). Improving outcomes for people with brain and other central nervous system tumours. Cancer service guideline [CSG10]. Available at: https://www.nice.org.uk/guidance/csg10/evidence (accessed 1 June 2016).

National Institute for Health and Care Excellence (NICE) (2011a). Spasticity in children and young people final scope. Available at: https://www.nice.org.uk/guidance/CG145/documents/spasticity-in-children-final-scope2 (accessed 1 June 2016).

National Institute for Health and Care Excellence (NICE) (2011b). Guidelines for treating convulsive status epilepticus in children. Available at: https://www.nice.org.uk/guidance/CG137/chapter/Appendix-F-Protocols-for-treating-convulsive-status-epilepticus-in-adults-and-children-adults-published-in-2004-and-children-published-in-2011#guidelines-for-treating-convulsive-status-epilepticus-in-children-published-in-2011 (accessed 1 June 2016).

National Institute for Health and Care Excellence (NICE) (2012). Spasticity in under 19s: management. NICE guidelines [CG145]. Available at: https://www.nice.org.uk/guidance/CG145/chapter/Introduction (accessed 1 June 2016).

National Institute for Health and Care Excellence (NICE) (2015). Draft scope for the proposed appraisal of APN311 for treating high risk neuroblastoma. Available at: https://www.nice.org.uk/Media/Default/About/what-we-do/NICE-guidance/NICE-technology-appraisals/Proposed-appraisals-no-wave/ID910-Neuroblastoma-(high-risk)-APN311-(1st-line)-draft-scope.pdf (accessed 1 June 2016).

New Scientist (2016). Evidence of 'shaken baby' questioned by controversial study. Issue 3099. Available at: https://www.newscientist.com/article/mg23230994-100-evidence-of-shaken-baby-questioned-by-controversial-study (accessed 11 November 2016).

NHS Choices (2015). Neurofibromatosis type 1: Symptoms. Available at: http://www.nhs.uk/Conditions/Neurofibromatosis/Pages/Symptoms.aspx (accessed 1 June 2016).

Oxford Vaccine Group (2016). Meningococcal disease. Available at: http://vk.ovg.ox.ac.uk/meningococcal-disease (last accessed 16 April 2018).

Tortora, G.J. & Neilsen, M.T. (2009). *Principles of Human Anatomy*, 11th edn. Wiley, Chichester.

Walker, L., Thompson, D., Easton, D., *et al.* (2006). A prospective study of neurofibromatosis type 1 cancer incidence in the UK. *British Journal of Cancer* 95, 233–238.

World Health Organization (WHO) (2015). Meningococcal meningitis. Fact sheet (last reviewed January 2018). Available at: http://www.who.int/mediacentre/factsheets/fs141/en/ (accessed 1 June 2016).

Chapter 9

Disorders of the cardiac system

Sheila Roberts

Aim

The aim of this chapter is for readers to develop their understanding of the anatomy and physiology of the cardiac system in order to appreciate various disorders of this system; to do this effectively the reader has also to understand pathophysiological mechanisms.

Learning outcomes

On completion of this chapter, the reader will be able to:

- Discuss the normal and consider the abnormal anatomy and physiology of the heart.
- Understand why some heart defects are considered cyanotic and some are acyanotic.
- Discuss the signs and symptoms of heart failure across the age ranges.
- Identify which heart conditions are congenital and which are acquired.

Keywords

- heart
- circulation
- congenital
- acquired
- disorders
- heart failure

Fundamentals of Children's Applied Pathophysiology: An Essential Guide for Nursing and Healthcare Students, First Edition.
Edited by Elizabeth Gormley-Fleming and Ian Peate.
© 2019 John Wiley & Sons Ltd. Published 2019 by John Wiley & Sons Ltd.
Companion website: www.wileyfundamentalseries.com/childpathophysiology

Chapter 9 — Disorders of the cardiac system

Test your prior knowledge

1. Draw and label the heart.
2. Draw the flow of blood through the heart.
3. Consider the adaptations required by the fetal circulation.
4. What is the difference between the pulmonary circulation and systemic circulation?
5. What is the difference between a congenital and an acquired disease?
6. Define heart failure.
7. Identify the signs and symptoms of heart failure.
8. Discuss the nursing care necessary for a child requiring oxygen therapy.
9. Discuss the impact of a congenital heart disorder on the child and family.
10. Discuss the long-term health outcomes for a child with a congenital heart defect.

Introduction

The cardiovascular system is responsible for providing the body with a continuous supply of oxygen and nutrients while also transporting the waste materials that need to be expelled from the body, such as carbon dioxide. The cardiovascular system includes:

- the heart, which pumps deoxygenated blood to the lungs, where gaseous exchange takes place, and oxygenated blood to the rest of the body;
- the veins, which are the blood vessels that transport the blood from the body back towards the heart;
- the arteries, which are the blood vessels that transport the blood away from the heart;
- the capillaries, which are very small blood vessels connecting the arteries to the veins.

This chapter will provide a brief overview of the anatomy of the heart. It will then consider a range of anomalies that can affect the heart and the impact that these may have on the infant, child or young person.

Anatomy of the heart

The heart is comprised of four chambers, the left atrium and left ventricle and the right atrium and right ventricle. Deoxygenated blood enters the heart from the superior and inferior vena cava directly into the right atrium. Contraction of the muscle of the right atrium causes an increase in pressure within the right atrium allowing the one-way valve, the right atrioventricular valve (also known as the tricuspid valve), situated between the right atrium and right ventricle, to open and allow the blood to pass through to the right ventricle.

As the atrium empties of blood and the ventricle fills the atrium relaxes and muscles of the right ventricle begin to contract increasing the pressure within the right ventricle. The atrioventricular valve closes and the blood is then forced through the pulmonary valve into the right and left pulmonary arteries. As the right ventricle empties of blood the pulmonary valve closes to prevent back flow of blood from the pulmonary arteries into the right ventricle.

The deoxygenated blood is transported via the right and left pulmonary arteries to the lungs where gaseous exchange takes place. Carbon dioxide is expelled and replaced with oxygen.

The oxygenated blood returns to the heart via the pulmonary veins directly into the left atrium. The left atrium fills with blood, the muscles of the left atrium contract and the resulting increase in pressure forces the blood through the left atrioventricular valve (also called the mitral or bicuspid valve) into the left ventricle.

Contraction of the left ventricle pumps the oxygenated blood through the aortic valve into the aorta for transportation round the body. Again the aortic valve closes to prevent

Disorders of the cardiac system   Chapter 9

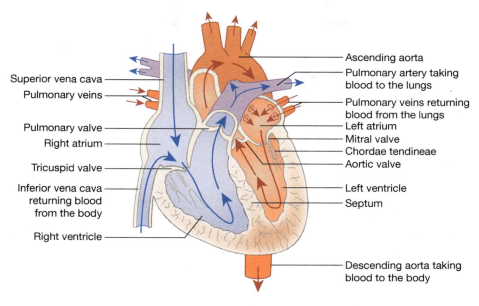

Figure 9.1 Diagrammatic representation of the blood flow through the heart. *Source:* Peate & Gormley-Fleming 2015. Reproduced with permission of Wiley.

back flow. Refer to Fig. 9.1 for a diagrammatic representation of the blood flow through the heart. For a more complete understanding of the anatomy and physiology of the heart refer to Roberts (2015).

Congenital disorders of the heart

A congenital heart defect (CHD) is an anatomical malformation of the heart and/or great vessels, which occurs during fetal development (Rao, 2015). A congenital heart defect is the most common of all defects that affects the newborn baby and is apparent in 8–10 of every 1000 live births (Siva *et al.*, 2016). This incidence increases in spontaneous miscarriage, still-born and premature babies. The reasons a baby may have a CHD are generally unknown, although there are situations where there is a known increased risk (Table 9.1).

Cardiac or heart failure

Cardiac failure (CF) occurs when the heart is unable to pump enough blood and therefore oxygen to meet the needs of the metabolising cells. Heart failure is a syndrome characterised by either or both pulmonary and systemic venous congestion generally leading to inadequate peripheral oxygen delivery. It is caused by cardiac dysfunction. Congenital heart defects are the most common reason for cardiac failure in infants; at what age this occurs depends on the severity of the defect. In the older child, cardiac failure may result from a range of problems (Table 9.2).

Cardiac failure can be categorised simply as caused by abnormal structures within the heart versus a normal heart, or more accurately according to the haemodynamic changes that occur:

- Preload increase or volume overload – commonly caused by large left-to-right shunts, such as ventricular septal defect and patent ductus arteriosus. Very rare before 6–8 weeks of age as pulmonary vascular resistance does not fall low enough to cause the large shunt before this age but then causes congestive cardiac failure (CCF) in the first 6 months of life.

Table 9.1 Possible causes for CHD

Risk factor	Possible congenital heart defect
Mother with type 1 or 2 diabetes	Transposition of the great arteries
Alcohol intake during pregnancy	Atrial septal defect Ventricular septal defect
Genetic conditions, e.g., babies with Down syndrome	Septal defect
Noonan syndrome	Pulmonary valve stenosis
Turner syndrome	Coarctation of the aorta
Exposure to rubella virus	Patent ductus arteriosus/pulmonary artery stenosis
Medication, e.g., benzodiazepines, (anti-convulsion medication) and ibuprofen (analgesic medication)	Atrial or ventricular septal defects
Mothers with phenylketonuria who do not adhere to a low-protein diet	Coarctation of the aorta and tetralogy of Fallot
Mother's exposure to organic solvents	Various

Source: Adapted from NHS Choices 2015.

Table 9.2 Possible causes of CF not associated with congenital heart defects

Approximate age of child	Aetiology leading to heart failure
Toddlers	Viral myocarditis
1–4 years	Myocarditis associated with Kawasaki disease
School-age children	Acute rheumatic carditis
Older children	Rheumatic valvular disease
Any age during childhood/adolescence	Cardiomyopathy
Newborns	Metabolic abnormalities, e.g., severe hypoxia, hypocalcaemia
Early infancy	Supraventricular tachycardia
Any age	Hyperthyroidism
Any age	Severe anaemia
School-age children	Acute systemic hypertension with glomerulonephritis

Source: Adapted from Park (2016).

- Excessive afterload or pressure overload – commonly caused by obstructive abnormalities, such as coarctation of the aorta or valve stenosis. The left ventricle is unable to generate sufficient pressure to overcome the fixed downstream obstruction and it cannot therefore maintain cardiac output (Panesar & Burch, 2016).
- Impaired contractility – the contractility is the ability of the myocardium (heart muscle) to contract. Impaired contractility is caused by any factor that affects the myocardium and its ability to contract, such as cardiomyopathy or myocarditis.
- Rhythm disturbances – arrhythmias can induce heart failure as a result of an inadequate heart rate. Tachycardia leads to inadequate filling of the heart chambers and therefore decreased cardiac output. Bradycardia leads to an increase in ventricular filling volume leading to ventricular dilatation.
- Distensibility disorders – distensibility refers to the ability of the chambers and vessels of the heart to increase in volume without a significant increase in pressure. When the heart is unable to do this cardiac output is affected.

- Ischaemia – relatively rare in children, it generally appears as a consequence of congenital coronary abnormalities or as a complication following surgical procedures for congenital heart disease. Acquired coronary disease in children is typically from Kawasaki disease (Dedieu & Burch, 2013).

Signs and symptoms

The severity of the symptoms will always depend on the severity of the heart condition. Symptoms also vary according to whether the left or the right side of the heart is primarily affected. Signs and symptoms include:

Infant

- Poor weight gain although the infant may be of average length – this is because the baby with CF has an increased metabolic rate and therefore needs additional calories; however, they tire easily and are unable to meet this calorific demand.
- Poor feeding due to fatigue.
- Diaphoresis (excessive sweating) especially when feeding due to a catecholamine (epinephrine and norepinephrine) surge that occurs when babies are challenged with feeding while in respiratory distress.
- Tachypnoea – left-sided heart failure causes congestion of the pulmonary veins and respiratory symptoms, such as breathlessness and grunting.
- Hepatomegaly (enlargement of the liver) is caused by congestion from right-sided heart failure.

Child

- Respiratory distress, tachypnoea and hepatomegaly persist.
- Increased shortness of breath during activities.
- Orthopnoea (shortness of breath when lying flat) may be evident in older children caused by increased distribution of blood to the pulmonary circulation.
- Tire easily.
- Oedema of the eyelids or feet along with jugular venous distension caused by congestion of the right side of the heart.
- Weight gain may be present due to oedema.
- Dizziness due to lack of blood supply and therefore oxygen to the brain.
- Abdominal pain, nausea and vomiting especially after eating due to mesenteric ischaemia; this is caused by poor blood supply to the mesentery.

General

- Tachycardia as the body attempts to pump more blood round the body.
- Gallop rhythm refers to an abnormal rhythm of the heart on auscultation. It includes three or even four sounds, thus resembling the sounds of a gallop. The normal heart rhythm contains two audible heart sounds the 'lub-dub' rhythm caused by the closing of the heart valves.
- Hypotension due to poor cardiac output.
- Cool peripheries with a weak, thready pulse due to decreased circulation combined with tachycardia.
- Decreased urinary output due to low circulatory output.
- Cardiomegaly seen on chest X-ray is nearly always present.

Table 9.3 Drugs that may be used in the treatment of heart failure (Joint Formulary Committee, 2015)

Drug	How it works	Possible side effects
Angiotensin-converting enzyme inhibitors (ACE), e.g., captopril	Prevents conversion of angiotensin I to angiotensin II. Dilate the blood vessels, making it easier for the heart to pump blood to the body	Hyperkalaemia in children with impaired renal function. Hypotension Persistent dry cough
Beta-blockers, e.g., atenolol	Decreases the activity of the heart by blocking the action of hormones such as epinephrine	May precipitate asthma Bradycardia Sleep disturbance in some instances
Diuretics usually loop diuretics, e.g., furosemide	Inhibits the body's ability to reabsorb sodium at the ascending loop (loop of Henle) in the nephron, which leads to an excretion of water in the urine	Hypokalaemia Dehydration
Aldosterone antagonists, e.g., spironolactone	Inhibits sodium resorption in the collecting duct of the nephron in the kidneys. This interferes with sodium/potassium exchange, reducing urinary potassium excretion and weakly increasing water excretion	Hyperkalaemia Hyponatraemia Dehydration
Positive inotropic drugs, e.g., digoxin	Increases the force of contraction of the myocardium	Dizziness Irregular heart beat
Anticoagulation, e.g., heparin	Interruption of the process involved in the formation of blood clots	Bleeding, which may cause, e.g., haematuria or nose bleeds

Management

The management of CF in children involves treating the underlying cause, such as correcting anaemia, surgically correcting congenital heart defects where possible or treating infections. Management also involves control of heart failure through the use of medication (Table 9.3), along with general supportive measures, such as rest and help with feeding. This may include high calorific feeds through a nasogastric tube and elimination of salt in the older child's diet. Too much salt in the body causes water to be retained, which in turn increases fluid retention further increasing oedema and breathing difficulties.

🚩 Red Flag

Many babies, children and young people with heart failure will require oxygen to be administered. It is important for healthcare professionals to remember that oxygen needs to be prescribed by a suitably qualified practitioner, such as a doctor or nurse prescriber, and oxygen use must be documented for each patient.

Oxygen concentrations will vary from patient to patient depending on their individual condition. However, it must be remembered that inappropriate concentrations can have serious implications ranging from lung damage, convulsions as the central nervous system is affected and retinal damage, particularly in neonates.

In patients who have long-term severe lung disease additional oxygen may slow their breathing sufficiently for carbon dioxide to build up to dangerous levels.

Healthcare professionals need to be aware of the dangers of administering too much oxygen. Saturation monitors and blood gases will provide a measure of blood oxygen levels, although it should be noted that while internal oxygen levels may under normal circumstances be 100% (see Fig. 9.3), oxygen saturation monitor readings taken peripherally on a child receiving additional oxygen should not be 100% as this may indicate that the child is receiving too much oxygen.

Classification of congenital heart defects

Congenital heart defects can be categorised into cyanotic and acyanotic defects. A baby or child with a cyanotic defect will present with a blue discolouring to their lips and extremities whereas the baby or child with an acyanotic heart defect will retain their normal colouring. However, a child with an acyanotic defect may become cyanosed and a child with a cyanotic defect may not show signs of cyanosis and therefore a more accurate classification involves blood flow (Fig. 9.2).

1. Increased pulmonary blood flow
2. Decreased pulmonary blood flow
3. Obstruction to blood flow out of the heart
4. Mixed blood flow.

Cyanosis occurs when there is an inadequate amount of oxygenated blood circulating in the body. The percentage of oxygen saturation varies through the heart chambers with the left side reaching 100% oxygen saturation as the blood returns from the lungs. Oxygen saturation on the right side of the heart is 75% as the deoxygenated blood returns from the body. The left side of the heart has higher pressure than the right side as the left ventricle is responsible for pumping blood throughout the body whereas the right ventricle is only pumping blood to the lungs. Where there are defects blood will flow from areas of higher pressure to lower pressure (Figs 9.3 and 9.4).

Cardiac investigations

Diagnosing a congenital heart defect involves:

- History taking
    - gestational and perinatal history
    - postnatal and present history
    - family history
- Physical examination
    - general appearance, e.g., respiratory state, colour including cyanosis, nutritional state
    - pulse including peripheral pulses and auscultation of the heart
    - blood pressure including four limb measurements

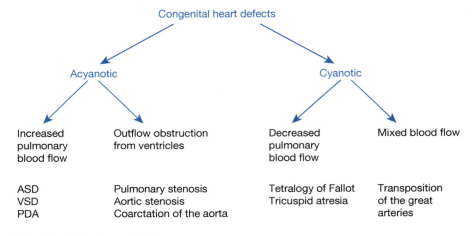

Figure 9.2   Classification of CHD.

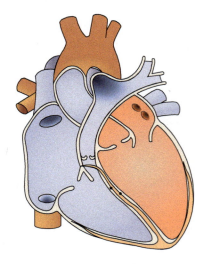

Right atrium 75%
Right ventricle 75%
Pulmonary artery 75%
Left atrium 100%
Left ventricle 100%
Aorta 100%

Figure 9.3 Diagram showing oxygen saturation levels within the heart.

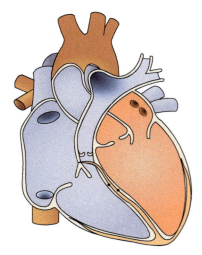

Right atrium 3–7 mmHg
Right ventricle 20 mmHg
Pulmonary artery 25/10 mmHg
Left atrium 5–10 mmHg
Left ventricle 100–110 mmHg
Aorta 100/70 mmHg

Figure 9.4 Diagram showing pressure in mmHg within the heart.

- Electrocardiogram
- Chest X-ray to consider heart size
- Echocardiogram
- Magnetic resonance imaging (MRI) and cardiac computed tomography (CT) may occasionally be required
- Cardiac catheterisation.

Investigation

Cardiac catheterisation is an invasive procedure that is used:

- to inject a contrast medium to show up veins in and around the heart
- to open or widen narrow or blocked blood vessels or valves with the use of a balloon on the end of the catheter with or without stents, e.g., in patent ductus arteriosus or pulmonary atresia

- to close holes or blood vessels, e.g., atrial septal defects
- to determine pressures within the heart
- to assess cardiomyopathy or myocarditis.

Depending on the age of the child a general anaesthetic is required or sedation in the older child. A needle is inserted into the femoral vein with a guide wire; the catheter is then threaded through the vein to the heart. X-rays are used to show the position of the catheter.

Children need to recover from the anaesthetic/sedation by resting, tolerating fluids and diet and passing urine before being discharged home. There is a very small risk of bleeding from the injection site and some discomfort may be experienced.

Red Flag

Cardiac catheterisation is not without risk; complications can range from mild bruising around the injection site to death, cerebral infarction (an obstruction of the blood flow to the brain typically from a thrombus). More minor complications include cardiac arrhythmias; however, the most frequently observed complication is arterial thrombosis (Krasemann, 2015).

Healthcare professionals need to be aware of the possibility of complications from cardiac catheterisation and ensure families are well informed prior to the procedure. Cardiac catheterisation involving an intervention rather than diagnostic is more prone to complications and the younger the child, the greater the risk.

Following any cardiac catheterisation procedure children should be carefully observed and monitored for any complications that may arise from the procedure itself and also from a general anaesthetic.

Children and families need discharge advice that is clear and understandable for them as individuals, with clear guidance on what to do if they are concerned.

ACYANOTIC CONGENITAL HEART DEFECTS
Increased pulmonary blood flow
Atrial septal defect (ASD)

The interatrial septum is the wall of tissue that separates the right atrium from the left atrium. It develops in stages during the first and second month of fetal development. During development a small section of the wall is left open covered by a small flap; this is the foramen ovale, which is a vital part of fetal circulation as it allows blood to bypass the lungs. During fetal circulation, blood entering the heart bypasses the right ventricle passing directly through the foramen ovale into the left atrium, through the left atrioventricular value to the left ventricle and is then pumped back to the body via the aorta. The fetus receives oxygen from the mother through the placenta. The flap of the foramen ovale closes at birth as the pressures within the heart adjust to normal circulation.

An atrial septal defect occurs when the interatrial septum fails to develop correctly leaving a hole in the atrial wall. Blood is forced back from the higher pressure left atrium to the lower pressure right atrium (Fig. 9.5).

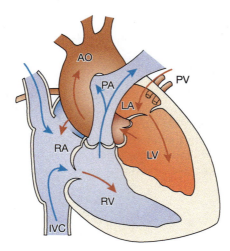

Figure 9.5 Diagram of ASD showing oxygenated blood flowing from the left atrium to the right atrium.

Types of ASD

- Secundum ASD – this is the most common type of ASD, accounting for 70% of all ASDs. It is in the centre of the atrial wall and is caused because the foramen ovale fails to close after birth, i.e., patent foramen ovale (PFO).
- Primum ASD – this accounts for about 25% of ASDs and arises from the lower end of the atrial septum.
- Sinus venosus ASD – this defect accounts for only 5% of ASDs and arises from the upper end of the atrial septum.

Pathophysiology

The slightly higher pressure within the left atrium causes oxygenated blood to flow from the left atrium through the septal defect to the right atrium, a left-to-right shunt, causing an increase in oxygenated blood through the right side of the heart. This additional flow is generally well tolerated although it can cause the right side of the heart to stretch and enlarge.

Signs and symptoms

Small defects are mainly asymptomatic, a murmur may be heard on auscultation of the chest and the defect may be detected during a routine health check.

Larger defects may cause symptoms of a left-to-right shunt with extra strain on the right-hand side of the heart. Babies may become breathless especially during feeding and therefore struggle to gain weight. Older children may have poor exercise tolerance. Frequent chest infections may be an additional indication. Left untreated cardiac failure or pulmonary hypertension may develop in later life.

Treatment

Eighty percent of small, secundum defects close spontaneously in the early years and may not require any treatment. A defect larger than 8 mm is unlikely to close spontaneously nor is spontaneous closure likely to occur after the age of 4 years (Park, 2016).

Larger defects may be closed though a cardiac catheterisation procedure using a septal occluder to cover the defect. A small catheter is inserted into a vein in the groin and fed through the vein to the heart. If this is not possible, open-heart surgery and cardiopulmonary bypass will be required.

Ventricular septal defect (VSD)

A ventricular septal defect is a congenital defect (hole) of the interventricular septum, which is the wall separating the right and left ventricles (Fig. 9.6). At 4–8 weeks' gestation, the previously single ventricular chamber of the heart is remodelled, and development of the septum occurs to form a four-chambered heart (Chamley et al., 2005), two ventricles and two atria. An error at this stage will result in a VSD.

Types of VSD

- Membranous VSD, which accounts for 80% of all ventricular septal defects.
- Muscular VSD.

Pathophysiology

Higher pressure in the left ventricle causes a left-to-right shunt of blood into the right ventricle and into the pulmonary artery. Increased blood volume in the right ventricle is pumped into the pulmonary artery and to the lungs. The increased blood flow to the lungs will over a period of time increase pulmonary vascular resistance. The increased pressure within the right ventricle and the increased pulmonary vascular resistance will cause the muscle of the right ventricle to hypertrophy. The right atrium may also enlarge as it attempts to overcome the resistance within the right ventricle.

Signs and symptoms

Infants and children with small VSDs may be asymptomatic. Larger defects will cause problems with growth and development as infants struggle to feed adequately. They may suffer from repeated chest infections, have a decreased exercise tolerance and develop cardiac failure. The degree and position of a murmur will depend on the severity of the defect and a chest X-ray may show cardiomegaly (enlargement of the heart).

Treatment

Small VSDs may spontaneously close in 30–40% of cases (Park, 2016). Surgical treatment is most likely to be required. Complete repair using sutures or a patch is common; this requires open heart surgery and cardiopulmonary bypass. Depending on size and location, it may be

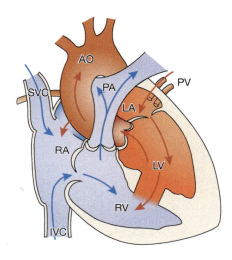

Figure 9.6 Diagram of VSD showing oxygenated blood flowing from the left ventricle to the right ventricle.

possible to close the VSD through a cardiac catheterisation procedure. Medical treatment for heart failure may be required prior to surgery. Surgery may be delayed in asymptomatic children until the age of 4 or 5 years. Those who respond well to medical treatment may have surgery delayed until approximately 18 months of age, whereas those with large defects and those who do not respond well to medical treatment should be operated on sooner.

Patent ductus arteriosus

Normal fetal circulation involves a small vessel, the ductus arteriosus, which connects the pulmonary artery to the aorta (Fig. 9.7). The fetal circulation bypasses the lungs due to oxygenation taking place at the placenta, blood is therefore diverted from the pulmonary artery directly into the aorta to return to the body. A patent ductus arteriosus is the failure of the vessel to close at or shortly after birth; it accounts for 5–10% of all congenital heart defects, excluding premature infants (Table 9.4).

Pathophysiology

Higher pressure within the aorta shunts the blood from the aorta into the pulmonary artery resulting in the blood being returned to the lungs and then back to the left side of the heart. This increases the volume of blood in the left side of the heart thus increasing the workload of the left side of the heart and pulmonary vascular congestion.

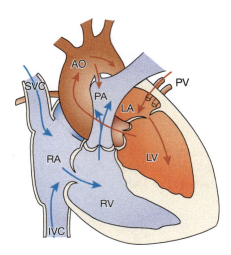

Figure 9.7 Diagram of PDA showing oxygenated blood returning to the heart from the aorta.

Table 9.4 Patent ductus arteriosus in the premature infant

- PDA appears in 45% of infants weighing less than 1.7 kg at birth and in about 80% of infants weighing less than 1.2 kg (Park, 2016).
- Additional problems are evident in infants with respiratory distress syndrome caused by the lack of surfactant in the lungs of premature infants. The pulmonary vascular resistance of the premature infant is reduced through improved oxygenation but the ductus arteriosus remains open because its response to oxygen remains immature. This results in the shunt of blood from aorta to pulmonary artery and the resulting increased blood volume through the immature lungs and left side of heart. Weaning an infant off ventilation becomes increasingly difficult.
- Episodes of bradycardia or apnoea may be evident in infants not requiring ventilation. A murmur and bounding peripheral pulses may be present.
- Pharmacological treatment for closure of a PDA may be achieved with intravenous ibuprofen or indomethacin.

Signs and symptoms

If the defect is small, infants may be asymptomatic; larger defects can increase the occurrence of chest infections, lead to heart failure and faltering growth. A murmur may be heard and an echocardiogram may show cardiomegaly.

Treatment

A PDA found incidentally though echocardiogram and causing no symptoms does not require closure. Closure via cardiac catheterisation is recommended when the PDA causes heart failure or concerns about the infant's growth and development. Surgical closure is indicated in some cases.

Outflow obstruction from ventricles

Outflow obstruction from the ventricles means that the blood leaving the heart from the ventricles, left or right, is met with an anatomical defect, a stenosis or narrowing. This causes an obstruction, which in turn causes an increase in pressure below the stenosis, usually in the ventricles, and a decrease in pressure beyond the stenosis in one of the great arteries. The stenosis is usually found near the valves.

Pulmonary stenosis

Blood leaves the right ventricular through the pulmonary artery, the entrance to which is guarded by the pulmonary valve. The valve consists of three semi-lunar cusps and their function is to prevent backflow of blood into the right ventricle. Pulmonary stenosis (Fig. 9.8) is narrowing of the pulmonary artery and accounts for 5–8% of all congenital heart defects (Park, 2016). Location of pulmonary stenosis may be:

- valvular – at the pulmonary valve (most common manifestation)
- subvalvular – narrowing below the valve
- supravalvular – narrowing of the pulmonary artery above the valve.

Pulmonary atresia is the most extreme form of pulmonary stenosis. There is no blood flow through the pulmonary artery and survival is only possible if there is also an interatrial defect, such as an ASD, present.

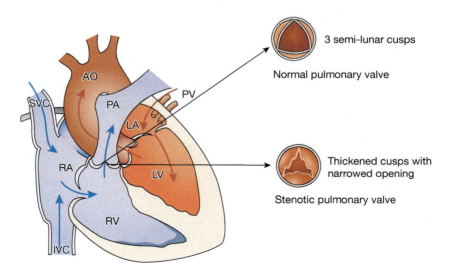

Figure 9.8 Diagram of pulmonary stenosis with right ventricular hypertrophy.

Pathophysiology

Resistance to blood flow into the pulmonary artery causes increased pressure within and hypertrophy of the right ventricle. As the right ventricle fails, the pressure within the right atrium will increase, which may cause the foramen ovale to re-open. As the pressure will be higher in the right atrium, deoxygenated blood will be shunted across the foramen ovale and into the left atrium to the left ventricle through the aorta to the body – systemic cyanosis will be present. Severe pulmonary stenosis will lead to heart failure.

Signs and symptoms

Depending on the degree of obstruction, an infant or child may be asymptomatic, have mild cyanosis or have signs and symptoms of heart failure. A heart murmur will be present and an echocardiogram will show a thickened pulmonary valve. The severity of the obstruction does not usually increase in mild cases but may progress with age in moderate to severe cases.

Treatment

Balloon valvuloplasty is the treatment of choice where possible. A catheter, with a small collapsed balloon at the end is inserted into the femoral vein and passed into the heart and the pulmonary artery. The balloon is then positioned in the narrowed valve, is inflated, stretching the valve open, before being deflated and removed. Surgery may be required if this procedure is unsuccessful or not indicated, for example, through position of the stenosis.

Aortic stenosis

The aorta is the body's largest artery. It begins in the left ventricle of the heart, ascends for a short distance before arching backwards and descending through the thoracic cavity, and on into the abdominal cavity. Blood is pumped from the muscular left ventricle through the aortic valve into the aorta and to the body. The aortic valve, formed of three semi-lunar cusps, guards the entrance of the aorta and prevents backflow of blood into the left ventricle. Aortic stenosis (Fig. 9.9) causes outflow obstruction from the left ventricle and accounts for 10% of all congenital heart defects (Park, 2016). Aortic stenosis location may be:

- valvular – at the aortic valve is the most common manifestation and is generally caused by malformation of the cusps resulting in bicuspid rather than tricuspid valve or from fusion of the cusps (Schroeder, Delaney & Baker, 2015). Many cases of bicuspid aortic valve go unnoticed in childhood (Park, 2016);
- subvalvular – narrowing of the aorta below the valve;
- supravalvular – narrowing of the aorta above the valve.

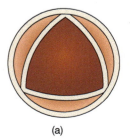 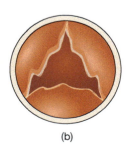 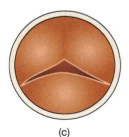

(a)   (b)   (c)

Figure 9.9 Diagram showing (a) normal tricuspid aortic valve; (b) stenotic tricuspid aorta valve; (c) abnormal bicuspid aorta valve.

Aortic atresia is the most extreme form of aortic stenosis. There is no blood flow through the aorta and survival is only possible if the ductus arteriosus remains open. Aortic atresia usually occurs in combination with other heart defects, typically hypoplastic left heart syndrome.

Pathophysiology

Resistance to blood flow into the aorta causes increased pressure within the left ventricle. The extra workload causes hypertrophy (thickening) of the left ventricle. As the left ventricle fails, the pressure within the left atrium will increase, which in turn causes increased pressure within the pulmonary veins, and leads to pulmonary oedema/congestion.

Signs and symptoms

Children with mild to moderate degrees of aortic stenosis may be asymptomatic although they may be exercise intolerant presenting with signs of chest pain and dizziness. Blood pressure is generally normal, as is an electrocardiogram (ECG). Diagnosis is confirmed with echocardiogram. In the case of aortic stenosis, the severity may worsen with time as a result of calcification (Park, 2016).

Neonates with severe aortic stenosis will show signs of reduced cardiac output, weak pulses, hypotension, tachycardia and poor feeding.

Treatment

The critically ill neonate will need medical treatment for heart failure, such as inotropic drugs and diuretics, along with prostaglandin to keep the ductus arteriosus open. Balloon valvuloplasty (see pulmonary atresia) of the aortic valve is the first line of treatment to stretch the aortic valve and increase blood flow. Surgical repair or replacement of the valve may be indicated if valvuloplasty is unsuccessful or as the condition worsens.

Medicine management

A newborn infant with a congenital heart defect that is reliant on the ductus arteriosus remaining open to provide some blood circulation, e.g., in the case of aortic atresia, is given prostaglandin E1 or prostaglandin E2, which are strong vasodilators.

Naturally occurring prostaglandin E2 is produced by both the placenta and the ductus arteriosus (DA) itself, and is the most potent of the E prostaglandins. It is what keeps the ductus arteriosus open in the unborn child. Prostaglandin E1 also has a role in keeping the DA open. Immediately after birth the levels of prostaglandin significantly reduce allowing the DA to close.

Prostaglandin is given intravenously and the dose is calculated according to body weight of the infant.

During the infusion the baby requires careful monitoring of heart rate, blood pressure, respiratory rate and core body temperature as the side effects of prostaglandin include apnoea, severe bradycardia, hypotension and fever. In the event of such occurrences the infusion may be stopped temporarily and restarted at a lower dose or the baby may require ventilator support in order for the prostaglandin to continue (Joint Formulary Committee, 2015).

Coarctation of the aorta

As the aorta arches backwards and begins its descent, there is a narrowing of the vessel. This is known as coarctation of the aorta (Fig. 9.10) and accounts for 8–10% of all congenital heart defects (Park, 2016). The most common manifestation is distal to the left subclavian artery and this may be before or after the ductus arteriosus.

Pathophysiology

As the narrowing of the aorta causes an obstruction to the blood flow, there is increased pressure proximal (before) to the defect and decreased pressure distal (after) to it. The increased pressure affects the head and upper extremities where the blood is supplied from the carotid and subclavian arteries, respectively, and also the heart as the blood is unable to move normally through the aorta. Decreased pressure affects the remainder of the body.

Signs and symptoms

Infants and children fall into one of two categories, symptomatic and asymptomatic.

Asymptomatic children may occasionally complain of chest pain, headaches, leg pains, and cramps with exercise or decreased exercise ability (O'Brien & Marshall, 2015). The pulse in the legs is weak or absent and the blood pressure is lower in the lower limbs than the upper limbs. ECG, chest X-ray are generally normal; however, an echocardiogram will reveal the altered blood flow.

Symptomatic infants often have additional heart defects, such as transposition of the great arteries, VSD or PDA, and they present with signs of heart failure with poor feeding, dyspnoea and oliguria. Heart murmurs are not usually present but a loud gallop is present along with weak and thread pulses. Chest X-ray shows signs of cardiomegaly and an echocardiogram confirms the site and size of the coarctation and any other defects.

Treatment

For the older infant and child, balloon angioplasty may be performed to widen the narrowing of the aorta. A catheter, with a deflated balloon, is passed through the femoral artery to the aorta; on reaching the narrowing the balloon is inflated to make the narrowing wider.

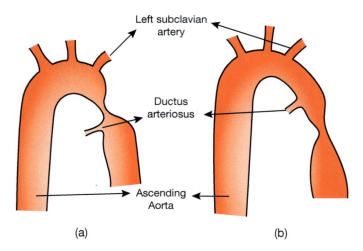

Figure 9.10 Diagram showing (a) preductal coarctation of the aorta; (b) postductal coarctation of the aorta.

An expendable stent may also be put in position at this stage, although this is generally used in children of at least 8 years of age.

Surgical correction of resection of the narrowed segment with an end to end anastomosis is the surgical treatment of choice.

CYANOTIC CONGENITAL HEART DEFECTS
Decreased pulmonary blood flow
Tetralogy of Fallot

Tetralogy of Fallot (TOF) accounts for about 10% of all congenital heart defects (Park, 2016) and occurs equally in boys and girls. It is associated with several genetic conditions, including trisomy 21 (Down syndrome), and may occur with other birth defects such as cleft lip and palate (O'Brien & Marshall, 2014). TOF (Fig. 9.11) consists of four defects:

1. ventricular septal defect – this is generally large
2. pulmonary stenosis – usually affecting the valve
3. overriding aorta – the aorta is positioned above the VSD
4. right ventricular hypertrophy.

Pathophysiology

Narrowing of the pulmonary valve causing outflow obstruction from the right ventricle causes the right ventricle to work harder and hence it becomes hypertrophied. The large VSD equalises the pressures in the two ventricles, although a shunt may still be evident depending on the pulmonary vascular resistance versus the systematic resistance; this will depend on the degree of pulmonary stenosis. A right-to-left shunt will be evident if the resistance is greater in the pulmonary arteries forcing unoxygenated blood into the overriding aorta and giving the child a cyanotic presentation.

Signs and symptoms

Children with an acyanotic TOF that is a left-to-right shunt demonstrating that the pulmonary resistance is not too high are often asymptomatic.

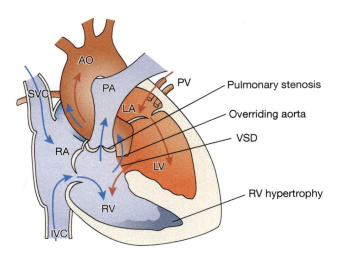

Figure 9.11   Diagram of tetralogy of Fallot.

Symptomatic infants may be acutely cyanosed at birth or develop worsening cyanosis over a period of time as the pulmonary resistance increases. The children may suffer from dyspnoea, clubbing and acute episodes of cyanosis and hypoxia (known as hypercyanotic spells). These occur when the body's oxygen requirement cannot be met, for example, during feeding or crying. The right-to-left shunt stimulates the respiratory centre to increase breathing, which in turn increases the venous return and further increases the right-to-left shunt. A heart murmur will be present, a chest X-ray will demonstrate a boot-shaped heart, caused by the right ventricular hypertrophy, although an echocardiogram will be the definitive diagnosis.

Treatment

Hypercyanotic spells during which the infant becomes acutely cyanosed with deeper and faster breathing, occur most frequently in the morning with crying, feeding, or when passing a stool. Treatment includes calming the baby and holding the baby in the knee-chest position, which increases systemic vascular resistance and therefore decreases the right-to-left shunting and aims to break the cycle. A severe hypercyanotic spell can lead to limpness, convulsions, risk of emboli or death (Park, 2016). If the hypercyanotic spell continues, medical treatment to suppress the respirations, for example, morphine may be administered, along with treatment of the acidosis with sodium bicarbonate.

Treatment of TOF includes medication to control hypercyanotic spells until surgery is indicated; dilation of the pulmonary artery may be performed as an interim step prior to full surgical correction.

🚩 Red Flag

Clubbing of the fingers and toes is characterised by a thickening and flattening of the tips of the digits. Clubbing is associated with cyanotic congenital heart defects and bacterial endocarditis. It is thought to occur because of chronic tissue hypoxaemia and polycythaemia – an overproduction of red blood cells due to low oxygen levels.

Healthcare professionals need to be aware that the presence of clubbing is known to significantly compromise the registration of SaO2 on the extremities with the result that readings are underestimated. Blood gases remain the gold standard for measuring blood oxygen levels, although this is an invasive procedure (Van Ginderdeuren, Van Cauwelaert & Malfroot, 2006).

Tricuspid atresia

The atrioventricular valves begin to develop between weeks 5 and 8 of gestation. Initially bicuspid the right atrioventricular valve develops a third cusp in the third month (Chamley et al., 2005). Failure of this tricuspid valve to develop results in tricuspid atresia (Fig. 9.12); blood is unable to flow from the right atrium to the right ventricle. However, blood will flow through the patent foramen ovale to the left atrium, through the left atrioventricular valve to the left ventricle and then through a VSD to the right ventricle and into the pulmonary artery for oxygenation in the lungs.

Pathophysiology

At birth it is imperative that the foramen ovale remains open and a VSD is required for circulation and therefore survival. The right ventricle and pulmonary artery are hypoplastic (underdeveloped) and there is often an associated transposition of the great arteries. All

Disorders of the cardiac system — Chapter 9

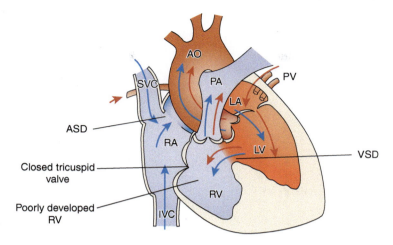

Figure 9.12 Diagram of tricuspid atresia.

blood entering the heart is shunted across from the right atrium to the left atrium causing dilation and hypertrophy of the right atrium. The left atrium and ventricle are enlarged as all blood, systemic and pulmonary, is shunted through the left side of the heart.

Signs and symptoms

Cyanosis is present at birth with associated tachycardia, dyspnoea and difficulty in feeding. Older children may have clubbing as a result of chronic hypoxia. A murmur is heard on auscultation, chest X-ray may show a boot-shaped heart while echocardiogram provides the diagnostic test.

Treatment

Intravenous prostaglandin is required to keep the ductus arteriosus open and a balloon septostomy may be performed to enlarge the shunt between the right and left atria. Staged surgery occurs over the first 1–2 years to correct abnormalities associated with tricuspid atresia.

Mixed blood flow
Transposition of the great arteries

Transposition of the great arteries (TGA) accounts for 5% of all congenital heart defects. In normal circulation the pulmonary artery leaves the right ventricle and goes to the lungs where blood is oxygenated. The aorta leaves the left ventricle and blood is delivered to the rest of the body. In TGA the pulmonary artery leaves the left ventricle and the aorta leaves the right ventricle. With no other defects, this provides two independent circulatory systems and is not compatible with life (Fig. 9.13).

Pathophysiology

For survival, additional defects such as ASD, VSD and PDA are required. A VSD is present in about 40% of cases, while in 40% of cases there is only a small ASD or PDA (Park, 2016). Hypoxia quickly progresses in neonates with minimal mixing of blood and early death can occur.

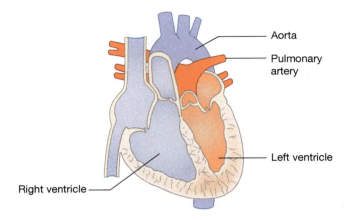

Figure 9.13 Transposition of the great arteries. The aorta takes blood from the right ventricle and the pulmonary artery takes blood from the left ventricle. *Source:* Peate & Gormley-Fleming 2015. Reproduced with permission of Wiley.

Signs and symptoms

Cyanosis is evident as blood returning from the body is recirculated to the body without oxygenation. Signs of heart failure may be seen as the heart attempts to overcome the defects especially when a VSD is present. There is no murmur if there is no VSD; however, a murmur will be present if there is an associated VSD. Chest X-ray shows cardiomegaly and an echocardiogram will demonstrate the extent of the problems.

Treatment

Prostaglandin infusion is required to keep the ductus arteriosus open and in the absence of a VSD, a balloon atrial septostomy is performed to increase the flow of oxygen-rich blood to the body. Signs of heart failure need treating with the appropriate medication. Surgery to swap the great vessels back to the correct position occurs within a few weeks of birth.

Case Study 1

Ben is newborn. He was delivered by normal vaginal delivery at 38 weeks' gestation after his mother, Sally, went into labour spontaneously. Sally has had a traumatic pregnancy as following her first ultrasound scan at 12 weeks' gestation concerns were voiced about the condition of her unborn baby's heart. Following a scan in the second trimester Sally received the news that Ben has hypoplastic left heart syndrome. As a result Ben was delivered in a specialist unit where he is now admitted to the cardiac unit for stabilisation. Hypoplastic left heart syndrome is a congenital defect of the heart characterised by underdevelopment of the left ventricle with associated stenosis or atresia of the aortic valve and also the mitral valves. The ascending aorta is also hypoplastic as there is restricted fetal blood flow through the aorta. Ben's in utero blood returning from the lungs entered the left atrium and was then diverted across the foramen ovale, into the right atrium to the right ventricle, into the pulmonary artery and through the ductus arteriosus to enter the aorta, and on to the rest of the body. See PEWS Fig. 9.14.

Vital signs

The following vital signs were noted and recorded immediately after birth:

Vital sign	Observation	Normal
Temperature	36.1 °C	36.5–37.5 °C
Pulse	160 beats per minute	100–170 beats per minute
Respirations	56 breaths per minute	40–60 breaths per minute
Blood pressure	52/31 mmHg	65/41 mmHg
Oxygen saturations	93%	98–100%
Colour	Mild cyanosis	Pink
PEWs score	0	

- Reflect and consider why immediately after birth Ben's vital signs of pulse, respiration and blood pressure fall within normal parameters.
- Without treatment what is the likely outcome for Ben?

Within 12 hours Ben is looking critically ill, the following vital signs were noted and recorded:

Vital sign	Observation	Normal
Temperature	37.1 °C	36.5–37.5 °C
Pulse	190 beats per minute	100–170 beats per minute
Respirations	75 breaths per minute	40–60 breaths per minute
Blood pressure	50/30 mmHg	65/41 mmHg
Oxygen saturations	86%	98–100%
Colour	Cyanosed	Pink
PEWs score	4	

Other signs include:
    Poor peripheral pulses
    Gallop rhythm
    Hepatomegaly
    Pulmonary crackles

- Reflect and consider what changes are occurring within Ben's heart causing him to deteriorate so rapidly.
- What investigations may be required?
- What immediate treatment will be required?

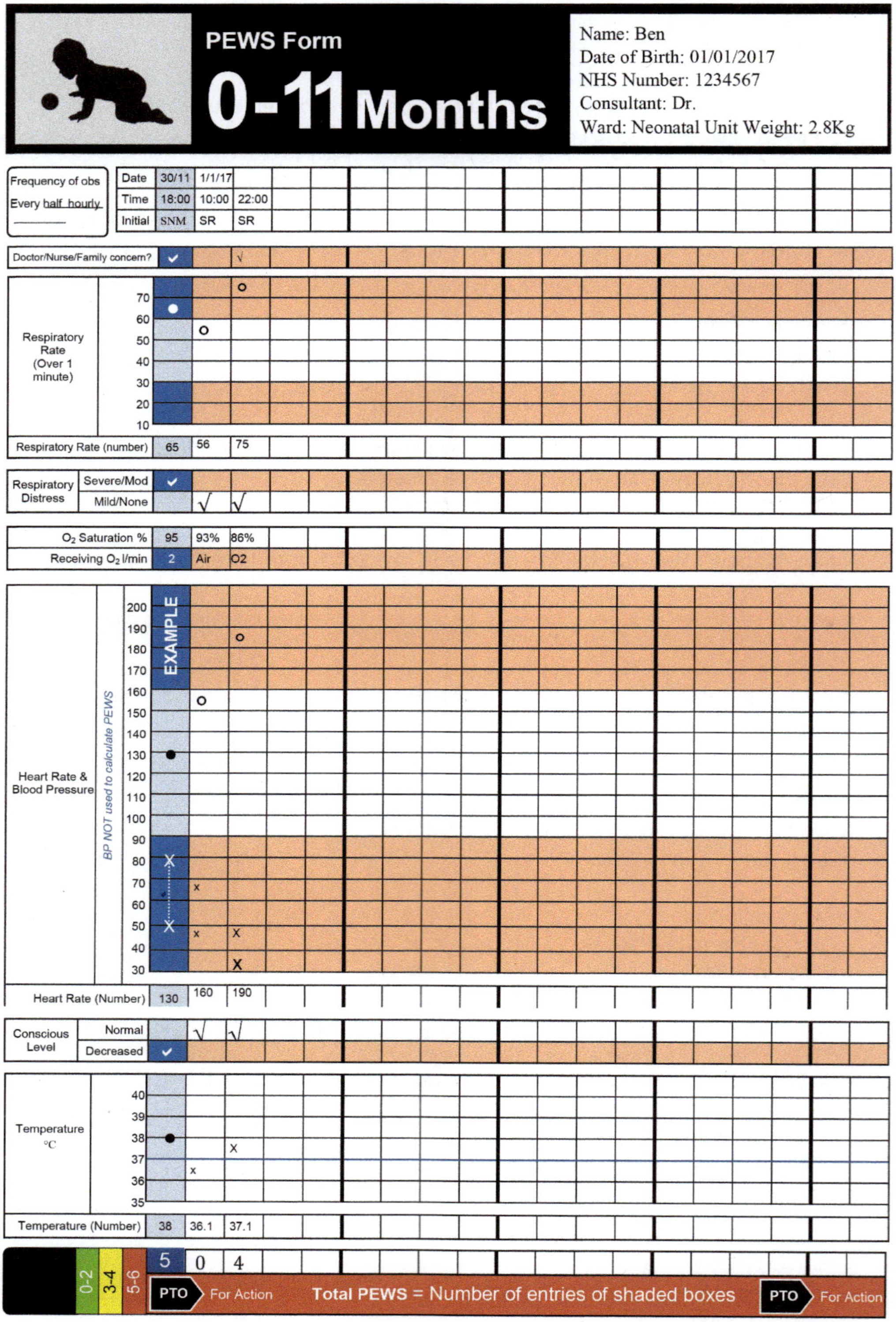

Chapter 9 — Disorders of the cardiac system

Figure 9.14 PEWS chart.

Disorders of the cardiac system Chapter 9

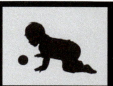

PEWS Form

0-11 Months

Name
Date of Birth
NHS Number
Consultant
Ward   Weight

PEWS Escalation Aid

S | **Situation:**
I am (name), a nurse on ward (X)
I am calling about (child X)
I am calling because I am concerned that…
(e.g. BP is low/high, pulse is XXX
temperature is XX, Early Warning Score is XX)

B | **Background:**
Child (X) was admitted on (XX date) with
(e.g. respiratory infection)
They have had (X operation/procedure/investigation)
Child (X)'s condition has changed in the last (XX mins)
Their last set of obs were (XXX)
The child's normal condition is…
(e.g. alert/drowsy/confused, pain free)

A | **Assessment:**
I think the problem is (XXX)
and I have…
(e.g. given O2 /analgesia, stopped the infusion)
OR
I am not sure what the problem is but child (X)
is deteriorating
OR
I don't know what's wrong but I am really worried

R | **Recommendation:**
I need you to…
Come to see the child in the next (XX mins)
AND
Is there anything I need to do in the meantime?
(e.g. stop the fluid/repeat the obs)

Download SBAR prompt cards and pads at
www.institute.nhs.uk/SBAR

Remember: If you feel you need more help at any time,
call for help – regardless of PEW Score

 0 1 Continue monitoring

2 Nurse in charge MUST review

3 Nurse in charge & Doctor MUST review

4 Nurse in charge & Doctor MUST review & inform Consultant

 5 6 Nurse in charge & Consultant MUST review

Record Call When PEWS 3 Or More				Record Time of Review, Who by & Plan		
Date	Time	PEWS	Print Name (nurse)	Time	Plan	Print Name
01/01/12	09:00	5	SN Morton	09:15	ED consultant called Anaesthetic review	Sister JACKS

NHS Institute for Innovation and Improvement

Download documents to use or edit at
www.institute.nhs.uk/PEWScharts

© NHS Institute for Innovation and Improvement 2012

Figure 9.14 (continued)

Investigations

- Full physical examination plus chest X-ray, which shows a mildly enlarged heart and pulmonary venous congestion
- Echocardiogram
- Electrocardiogram

Investigations

Electrocardiogram:

An electrocardiogram (ECG) is used to check the heart's rhythm and electrical activity. Leads are attached to the patient and a trace recorded on the monitor. The normal P, QRS and T waves are representative of the electrical activity within the heart during one full cardiac cycle. In normal sinus rhythm the P wave represents atrial contraction, the QRS complex represents the depolarisation of the ventricles causing them to contract, and the T wave is the repolarisation or relaxation of the ventricles.

The procedure involves the healthcare professional washing their hands to prevent cross-infection and collecting together the required equipment: the ECG monitor, leads, electrodes and alcohol swabs; the skin needs to be clean and dry. The child and family need to be fully informed and prepared for the procedure. An ECG may be recorded with 3, 6 or 12 leads. The electrodes are placed on the child (see Fig. 9.15):

Chest:

- V1 – 4th intercostal space to right of sternum
- V2 – 4th intercostal space to left of sternum
- V3 – midway between V2 and V4
- V4 – 5th intercostal space at mid-clavicular line
- V5 – 5th left intercostal space, midway between V4 and V6
- V6 – 5th left intercostal space

Limbs:

- One on each arm at level of wrists
- One on each leg just above the ankle

Treatment

Initial treatment for hypoplastic left heart syndrome is stabilisation of the infant including ventilation and inotropes to correct heart failure. Prostaglandin infusion is required to keep the ductus arteriosus open and ensure adequate systemic circulation. A balloon atrial septostomy may be performed to ensure the patency of the left and right atria.

It is not possible to correct hypoplastic left heart syndrome but surgery can be carried out to allow the heart to function more adequately. Surgery is done in stages and is either the Norwood procedure or the hybrid approach. Heart transplantation is an alternative option.

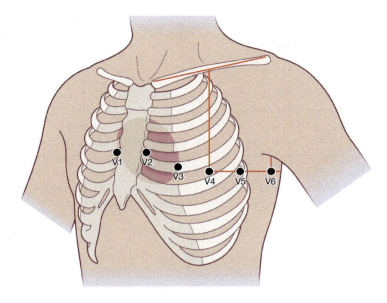

Figure 9.15 Position of chest ECG leads. *Source:* Nair & Peate 2017. Reproduced with permission of Wiley.

Acquired heart disease

Acquired heart disease in children refers to conditions that occur after birth or which affect an otherwise normal heart. They occur for a variety of reasons, such as infection, autoimmune responses or environmental factors.

Kawasaki disease

Pathophysiology

Kawasaki disease predominantly affects infants and young children, although it can occasionally affect older children and adolescents. It is an acute, self-limited disease causing vasculitis of small- and medium-sized vessels. Initially affecting the small capillaries, it progresses to affect the medium-sized vessels including the coronary arteries. Left untreated approximately 20% of children will develop dilation of the coronary arteries and formation of coronary artery aneurysms (Newburger, Takahashi & Burns, 2016), making Kawasaki disease the commonest cause of acquired heart disease in children. The precise cause of Kawasaki disease is unknown although one or a multiple of infectious triggers is most likely, combined with potential abnormalities of the immune system. Other arteries, such as the iliac, femoral, axillary and renal, may also be affected but with less frequency.

Signs and symptoms

- Fever >39 °C, for at least 5 days not responding to antipyretic medication or antibiotics
- Bilateral conjunctivitis
- Red cracked lips
- Strawberry tongue – the normal coating of the tongue comes off leaving the large papillae exposed

- Oedematous hands and feet
- Erythema of palms and soles leading to desquamation (peeling) of skin on the fingers and toes in the later stages.

Cardiac involvement

Tachycardia, gallop rhythm, cardiomegaly and other signs of cardiac failure may be present. When coronary artery aneurysms appear (rarely before 10 days of onset of illness (Park, 2016)), they vary in size; the larger aneurysms can thrombose or clot causing myocardial infarction. Aneurysms that heal do so with stenosis (narrowing) causing myocardial ischaemia months or even years later. Symptoms of myocardial infarction in children include abdominal pain, pallor, restlessness and shock. Younger children rarely complain of chest pain. Additionally children may develop myocarditis, valvular regurgitation or pericardial effusion, all of which lead to poor cardiac function.

Treatment

The aim of the treatment is to reduce inflammation within the coronary arteries and to prevent thrombosis by inhibiting platelet accumulation (Park, 2016).

- Intravenous immunoglobulin reduces the incidence of coronary artery aneurysms from about 20% to less than 5% (Harnden, Tulloh & Burgner, 2014).
- Aspirin is used for its antiplatelet affect.
- Corticosteroids – anti-inflammatory medication.

Medicine management

Aspirin (acetylsalicylic acid) is unlicensed for children under the age of 16 years. An unlicensed drug is a medication that does not have a marketing authorisation provided by the Medicines and Healthcare products Regulatory Agency (MHRA). The MHRA is responsible for ensuring medicines are safe. Prescribing unlicensed medicines to children, increases the prescriber's potential liability, the prescription must therefore be justified and the child (if age appropriate) and the child's carer must be informed (Joint Formulary Committee, 2015).

Infective endocarditis

Infective endocarditis is an infection of the valves and inner lining of the heart which can lead to valve damage and varying degrees of morbidity or even mortality (Schroeder et al., 2015). Children who have undergone surgery for major congenital heart defects are most at risk, and children with a prosthetic heart valve are at particularly high risk. However, it can also occur spontaneously.

Various organisms are responsible for causing infective endocarditis including streptococcus, most commonly seen following dental procedures. Enterococci found following genitourinary or gastrointestinal surgery and staphylococcus found in post-operative endocarditis can also cause infective endocarditis.

Pathophysiology

The micro-organisms grow on a section of the endocardium where there is or has been an abnormal flow or pressure of blood. The change in the endocardium makes it susceptible to the growth of invading organisms, which form a vegetation. These lesions may invade surrounding heart tissue such as the valves or myocardium or they may break off and cause an embolism somewhere within the body.

Signs and symptoms

Signs and symptoms include a low-grade prolonged pyrexia along with other non-specific symptoms such as malaise, headaches and weight loss. A heart murmur is likely to be heard and splenomegaly is common. Petechiae may be seen on the skin or mucous membranes, and signs that result from embolus formation elsewhere in the body may be present.

Routine blood tests including full blood count (FBC) and C-reactive protein (CRP) are required; however, it is positive blood cultures, raised erythrocyte sedimentation rate (ESR) and anaemia, along with changes seen on ECG and an echocardiogram, that will aid diagnosis.

Treatment

High doses of intravenous antibiotics are required for a prolonged period of time; these should be modified as blood culture results become available. Early treatment of infective endocarditis generally has a successful outcome, but when treatment is delayed, emboli are present or heart valve involvement has occurred prognosis may be less favourable. Death occurs as a result of heart failure or myocardial infarction.

Rheumatic fever

Rheumatic fever is caused by group A haemolytic streptococcal infection of the pharynx. The child, between the ages of 6–15 years will present with a history of a streptococcal throat infection between 1 and 5 weeks previously. Rheumatic fever causes the body to attack its own tissues causing widespread inflammation, it affects the joints, the skin and the brain with the most serious complication being cardiac valve damage.

Signs and symptoms

Signs and symptoms are described as major or minor (Table 9.5) and are accompanied by a history of streptococcal throat infection or elevated streptococcal antibody titre. The streptococcal antibody titre is a blood test that detects the presence and measures the

Table 9.5   Manifestations of rheumatic fever

Major manifestations	Minor manifestations
Arthritis, swelling, pain, redness and heat, involving one or several of the large joints	Fever, low grade but may spike in early evening
Carditis resulting in tachycardia, a heart murmur, pericarditis, cardiomegaly and signs of heart failure	Arthralgia or joint pain
Erythema marginatum is a type of erythema (redness of the skin or mucous membranes) involving pink rings on the trunk and inner surfaces of the limbs. The rash disappears in the cold and reappears in the warm.	Blood results reflect inflammatory responses, raised erythrocyte sedimentation rate (ESR) and C-reactive protein (CRP)
Subcutaneous nodules are small non-tender swellings, which may be found singularly or in crops over bony prominences, such as feet, hands, elbows or scalp.	An ECG would demonstrate a prolonged PR interval indicating some degree of heart block
Sydenham chorea is a disorder characterized by rapid, uncoordinated jerking movements primarily affecting the extremities and reflects the involvement of the central nervous system	

amount of antibodies within a person's blood, an elevated level is diagnostic of a recent streptococcal infection. Diagnosis requires the presence of two major or one major and two minor manifestations plus the evidence of a recent streptococcal infection (Markham & Tulloh, 2015).

Treatment

Following diagnosis, benzathine penicillin is the antibiotic of choice. Anti-inflammatory medication is also indicated for treatment of arthritis and carditis. Bed rest is indicated in all cases ranging from a week or two for mild symptoms to a couple of months for severe symptoms. Prophylactic antibiotics are recommended for all children who have had rheumatic fever, the duration of which depends on the severity of the condition but may be lifelong.

Medicine management

Penicillin refers to a group of antibiotics that includes benzylpenicillin (penicillin G) and phenoxymethylpenicillin (penicillin V). They are bactericidal and act by interfering with the bacterial cell wall synthesis. Penicillins diffuse into the body tissues and are excreted in the urine (Joint Formulary Committee, 2015).

Penicillin is commonly associated with an *allergic reaction* and patients need to be asked if they have a history or family history of allergy to penicillin. Common signs and symptoms of penicillin allergy include urticaria, diarrhoea and fever. Severe reactions include anaphylaxis, a life-threatening condition that affects multiple body systems.

Patients who are allergic to one penicillin will be allergic to them all because the hypersensitivity is related to the basic penicillin structure.

Cardiomyopathy

Cardiomyopathy is a chronic and sometimes progressive disease in which the heart muscle (myocardium), is abnormally enlarged and thickened. Cardiomyopathy generally begins in the ventricles and progresses to affect the atria. The muscle cells become damaged, the heart weakens and is unable to pump blood efficiently, and heart failure develops. In approximately 50% of cases, the cause of cardiomyopathy is unknown, although some known causes include:

- myocarditis, which is the most known cause of dilated cardiomyopathy
- familial of which the common inheritance mode is autosomal dominant and accounts for around 30% of cases (Day & Fenton, 2013)
- infections – predominantly viral but can also be bacterial and fungal
- arrhythmias, such as supraventricular tachycardia or bradycardia
- endocrine disorders, such as hyper/hypothyroidism or congenital adrenal hyperplasia
- storage disease, such as glycogen storage disease
- nutritional deficiencies, such as protein, thiamine or vitamin E/D
- ischaemia, such as hypoxia, birth asphyxia or drowning
- toxins, such as radiation, penicillin sensitivity, iron or copper
- systemic disorders, such as systemic lupus, juvenile idiopathic arthritis or osteogenesis imperfecta.

Cardiomyopathy in children can be divided into three categories according to the type of abnormal structure and the dysfunction present: dilated cardiomyopathy, hypertrophic cardiomyopathy, and restrictive cardiomyopathy (Schroeder et al., 2015).

Dilated cardiomyopathy

Dilated cardiomyopathy is rare but the most common type of cardiomyopathy in children.

Pathophysiology

A weakening of the systolic contraction, that is the contraction of the ventricles and specifically the left ventricle, is associated with dilation of all four heart chambers. Thrombus formation is common in the apical portion of the ventricles or in the atrial appendages which may lead to pulmonary and systemic embolization (Park, 2016).

Signs and symptoms

The signs and symptoms include tiredness and general signs of heart failure, see previous section on heart failure. An echocardiogram will be diagnostic, although cardiac catheterisation may give a more complete aetiology.

Treatment

Treatment is that associated with heart failure, along with treating the underlying cause if known. Children may progress to needing a heart transplant.

Hypertrophic cardiomyopathy

Hypertrophic cardiomyopathy is the second most common form of the heart disease affecting the heart muscle. It is genetically transmitted in many cases and sporadic in the remainder. Hypertrophic cardiomyopathy is the most common cause of sudden cardiac death in adolescents (Park, 2016).

Pathophysiology

An abnormal growth of muscle fibres leads to thickening (hypertrophy) of the heart walls, typically the left ventricle and specifically the septum is most often affected, this is known as asymmetric septal hypertrophy. However, the distribution, location and degree of hypertrophy may vary, symmetric ventricular hypertrophy refers to evenly distributed hypertrophy throughout the ventricles and apical hypertrophy refers to thickening at the apex of the heart. The thickened muscle walls cause the heart to be stiff and small leading to difficulties with blood flow. Progressive hypertrophy leads to obstruction of blood flow.

Signs and symptoms

Dyspnoea, tiredness, palpitations and chest pain are often the presenting signs and symptoms. Heart murmurs are heard, ECG abnormalities are common and echocardiograms will demonstrate varying degrees of hypertrophy. Sudden death may occur during exercise and atrial fibrillation may cause a stroke.

Treatment

Treatment includes reducing the left ventricular outflow obstruction and increasing the ventricular compliance. Beta-blockers reduce the degree of obstruction, decrease the incidence of angina pain and have anti-arrhythmic actions (Park, 2016).

Restrictive cardiomyopathy

Restrictive cardiomyopathy is extremely rare in children and it is generally idiopathic with a poor outlook.

Pathophysiology

The ventricles are normal in size and pumping (systolic) function but have abnormal diastolic filling due to the stiff ventricle walls and an inability to expand. As a result the atria are dilated and as the disease progresses blood flow is restricted.

Signs and symptoms

Exercise intolerance, tiredness, dyspnoea and chest pain may be present. Heart murmurs are audible on auscultation and hepatomegaly may be present. An echocardiogram will demonstrate dilation of the atria.

Treatment

Treatment is to alleviate symptoms with the use of drugs. A pacemaker may be indicated for permanent heart block and heart transplant may be considered before pulmonary hypertension develops.

Cardiac arrhythmias

Normal heart rates vary with age, the younger the child the faster the heart rate (Park, 2016). Cardiac arrhythmias occur in children:

- with or without a congenital heart defect
- following surgical repair of a heart defect
- with cardiomyopathy
- who have a cardiac tumour
- secondary to metabolic or electrolyte imbalance.

Regular sinus rhythm refers to a normal heart rhythm at an age-related normal rate. Sinus tachycardia refers to a normal heart rhythm at an age-related elevated rate. Sinus bradycardia refers to a normal heart rhythm at an age-related low rate.

Cardiac arrhythmias generally arise in the right atrium due to abnormalities in impulse generation (Schroeder et al., 2015); some are self-limiting while others cause poor cardiac output, with associated symptoms. Treatment of arrhythmias depends on the cause, for example, correcting electrolyte imbalance will correct the arrhythmia; others may require medication or even pacemaker placement.

Case Study 2

Lara is 12 years old, she has recently become interested and keen to participate in hockey. Having never been particularly interested in sport she is pleased that something has sparked her interest. However, when she plays she is aware of her heart beating very fast but has put this down to being unfit. During one particularly hard match Lara experiences the same feelings of a very fast heart rate, she also feels dizzy and faints. The school call an ambulance and she is taken to the children's emergency department of her local hospital. Her parents arrive shortly afterwards.

Reflect on this brief history and consider the following:

Vital signs

The following vital signs were noted and recorded:

Vital sign	Observation	Normal
Temperature	36.8 °C	36.3–37.5 °C
Pulse	116 beats per minute	70–120 beats per minute
Respirations	22 breaths per minute	20–30 breaths per minute
Blood pressure	112/62 mmHg	100–130 mmHg

A full blood count was performed: no abnormalities found
An ECG shows a normal sinus rhythm

1. With all current investigations within normal limits being normal, what additional tests may be required?
2. Lara and her parents are understandably feeling anxious, what steps will the healthcare professional take to provide reassurance?

Lara is fitted with a Holter monitor, which will provide a 24-hour ECG. During this time she is advised to sleep, play and exercise as normal. Results of the 24-hour ECG demonstrated one episode of:

- Pulse: 240 beats per minute
- ECG: an earlier than normal deflection of the QRS complex

Wolff-Parkinson-White syndrome

Wolf-Parkinson-White (WPW) syndrome is a disorder of the conduction system of the heart. It is caused by the presence of an abnormal accessory conduction pathway between the atria and the ventricles (Mathur, Kapoor & Baj, 2014). The accessory pathways are congenital and in children with WPW the electrical signals in the heart do not travel along the normal route because of the extra (accessory) pathway, known as the bundle of Kent. The accessory pathway directly connects the atrium to the ventricle and therefore this pathway allows atrial activity to bypass the normal bundle of His and Purkinje system, allowing the ventricle to become excited before it would normally do so, resulting in an abnormal ECG. This also gives rise to the alternative name for WPW of 'pre-excitation syndrome'. Type 'A' pre-excitation pathway refers to the left atrium and left ventricle, and type 'B' pre-excitation pathway exists between the right atrium and right ventricle.

WPW syndrome can occur on its own, although in some cases it is associated with additional congenital cardiac defects, such as Ebstein anomaly or transposition of the great arteries.

Signs and symptoms

- There are two arrhythmias associated with WPW syndrome:
  - supraventricular tachycardia (SVT);
  - atrial fibrillation (AF) – although atrial fibrillation is rare in children, when it does occur the accessory pathway will send fast irregular signals from the atria to the ventricle causing ventricular fibrillation, which is potentially life threatening.
- Chest pain
- Palpitations
- Dyspnoea
- Tachycardia
- Dizziness
- Syncope

Treatment

Treatment consists of stopping the acute episode of supraventricular tachycardia and prevention of further episodes.

Acute episodes of SVT:

- Vagal manoeuvres are techniques designed to stimulate the nerve that slows down the electrical signals in your heart. Techniques include:
  - Valsalva manoeuvre – this is a moderately forceful attempt at exhalation against a closed airway, usually done by closing the mouth, pinching the nose shut and pressing out as if blowing up a balloon.
  - Carotid sinus massage – this involves massaging the neck in the region of the carotid sinus in an attempt to stimulate the vagus nerve.
  - Splashing cold water or ice water on the face may have a similar affect to the Valsalva manoeuvre.
- Medication – adenosine is the drug of choice for terminating supraventricular tachycardia, including those associated with WPW syndrome (Joint Formulary Committee, 2015).
- Cardioversion may be required if neither of the above work.

Preventing further episodes:

- Medication – an anti-arrhythmic drug such as amiodarone slows down the electrical impulses in the heart.
- Catheter ablation – a procedure where a catheter is guided from the femoral vein to the heart. The catheter records the electrical activity of the heart in order to pinpoint the exact location of the problem. High-frequency radio waves are used to destroy the tissue that causes the arrhythmia. It is effective in around 95% of cases.

Red Flag

A diagnosis of a heart defect either during pregnancy or after the baby has been born, or the diagnosis of heart disease in a child or young person is devastating for the family. Fear of the unknown, concerns as to whether the child will survive and questions relating to long-term health will affect the family. Healthcare professionals caring for a child with congenital or acquired heart disease need to be mindful of the need for holistic care. Up-to-date evidence-based care needs to be applied to the assessment, planning and care of the child to ensure the best possible outcome.

Consideration must be given to the child's need for rest, sleep and nutrition along with the more procedural aspects of care, such as monitoring the child's condition and response to treatment. Family-centred care is fundamental when caring for a baby, child or young person and should be considered at all times

Conclusion

Although congenital heart defects are the most common of congenital problems to affect babies, it is important to remember that each individual condition is rare. The heart is a vital but complex organ. This chapter has considered a range, but not a complete list of the diseases and defects that affect the heart. There are other congenital and acquired conditions which the reader needs to be aware of. Understanding the anatomy and physiology of the heart is essential to the understanding of heart disease.

References

Chamley, C., Carson, P., Randall, D. & Sandwell, M. (2005). *Developmental Anatomy and Physiology of Children*. Churchill Livingstone, London.

Day, T. & Fenton, M. (2013). Dilated cardiomyopathy in children. *Paediatrics and Child Health* 23(2), 59–63.

Dedieu, N. & Burch, M. (2013). Understanding and treating heart failure in children. *Paediatrics and Child Health* 23(2), 47–52.

Harnden, A., Tulloh, R. & Burgner, D. (2014). Easily missed? Kawasaki disease. *British Medical Journal* 349, g5336.

Joint Formulary Committee (ed.) (2015). *British National Formulary for Children 2015–2016*. BMJ Group and Pharmaceutical Press, London.

Krasemann, T. (2015), Complications of cardiac catheterisation in children. *Heart* 101, 915.

Markham, R. & Tulloh, R. (2015). Fifteen-minute consultation: rheumatic fever. *Archives of Disease in Childhood. Education and Practice Edition* 100(4), 176–179.

Mathur, V., Kapoor, S. & Baj, B. (2014). Wolf-Parkinson-White syndrome: current concepts in anaesthetic practice. *British Journal of Medicine & Medical Research* 4(8), 1604–1611.

Nair, M. & Peate, I. (2017). *Fundamentals of Anatomy and Physiology: For Nursing and Healthcare Students*, 2nd edn. Wiley, Oxford.

Newburger, J., Takahashi, M. & Burns, J. (2016). Kawasaki disease. *Journal of the American College of Cardiology* 67(14), 1738–1749.

NHS Choices (2015). Congenital heart disease: Causes. Available at: http://www.nhs.uk/Conditions/Congenital-heart-disease/Pages/Causes.aspx (last accessed 16 April 2018).

O'Brien, P. & Marshall, C. (2014). Tetralogy of Fallot. *Circulation* 130, e26–e29.

O'Brien, P. & Marshall, A. (2015). Coarctation of the aorta. *Circulation* 131, e363–e365.

Panesar, D. & Burch, M. (2016). Understanding and treating heart failure in children. *Paediatrics and Child Health*.

Park, M. (2016). *Park's The Pediatric Cardiology Handbook*, 5th edn. Elsevier Saunders, Philadelphia.

Rao, A. (2015). An understanding of congenital heart disease in children. A review article. *Indian Journal of Research* 4(9). ISSN 2250-1991.

Roberts, S. (2015). The cardiac system In: Peate, I. & Gormley-Fleming, E. (eds). *Fundamentals of Children's Anatomy and Physiology*. Wiley, Oxford.

Schroeder, M., Delaney, A. & Baker, A. (2015). The child with cardiovascular dysfunction. In: Hockenberry, M. & Wilson, D. (eds). *Wong's Nursing Care of Infants and Children*, 10th edn. Elsevier, Missouri.

Siva, P., Senthilvelan, B., Gopalakrishnan, H. & Subramanian, S. (2016). Role of pulse oximetry in screening newborns for congenital heart disease at 1 hour and 24 hours after birth. *International Journal of Contemporary Pediatrics* 3(2), 631–634.

Van Ginderdeuren, F., Van Cauwelaert, K. & Malfroot, A. (2006). Influence of digital clubbing on oxygen saturation measurements by pulse-oximetry in cystic fibrosis patients. *Journal of Cystic Fibrosis* 5, 125–128.

Chapter 10

Disorders of the respiratory system

Elizabeth Mills, Rosemary Court and Susan Fidment

Aim

To understand the pathophysiology of the respiratory system during an acute illness phase, and the care and management required by the child and family.

Learning outcomes

On completion of this chapter, the reader will be able to:

- Explain the process of respiratory assessment.
- List common signs and symptoms of respiratory illness.
- Describe the altered physiology that occurs in common childhood respiratory disorders.
- Explain the nursing care and management that children and families require during an acute respiratory illness.

Keywords

- airway
- internal and external respiration
- ventilation
- oxygen
- carbon dioxide
- transportation of gases
- hypoxia
- apnoea
- dyspnoea

Fundamentals of Children's Applied Pathophysiology: An Essential Guide for Nursing and Healthcare Students, First Edition.
Edited by Elizabeth Gormley-Fleming and Ian Peate.
© 2019 John Wiley & Sons Ltd. Published 2019 by John Wiley & Sons Ltd.
Companion website: www.wileyfundamentalseries.com/childpathophysiology

- inspiration
- expiration
- upper and lower respiratory tract
- chemoreceptors
- respiratory disorders

Test your prior knowledge

1. State the normal respiratory rate range for the following age ranges: Newborn, 1 year, 5 years, 12 years.
2. List four components of a respiratory assessment.
3. List three causes of upper airway obstruction.
4. List three causes of lower airway obstruction.
5. Describe the difference between a wheeze and a stridor.
6. Name three common causative organisms of bronchiolitis.
7. Name four triggers that may initiate an asthmatic episode.
8. Name two respiratory illnesses which are preventable by vaccination.
9. List four reasons why infants are more susceptible to respiratory illness and respiratory distress.
10. Why are antibiotics not recommended in the treatment of bronchiolitis?

Introduction

Respiratory illness is very common in infants and children, and is the most frequent reason for children to attend the GP or be admitted to hospital. Different types of respiratory illness and conditions range from mild and self-limiting, to severe and life threatening, and if the child has other medical issues, such as a long-term, complex condition, then an acute respiratory illness can have a very serious effect on the child's health (ALSG, 2016).

Infants and young children have an increased susceptibility to respiratory illnesses and subsequent respiratory distress and progressive failure, potentially leading to respiratory arrest. This is due to a number of important factors (ALSG, 2016; Akers, 2015):

- Immaturity of the immune system makes babies and young children vulnerable to infections.
- Upper and lower airways are narrow and small making them easily blocked with mucous and restricted by swelling and oedema; this is particularly important in infants aged 0–6 months, who tend to be obligatory nose breathers and unable to breathe through their mouth.
- Infants have a particularly soft, compliant chest wall, which is easily sucked in during respiratory distress and increases the work of breathing, causing the classic sign of recession. Along with this, infants have a round-shaped rib cage and horizontal-positioned ribs, which have a limited effect in assisting with increasing chest expansion.
- Smaller number of alveoli, as the lungs are not fully mature until approximately 8 years of age, by which time the lungs will contain around 500 million alveoli, and a large surface area for gaseous exchange.

Respiratory assessment

Respiratory assessment is a fundamental skill of the nurse caring for the sick child. Assessing differing elements of respiratory function will give you an overall indication of the child's respiratory status.

A full respiratory assessment will include the following observations:

- Respiratory rate – an increased respiratory rate usually indicates an increased demand for oxygen within the body, therefore it is important to know the 'normal' expected respiratory rate of different age groups, as respiratory rates vary widely from birth to 16 years of age. Best practice states that a respiratory rate should be measured for a full minute, to identify breathing irregularities in rhythm and rate (RCN, 2013). During this time it is useful to be able to observe other aspects of the respiratory assessment, for example, chest movement.

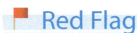

Apnoea is a brief period of time with no breathing activity, which lasts for approx. 10–20 seconds

Infants are particularly prone to apnoeas as they become exhausted from respiratory distress and the increased work of breathing. Seek senior help immediately if you think an infant or child is having apnoeas, as this is a sign that respiratory arrest may be imminent.

- Observe chest movement – observe the chest movement during the respiratory cycle; if possible you should undress the child to visualise the chest wall. Check for equal movement on both sides of the chest, unequal lung expansion could indicate an area of collapse or consolidation within the lung fields, or a pneumothorax. Look for other indications of respiratory distress, observe for any recession, and use of other accessory muscles. Recession occurs when a child has increased work of breathing due to the compliant (soft) chest wall. In babies and young children, recession can occur at lower levels of respiratory distress and in-drawing of the chest wall will increase as respiratory distress increases. Recession can be seen in different areas of the chest wall:
  - intercostal recession – in-drawing between the rib spaces
  - subcostal recession – in-drawing underneath the rib cage
  - suprasternal recession – in-drawing above the rib cage
  - sternal recession – in-drawing of the sternum, which is the large flat bone on the front of the ribcage, which indicates significant respiratory distress, in any age group.
- As children increase in age the chest wall and rib cage become more calcified and rigid, and less likely to be sucked in during increased respiratory effort. Therefore an older child with recession is a sign of more severe respiratory distress.
- Accessory muscle use – in addition to recession, children may show other signs of increased respiratory effort:
  - head bobbing – infants have a tendency to head bob in an attempt to increase respiratory effect;
  - diaphragmatic breathing – infants use the diaphragm as a major muscle in the respiratory cycle; the diaphragm and abdominal muscles will be working extra hard at times of respiratory distress, and therefore a 'see-saw' breathing pattern may be observed (paroxysmal breathing);

- tracheal tug – the soft tissue around the trachea will be indrawn in respiratory distress and is a sign in all age groups;
- nasal flaring – a sign of respiratory distress, seen particularly in infants, because below 6 months of age, infants are primarily nose breathers and do not know how to mouth breathe.

Respiratory noises

Listen for audible noises made during the respiratory cycle (inspiration and expiration). Types of noises you may hear are:

- Stridor – this is a 'harsh' respiratory noise made on inspiration and usually indicates a partial upper airway obstruction. It is typically heard in conditions such as croup or foreign body obstruction.
- Wheeze – this is a softer 'musical' sound, usually heard on expiration and is produced in the lower respiratory tract, often due to air being trapped in the alveoli and small airways. It is the typical noise heard in asthma.
- Grunting – a sound produced by infants in severe respiratory distress. It is a noise produced when the epiglottis is used to partially close the trachea on expiration to stop the alveolar collapsing and ease the work of breathing. It is an indication of severe respiratory distress and help should be sought immediately.

Measuring oxygen saturations

Using an oxygen saturation monitor with an infrared probe enables a measurement of the amount of oxygen dissolved in the blood to be made. Normal oxygen saturation levels should be 95% and above. In some groups of children, however, a lower measurement is acceptable, for example, children with certain cardiac conditions – please refer to local guidelines and policies.

Skin colour

Pale skin colour can be an indication of inadequate oxygen delivery to the cells and/or inadequate circulatory perfusion to the skin. However, it is always best to seek clarification from parents or carers on the child's normal skin colour, as some children are usually pale. This can also be difficult to detect in the child with a darker skin tone, and you will need to carefully observe the mucous membranes (inside the mouth and eye lids etc.).

Heart rate

 Red Flag

Cyanosis is the blue tinge that appears in mucous membranes and skin when children are severely hypoxic. This is a severe warning sign, and help should be sought immediately.

Children in respiratory distress will have a raised heart rate too, due to the circulatory system compensating for a lack of oxygen. However, check that the heart rate is increased in a comparable amount as a hugely increased heart rate may be indicating other issues such as a cardiac condition, which could be causing the respiratory distress, or another diagnosis.

Red Flag

Bradycardia is a severe warning sign, and could be indicating that cardio respiratory arrest is imminent, therefore immediate senior help is required.

Mental status

The effect of hypoxia on the brain is to alter the mental status; this could mean that a child becomes floppy or irritable and then more drowsy as the hypoxia progresses. Using a neurological assessment tool is useful, for example, AVPU or the Glasgow Coma Scale to objectively measure mental status.

Case Study

Rosie is a 4-week-old baby, who is being admitted onto a medical ward with respiratory distress and poor feeding. She is waiting to be reviewed by the medical staff, when Rosie's mum comes to find you and says that Rosie has gone a 'funny colour'.

When you assess Rosie:
Respiratory rate – 65 bpm
Severe intercostal and subcostal recession, and diaphragmatic breathing. Nasal flaring
Oxygen saturations – 90% in air
Heart rate – 185 bpm; capillary refill time – 2 seconds; BP – 80/55
Skin colour – pale
Mental status – responds to mum's voice (AVPU)
Investigations – nasopharyngeal aspirate (NPA) taken in A&E result is RSV + ve

Oxygen therapy

Due to the low levels of oxygen in Rosie's blood, delivering oxygen is the first priority. In this emergency situation, use a non-rebreathe oxygen mask, with the oxygen flow meter turned to 15 L. The non-rebreathe mask has a reservoir bag which will fill with oxygen and deliver a high concentration of oxygen.

However, once Rosie becomes more stable it may be more appropriate to use an oxygen mask, which will deliver a lower concentration of oxygen, or nasal prongs. If Rosie continues to require a high level of oxygen to maintain her oxygen blood levels then she would need to be nursed in an area that can deliver high-flow nasal cannula oxygen therapy or non-invasive CPAP or that can potentially intubate and ventilate (e.g., high-dependency area, children's critical care or intensive care).

Clearance of nasal and oral secretions

While observing the effect of the oxygen, Rosie appears to have white bubbly secretions coming from her nostrils and in her mouth. Because of the small size of an infant's nostrils and airways, these can easily become blocked with secretions produced during a respiratory illness such as bronchiolitis. This can be a problem for infants particularly as they like to nose breathe, which is difficult once the nostrils become blocked. Often these secretions can be wiped away with a tissue. Some babies benefit from saline nose drops to keep the mucous loose and easily cleared from the nostrils.

In a clinical ward, it may be appropriate to use gentle suctioning to clear secretions in the nostrils and mouth. This is a clinical skill which should only be performed when the need for it has been assessed, such as in respiratory distress or feeding difficulties, and it should not be performed routinely on infants with bronchiolitis (NICE, 2015). Refer to local guidelines and policies when performing suction, and only undertake this skill when you have been assessed as competent, or under direct supervision with a qualified healthcare professional.

Infection control precautions

Bronchiolitis is highly infectious and infection control measures must be undertaken with regard to local policies and guidelines. In particular, good hand hygiene and grouping (cohorting) of infectious patients in restricted areas. Parents managing infants at home with bronchiolitis, should be advised on hand hygiene and washing of toys and equipment.

Bronchiolitis

Bronchiolitis is a common lower respiratory tract illness affecting children under the age of 2 years. It is most commonly seen in those under 1 year and peak incidence is age 3–6 months. It is estimated that a third of all children in the UK will have had bronchiolitis in their first year of life, and approximately 3% of children with bronchiolitis will need hospitalisation for supportive care.

What is bronchiolitis?

The disease is caused by a viral infection; approximately 80% of cases are caused by respiratory syncytial virus (RSV) but bronchiolitis can also be caused by other viruses, such as adenovirus and rhinovirus.

The infection causes inflammatory obstruction of the lower airways and alveoli, due to necrosis of the cell lining. Ciliary damage impedes secretion clearance of the lower lung fields combined with increased mucous production. Air becomes trapped below the obstruction of secretions, and it becomes more difficult for the infant to exhale, hence a wheezy noise develops and respiratory distress follows. In severe cases, a consolidation or collapse occurs in the affected area of lung, and gaseous exchange may be impaired (Glasper & Richardson, 2010).

Bronchiolitis normally presents as a cough with increased effort in breathing; it often affects the infant's ability to feed. It can be confused with the 'common cold' as there are common features. However, the presence of lower respiratory tract infection, such as a wheeze or crackles, can be heard on auscultation. The symptoms are usually mild, but in some cases will be severe, particularly if the infant has associated risk factors, such as chronic lung disease, congenital heart disease, premature birth, neuromuscular disorder or an immunodeficiency disorder (NICE, 2015).

Very young infants, for example, those under 6 weeks of age, may have apnoea (periods of no respiratory effort, which may or may not be self-resolving). Symptoms usually peak at 3–5 days of the disease trajectory and the cough normally resolves within 3 weeks. Some children can be left with a residual wheeze.

Treatment

Treatment for bronchiolitis is mainly supportive. It may include giving oxygen therapy for low oxygen saturation (usually 92% and below), which may be via nasal cannulae or in a head box. Ideally, oxygen should be given humidified and warmed if it is given for any prolonged length of time. The amount of oxygen given should be titrated to the level of oxygen saturations of the infant to avoid over-delivery of oxygen, which has been shown to have harmful effects if given in excess over a prolonged period of time.

Support with hydration and feeding may be required for infants with severe infection. This may include intravenous fluids to correct dehydration and/or nasogastric feeding. Due to respiratory distress infants can have difficulty feeding adequately; this needs to be assessed on an individual basis. Secretion clearance from the nostrils, either with suction or saline nose drops, can often facilitate more effective feeding.

No medication is recommended to treat bronchiolitis, although the use of paracetamol and ibuprofen may be used if the child is old enough, to treat discomfort. The use of antibiotics is not recommended for bronchiolitis; however, it may be required if the child develops a post-viral, bacterial infection. Risk factors for severe illness include infants under the age of 2 months, prematurity, congenital heart disease and chronic lung disease.

Parental/carer support is required, as this can be a frightening experience for parents and may be the first illness for their infant. Parents/carers at home with a child with bronchiolitis should be given advice about what to expect and when they need to call for advice or help (NICE, 2015).

Upper airway disorders

Babies and young children are vulnerable to upper airway problems because of the small size of their anatomy, as discussed previously.

Croup

Croup is a common condition, also known as acute viral laryngotracheobronchitis, often caused by the parainfluenza virus. The peak incidence for croup is 2 years of age; however, it can occur from 6 months up to 5 years of age.

Children with croup have the distinctive 'croup' sound on inspiration, called a stridor; this is due to swelling and oedema of the upper airway causing a partial obstruction. They may also have a barking cough, a mild fever and hoarse voice.

Inhalation of warm moist air is often recommended; however, there is little evidence of benefit. Oral or nebulised steroids may be given to reduce the severity and length of the illness.

Epiglottitis

Epiglottitis is swelling of the epiglottis and surrounding tissues due to infection. It is treated as a potentially life-threatening emergency as total obstruction of the larynx can occur. Urgent hospital admission is required for a child with suspected epiglottitis.

This condition has become much rarer in children since the introduction of the HIB vaccination as it is primarily caused by the *Haemophilus influenzae* bacteria. The most common age occurrence is 2–6 years.

Children presenting with epiglottitis typically may be drooling, have a muffled voice and look very unwell, due to the overwhelming infection and pyrexia. It is very important not to upset the child who you may suspect has epiglottitis, do not insist that they lie flat, as they often find their own most effective position for breathing, which will often be leaning forward and they may prefer to sit on a parent's lap. Causing the child unnecessary distress, for example, attempting cannulation, may invoke a complete obstruction of the upper airway and require emergency airway management.

Antibiotic therapy will be required once the airway has been secured, and this will usually be with intubation. After antibiotic therapy has been established, recovery is normally rapid.

Aspiration of a foreign body

This is an uncommon occurrence in children; however, because infants and children are inquisitive and put objects in their mouth or are learning to eat different types of food, then aspiration of a foreign body is a possibility.

Children often have sudden onset of respiratory distress and a history of choking. Children with suspected aspiration of a foreign body will need a laryngo-bronchoscopy to remove the object from the airway.

Children who present with an acute choking episode need to be treated with the choking algorithm (ALSG, 2016) (Fig. 10.1).

Pneumonia

Pneumonia is globally recognised as the leading cause of death from infection in the under-fives, accounting for approximately one-fifth of childhood deaths worldwide (World Health Organization, 2014).

Pneumonia is an infection affecting the lower respiratory tract and can be caused by viral or bacterial pathogens. Infants, children and young people are affected by different organisms. Infection can occur via the bloodstream or through inhalation via the airway epithelium. It is characterised by inflammation of the lung parenchyma leading to consolidation of alveoli. There are different classifications of pneumonia, which can relate to the anatomical distribution of the disease, the infective pathogen responsible for the disease, or whether the disease is community-acquired or hospital-acquired (nosocomial).

According to Glasper and Richardson (2010), pneumonia can be classified by the site of its anatomical distribution:

Lobar pneumonia involves a large portion of an entire lobe of a lung and is predominantly caused by *Streptococcus pneumoniae*.

Bronchopneumonia begins in the terminal bronchioles, which become congested with exudate and form patches of consolidation involving several lobes of the lungs; it usually follows another respiratory illness, such as whooping cough or bronchiolitis.

Interstitial pneumonia involves the walls surrounding the alveoli and bronchioles and is usually caused by viral or mycoplasma infections. The inflammatory process is confined within the alveolar walls and the peribronchiolar and interlobular tissues.

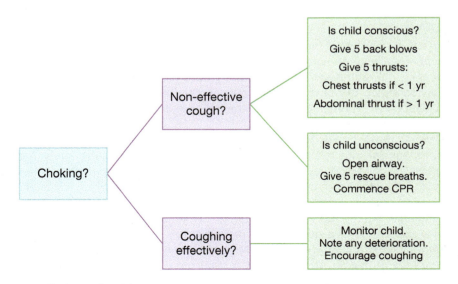

Figure 10.1 Choking algorithm.

Altered physiology
Bacterial pneumonia

Infectious organisms are spread to the lower respiratory tract either via the bloodstream or the upper respiratory tract. The body responds to the pathogen by triggering an immune response in the lungs. The lung capillaries begin to leak plasma proteins, red blood cells, and inflammatory and immune response mediators into the alveoli resulting in a reduced functional area for gaseous exchange. As a result the rate of breathing increases to meet the rising demand for oxygen and to combat the rising carbon dioxide levels. Mucus production increases and fluid continues to fill the alveoli. As the disease progresses the alveoli further fill with fluid and debris caused by the large number of white blood cells being produced to fight the infection. Ultimately some alveoli become solid as the normally hollow air space is filled with fluid and debris. This results in an area of consolidation within the lung where gaseous exchange is severely impaired.

Viral pneumonia infects the walls of the alveoli and the parenchyma of the lung. The ciliated epithelial cells become damaged as the virus replicates in the alveolar epithelial cells, leading to rupturing of the walls of the alveoli and the bronchioles.

Diagnosis

Distinguishing between viral and bacterial infection can be difficult and it can also be hard to obtain a definitive diagnosis of bacterial infection in babies and young children. Recommendations suggest that in children where there is persistent or repetitive fever greater than 38.5 °C together with chest wall recession and a raised respiratory rate, a diagnosis of bacterial pneumonia should be considered (Harris et al., 2011).

Chest X-ray is only indicated when a child fails to respond to treatment or if complications are suspected.

Signs and symptoms

Signs and symptoms are often non-specific and vary according to the age of the child and the causative pathogens. Respiratory assessment is the most important diagnostic tool.

- Neonates and infants may present with cough, fever, lethargy, poor feeding.
- Pre-school children may present with cough, fever, chest pain, abdominal pain, vomiting.
- Older children may present with fever, cough, chest pain and dyspnoea.
- Children with community-acquired pneumonia may present with fever, tachypnoea, breathlessness or difficulty in breathing, cough, wheeze or chest pain. They may also present with abdominal pain and/or vomiting and may have headache.

Investigations

Chest X-ray is only necessary if there is failure to respond to treatment or if complications are suspected.

Full blood count, C-reactive protein and blood cultures should be performed, and a blood gas to assess respiratory function may be indicated if there is acute respiratory distress.

Nasopharyngeal aspirate for viral immunofluorescence and/or sputum specimen for microscopy, culture and sensitivity may also be considered.

Assessment and treatment

The priority for managing a child with pneumonia is prompt identification and treatment of respiratory distress. Full respiratory assessment should be undertaken, including pulse oximetry and supplementary oxygen administered if the oxygen saturation reading is below 92%.

Children demonstrating signs of severe respiratory distress and decreasing levels of consciousness may require tracheal intubation and artificial ventilation in order to maintain adequate oxygenation.

Assessment of the nutritional status of the child is important in preventing dehydration (see red flag box, next section). Symptoms of respiratory distress, such as tachypnoea and recession, can impede the ability to swallow and children should be assessed for dehydration. Dependent upon the severity of the respiratory distress it may be necessary to commence intravenous fluids or enteral feeding via a nasogastric tube. Presence of a nasogastric tube, however, can exacerbate respiratory distress if it occludes too much of the airway.

Antimicrobial therapy is usually started with a diagnosis of bacterial pneumonia and the type of drug and route of administration will depend upon the age of the child, the severity of the illness and the causative pathogen (if known).

Children who are not requiring oxygen and are drinking adequately can be managed at home with a course of oral antibiotics.

Complications

If the pneumonia fails to respond to treatment there is a risk of developing empyema. Empyema is a serious respiratory condition which is caused by the pleural fluid within the pleural space becoming infected. Left untreated the pus thickens and causes sections of the pleura to stick together forming pockets of pus. The thickening deposits can extend to the outer layer of the lung, which prevents adequate lung expansion. Empyema is treated with insertion of a small chest drain connected to an underwater seal to allow the infected fluid to drain.

🚩 Red Flag

Dehydration

Dehydration can be a common adjunct to respiratory infection as a result of difficulties in coordinating breathing and swallowing mechanisms. In addition, paroxysmal coughing can result in episodes of vomiting. Infants and children should be assessed for signs of dehydration and managed accordingly. Parents of children who are diagnosed with a respiratory infection but who are not admitted to hospital should be informed about what symptoms to look out for and advised when to contact a healthcare professional should symptoms persist.

Signs of clinical dehydration as identified by the National Institute for Health and Care Excellence (NICE) (2009) appear in the following table:

Altered responsiveness, for example, irritable or lethargic	Decreased urine output
Normal skin colour	Sunken eyes
Warm extremities	Tachycardia
Dry mucous membranes	Tachypnoea
Normal peripheral pulses	Normal capillary refill time
Reduced skin turgor	Normal blood pressure

Whooping cough (pertussis)

Pertussis is a highly contagious acute respiratory infection, which is predominantly caused by the bacterium *Bordetella pertussis*. Incidence of the disease is relatively low as a result of the 5-in-1 vaccine given as part of the routine vaccination schedule to infants at 8 weeks, 12 weeks and 16 weeks of age (see 'Vaccinations' box later). It is reported that overall pertussis activity in England is at raised levels in comparison to the years preceding the most recent outbreak in 2012 (Health Protection Report, 2015). Young unimmunised infants, particularly premature babies, babies under 3 months of age and babies born to unimmunised mothers, are identified as the most vulnerable group, with the highest rates of complications and death (Public Health England, 2016a).

Presenting symptoms in the catarrhal stage include mild fever, runny nose and occasional cough lasting 7–10 days. The paroxysmal stage can last for up to 10 weeks and during this stage the cough gradually develops into a paroxysmal cough causing a characteristic inspiratory 'whoop', vomiting and exhaustion. The convalescent stage involves a general recovery with a gradual resolution of the cough over a 2–3-week period. Diagnosis can often be delayed in older children who present with a persistent cough rather than a 'whooping' cough. The infection can be more serious in infants as paroxysms of coughing can result in episodes of apnoea. Vigorous persistent coughing can cause nosebleeds and subconjunctival haemorrhage.

Whooping cough (pertussis) is spread person to person by droplet infection and the incubation period is 7–10 days. A case is infectious from 7 days following exposure up to 3 weeks after the onset of paroxysmal cough, and symptoms can persist for 3 months. A single attack confers lifetime immunity.

Management

Pertussis is treated by administration of an antimicrobial therapy in order to reduce the period of infectivity. Antimicrobial therapy, however, does not shorten the course of the illness or manage other associated symptoms. Close contacts and other household members also require treating with antimicrobial therapy (Public Health England, 2016a).

Infants and children can become very anxious during episodes of coughing and require supportive care in managing their fear and distress. Fluid intake and nutrition need to be carefully monitored as paroxysmal coughing often causes vomiting of mucus.

Complications

Complications of whooping cough include lobar pneumonia, atelectasis and bronchiectasis. In addition, prolonged episodes of coughing can result in nosebleed, subconjunctival haemorrhage and inguinal hernia.

Notifiable diseases

Pertussis is a notifiable disease in accordance with the Health Protection Legislation (England) Guidance 2010. Suspected cases should be notified by telephone, to the local health protection team as soon as is practicable and written notification sent within 3 days (Department of Health, 2010).

Vaccinations

The following vaccines form part of the routine vaccinations schedule that is freely available through the NHS to all babies and children in the United Kingdom. Significant protection against respiratory infections is provided within this schedule and the importance of having babies and children vaccinated should be discussed with parents.

5-in-1 vaccine:
Protects against: diphtheria, tetanus, whooping cough, polio and Hib (*Haemophilus influenzae* type b)
Given at: 8, 12 and 16 weeks of age
4-in-1 pre-school booster:
Protects against: diphtheria, tetanus, whooping cough, polio and Hib (*Haemophilus influenzae* type b)
Given at: 3 years 4 months of age
Pneumococcal conjugate vaccine (PCV) or pneumo jab:
Protects against: some types of pneumococcal infection
Given at: 8 weeks, 16 weeks and 1 year

The following is an optional vaccination offered in addition to the routine vaccinations to 'at risk' groups of babies or children.

BCG (Bacillus Calmette-Guérin) tuberculosis vaccine:
Protects against: tuberculosis (TB)
Given to: babies and children who have a high chance of coming into contact with TB
Given at: birth to 16 years of age

The BCG vaccine is not currently part of the routine NHS vaccination schedule. It is only given to a child or adult thought to have an increased risk of coming into contact with TB.

Universal vaccination at birth is recommended for infants living in high TB incidence and there are 11 high incidence areas identified in the UK (Public Health England, 2016b).

Current information on vaccines and vaccination procedures in the United Kingdom can be found in 'Immunisation against infectious disease' (UK Immunisation Schedule, 2016).

Tuberculosis

It is reported that the incidence of TB in England over the past 4 years demonstrates a year on year decline, down to 5658 cases in 2015, and an overall reduction of one-third, since the peak of 8280 cases in 2011 (Public Health England, 2016b). Tuberculosis is a chronic specific inflammatory infectious disease caused by the slow-growing bacillus *Mycobacterium tuberculosis*. It generally targets the lungs but can also affect any part of the body. Pulmonary TB accounts for approximately 60% of all cases of TB in the UK (Public Health England, 2014). Children are usually infected by inhalation of infected droplet nuclei from infected individuals who are immediate family or regular contacts. Children with the disease are themselves nearly always non-infectious, therefore if a child is diagnosed with TB, public health should be notified to initiate contact tracing to find the source.

Inhaled bacilli implant in the distal airspaces of the lower part of the upper lobe or the upper part of the lower lobe of the lungs. In many cases the infection is contained by the immune system and does not cause the disease; however, there is residual area of infection present in the lung called the Ghon focus and enlargement of the mediastinal lymph nodes referred to as the *primary complex*. Infection may be spread via the bloodstream distributing the infection to other parts of the body where it may lodge. The organism may remain inactive indefinitely or may reactivate at a later stage to cause pulmonary or extra-pulmonary TB dependent upon the site of the infection.

Extra-pulmonary TB can present as cervical lymph node enlargement, spinal TB, TB meningitis, TB arthritis and less commonly in children abdominal TB and genitourinary TB (Smyth, 2013).Clinical features depend upon the level of immune response varying from local containment and dormancy of the infection to overwhelming and disseminated infection.

The majority of infants and children, who become infected with *Mycobacterium tuberculosis*, do not progress to develop TB and therefore remain asymptomatic. Common presenting symptoms are very gradual in onset and include cough and respiratory symptoms, weight loss, failure to thrive and anorexia, dyspnoea and fever. Approaches to diagnosis will depend upon whether the infection is detected through passive or active case finding. Active case finding will detect infection through contact tracing or routine immigration screening. Passive case finding detects infection through examination of children presenting with signs and symptoms. Diagnosis is based upon chest X-ray, tuberculin testing, sputum testing and gastric aspiration.

Early diagnosis is essential in relation to identification of the primary case that spread the disease to the child, and for starting long-term antituberculosis drug therapy. Treatment and preventative therapy is under the care of a specialist clinician and can involve taking antituberculosis drugs for a period of 3–6 months. Concordance with treatment is essential in order to adequately treat the disease and reduce the risk of drug resistance. Without appropriate advice, as children may become symptom free after only a few weeks, continuing to take long-term, preventative medications can be problematic. For infants and children with active disease, multiple medications will be required over a long period of time.

Tuberculosis is a notifiable disease in accordance with the Health Protection Legislation (England) Guidance 2010. Suspected cases should be notified by telephone, to the local health protection team as soon as is practicable and written notification sent within 3 days (Department of Health, 2010).

Red Flag

Parents need to be alerted to the following signs and seek immediate hospital treatment should any be present:

- worsening effort of breathing (e.g., grunting, nasal flaring, marked chest recession)
- fluid intake is 50–75% of normal or no wet nappy for 12 hours
- apnoea or cyanosis
- exhaustion (e.g., not responding normally to social cues, wakes only with prolonged stimulation)

(NICE, 2009)

Chapter 10
Disorders of the respiratory system

Case Study

Olivia is a 13-year-old girl, who has visited her GP on several occasions over the past month with a history of persistent cough, wheeze and shortness of breath. She has been treated for a viral respiratory tract infection. During PE she became distressed and finding it difficult to breath. The school rang the emergency services for an ambulance. Olivia has no further medical history and school have contacted her mum to let them know what has happened.

Vital signs

Physical and bloods
The following vital signs where noted and recorded:

Pulse	120
Respiratory rate	30
SaO2	92%
Blood pressure	110/70
Temperature	36.8 °C

A full blood count was performed.

Test	Result	Guideline normal values
White blood cells (WBC)	6×10^9/L	$4–11 \times 10^9$/L
Neutrophils	4.4×10^9/L	$2.0–7.5 \times 10^9$/L
Lymphocytes	2.8×10^9/L	$1.3–4.0 \times 10^9$/L
Red blood cells (RBC)	5.1×10^9/L	$4.5–6.5 \times 10^9$/L
Haemoglobin (Hb)	14 g/dL	11.5–16.5 g/dL
Platelets	320×10^9/L	$150–440 \times 10^9$/L

Reflect on this case and consider the following:

1. What could be the most likely diagnosis?
2. What further information do you require from Olivia and her mum in order to ensure that safe and effective family-centred care is provided for her?
3. List any further investigations that Olivia might require.
4. What treatment options are available for Olivia?

Investigations

Chest X-ray

An X-ray is a diagnostic test that uses small amounts of radiation to generate a picture of organs, tissues and bones of the body. When an X-ray is taken of the chest it can help to identify abnormalities or disease of the airways, heart, lungs, blood vessels and bones. Chest X-rays can also be used to identify the presence of fluid in the lungs or fluid and air around the lungs. A chest X-ray can be requested for a variety of reasons, including to assess injury after an accident or to monitor the progression of a disease (cystic fibrosis).

A chest X-ray is a quick, easy and effective test that has been used for decades in the assessment and treatment of patients.

⚑ Red Flag

Prolonged increased effort of breathing
Increased effort of breathing is tiring and the body cannot maintain this for long periods of time. Identifying this early can reduce the risk of respiratory arrest. Early indicators that the body is starting to get into difficulty can be easily identified. These include:

- **Altered neurological state:** vacant look, restless, irritable, sitting very still
- **Increased effort of breathing:** nasal flaring, shoulder bobbing, clavicle or tracheal tug, intercostal and subcostal recession (using the small muscles within the rib cage to assist with breathing)
- **Tripoding:** using arms to alter position to enable more chest expansion to try and assist/ease effort of breathing
- **Respiratory arrest:** Breathing stops and does not spontaneously restart.

Asthma

Due to its nature, there is no clear definition of asthma, which makes it difficult to provide recommendations for a diagnosis of asthma that is evidence-based (BTS/SIGN, 2014). The recognised symptoms of asthma can include wheeze, breathlessness, chest tightness, cough and variable airway obstructions. However, the symptoms of asthma are individual to each patient, which can increase the difficulty of diagnosis. The presenting symptoms are usually reversible with drug therapy or can be spontaneously reversed without.

In the airways of an asthmatic, there is increased inflammation and hyper-responsiveness to identified stimuli or triggers (Fig. 10.2); these can include exercise, stress and allergens (pollen, dust, pet dander). The airways present with a bronchospasm, which is the narrowing of the bronchial walls due to an uncontrolled smooth muscle contraction as a result of hyper-responsiveness to an identified stimulus. At the same time, inflammation within the airways occurs causing the airways to become hyper-responsive and narrow easily in reaction to the stimulus. There is further narrowing of the airways through invasion by the inflammatory cells, as the body responds to protect itself. Inflammatory cells contain chemical mediators, including histamine, prostaglandins and leukotrienes, which cause vasodilation and increased capillary permeability. This results in mucus production and oedema occurring within the airways (Kelsey & McEwing, 2010).

Altered pathophysiology

Within a normal airway structure the bronchial wall and basement membrane are thin, with a thin viscous layer of fluid covering the epithelial surface. The smooth muscle is relaxed leaving the airway wide open for good air flow. In an asthmatic airway structure, however, the bronchial walls and basement membrane are inflamed and thickened, with inflammatory exudate covering the lumen of airways. The smooth muscle is constricted and in spasm leading to bronchospasm and airway obstruction. This reduces the size of the airway leading to poor airflow and a wheeze being produced.

Chapter 10   Disorders of the respiratory system

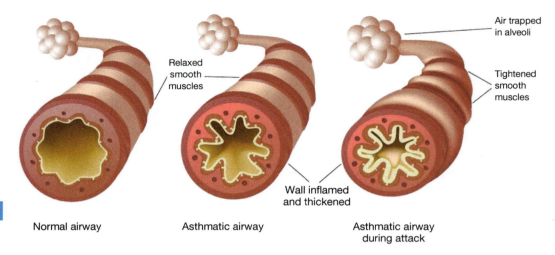

Figure 10.2 Difference between a normal airway and an asthmatic airway.

🚩 Red Flags

Medication

Salbutamol (Blue inhaler): can cause fine muscle tremors throughout the body; this includes the heart muscle, leading to tachycardia and palpitations.

Becotide/Beclomethasone (Brown inhaler): can cause a dry mouth and oral thrush. To reduce the incidence of this happening, encourage the child to brush their teeth after using their inhaler.

Inhaler technique: ensuring correct inhaler technique is the cornerstone to effective asthma management and treatment. All patients (and parents) need to have regular checks that they are using the inhaler correctly.

Oral steroids: Long-term use of oral steroids can lead to poor bone health, cataract development (Bhatt, Vyas & Forster, 2013).

Assessment

When undertaking a nursing assessment of a child with a suspected or known asthma attack there are some specific questions that need to be answered to assist in their treatment. These include the following:

- What symptoms has the child got?
- Do they have a cough? If so, is it persistent, nocturnal, productive or episodic?
- Do they have a wheeze? If so, is it inspiratory/expiratory, nocturnal, and is it caused by anything specific like exercise, emotions or feeding, for example?
- Are they breathless? If so, is it persistent or variable (e.g., can they complete a sentence without becoming breathless if they are talking to you)?
- How long have they had the symptoms and when did the symptoms begin?
- How long do the symptoms last for?

- Does the child look distressed or are they in distress?
- Is there any family history of asthma, eczema or hayfever in the family?

Care and treatment

When planning the nursing treatment for an asthmatic child, the ultimate goal is to restore a normal breathing pattern as asthma is a reversible condition. The use of continuous monitoring of vital signs until the child is stabilised is paramount, to monitor the effectiveness of the inhaled medication. The maintenance of oxygen saturation levels above 92% is essential to ensure adequate oxygenation, but also to assist in the effort of breathing. This is done through the safe administration of prescribed oxygen via a non-rebreathe mask. The administration of prescribed bronchodilators and oral steroids is the most effective way to get asthma back under control. When administrating medication it is important to follow the Nursing Midwifery Council (NMC) (2007) Standards for Medicine Management. During care delivery it is important that comfort and reassurance is given to both the child and parent as dyspnoea (shortness of breath) is very frightening to both the child and parent. Giving reassurance to a parent will help to reduce their own anxiety, which in turn will help the child to relax and breathe more easily.

Once the child's asthma is under control the next step is to develop or review the child's asthma plan; this is best done by an asthma specialist nurse who will work with the child and their family to discuss their educational needs, support and care pathway (Bhatt, Vyas & Forster, 2013). As part of this ongoing support and treatment, if it is felt to be appropriate, the introduction of regular peak expiratory flow rate (PEFR) measurement will be considered and implemented.

Investigations

Peak flow readings:
These are objective lung function measurements of the peak expiratory flow (PEF). This is the maximum flow of air achieved during expiration, delivered with the maximum force. The PEF is recorded in litres per minute (L/min). It is done using a simple and portable device that can be used in the home and in hospital, and which is suitable for children over the age of 6 years.

The negative side is that they are not as sensitive as spirometry readings, which require more sophisticated equipment that is usually non-portable and requires specialist training to undertake the procedure and interpret the readings.

What are peak flow zones?
Peak flow zones are based on the traffic light concept: red means danger, yellow means caution, and green means safe. Based on the patient's personal best, the three peak flow zones include:

Green: 80–100 % of your personal best PEFR; asthma is under control.
Yellow: 50–79 % of your personal best PEFR; asthma is getting worse; you may need to use quick-relief medications.
Red: below 50% of your personal best PEFR; medical alert, take quick-relief medication; GET medical help *immediately*.

Table 10.1 Features of acute/severe and life-threatening asthma

Main symptoms of asthma	Features of acute/severe asthma	Features of life-threatening asthma
Cough which may become productive	Peak flow less than 50% of predicted or best	Peak flow less than 33% of predicted or best
Dyspnoea and chest tightness	Dyspnoea – unable to complete a sentence in one breath	Oxygen saturation less than 92%
Wheeze	Tachypnoea	Silent chest
Peak Flow less than predicted or best	Tachycardia	Week and feeble respiratory effort
		Cyanosis
		Bradycardia or hypotension
		Confusion, exhaustion or coma

Management of acute/severe or life-threatening asthma (see Table 10.1)

Asthma treatment protocols are subject to regular review. Clear guidelines have been produced in relation to (BTS/SIGN, 2014):

- the management of acute asthma in children in the emergency department
- the management of acute asthma in children in hospital
- the management of acute asthma in infants aged <2 years in hospital.

Difficult asthma

Asthma that is not under control may be a result of several different reasons, which need to be considered. These reasons include the individual not getting the right level of support or not accessing care when they need it. This could be a result of lack of information or understanding about asthma, or a lack of services available to the individual. Concordance with medication can be an issue. This is where the rule of thirds applies: one-third will take medication as directed, one-third will partially follow instructions, and one-third do not take medication at all (Tate, 2010). People may not understand what their medicines are for and how to take them, or they may not be taking their medicines as prescribed. Some people do not have access to effective healthcare or medicines because of financial, language, cultural or social barriers, whereas others are unable, unwilling or unaware of the need to avoid persistent exposure to triggers such as cigarette smoke or exposure to workplace substances. People may have other underlying health conditions that have not been identified and which may make their asthma symptoms worse or they may be misdiagnosed with asthma and thus asthma medicines will not help their symptoms. The National Review of Asthma Deaths (NRAD) (2014) found deficiencies in both the routine care of people with asthma and the treatment of attacks (Royal College of Physicians, 2015). In many instances, neither doctors nor patients recognised the signs of deteriorating asthma; they also did not react quickly enough when these were seen.

Conclusion

Respiratory illnesses in children are common as a result of developmental differences in the respiratory systems of infants and young children. Effective respiratory assessment enables early detection and appropriate care and management of the sick child.

References

Akers, E. (2015). The respiratory system. In: Peate, I. & Gormley-Fleming, E. (eds). *Fundamentals of Children's Anatomy and Physiology*. Wiley, Oxford, Chap. 10.

ALSG (2016). *Advanced Paediatric Life Support: A Practical Approach to Emergencies*, 6th edn. Wiley, Oxford.

Bhatt, J., Vyas, H. & Forster, D. (2013). Management of asthma and allergy. In: Mighten, J. (ed.). *Children's Respiratory Nursing*. Wiley, Oxford.

British Thoracic Society/Scottish Intercollegiate Guidelines Network (BTS/SIGN) (2014). *British Guidelines on the Management of Asthma*. A National Clinical Guideline. British Thoracic Society, London.

Department of Health (2010). *Health protection legislation guidance 2010*. Public Health England, London.

Glasper, A. & Richardson, J. (2010). *A Textbook of Children's and Young People's Nursing*, 2nd edn. Churchill Livingstone, Oxford.

Harris, M., Clark, J., Coote, N., et al. (2011). British Thoracic Society guidelines for the management of community acquired pneumonia in children: update 2011. Available at: http://thorax.bmj.com/content/66/Suppl_2/ii1 (last accessed April 2018).

Health Protection Report (2015). Laboratory confirmed pertussis in England: data to end-June 2015. Available at: https://www.gov.uk/government/publications/health-protection-report-volume-9-2015/hpr-volume-9-issue-30-news-28-august (last accessed 17 April 2018).

Kelsey, J. & McEwing, G. (2010). Respiratory illness in children. In: Glasper, A. & Richardson, J. (eds). *A Textbook of Children and Young People's Nursing*, 2nd edn. Elsevier, London.

National Institute for Health and Care Excellence (NICE) (2009). Diarrhoea and vomiting caused by gastroenteritis in under 5s: diagnosis and management. Clinical guideline [CG84]. Available at: https://www.nice.org.uk/guidance/cg84/chapter/1-guidance#assessing-dehydration-and-shock (last accessed 17 April 2018).

National Institute for Health and Care Excellence (NICE) (2015). Bronchiolitis in children: diagnosis and management. NICE guidelines [NG9]. Available at: https://www.nice.org.uk/guidance/ng9 (last accessed 17 April 2018).

Nursing & Midwifery Council (NMC) (2007). Standards for medicines management. NMC, London. Available at: https://www.nmc.org.uk/standards/additional-standards/standards-for-medicines-management/ (last accessed 17 April 2018).

Public Health England (2014). The Green Book. Available at: https://www.gov.uk/government/collections/immunisation-against-infectious-disease-the-green-book (accessed October 2016).

Public Health England (2016a). Pertussis: guidelines for public health management. Available at: https://www.gov.uk/government/uploads/system/uploads/attachment_data/file/541694/Guidelines_for_the_Public_Health_Management_of_Pertussis_in_England.pdf (accessed October 2016).

Public Health England (2016b). Tuberculosis in London. Annual review (2015 data). Data from 2000 to 2105. Available at: https://www.gov.uk/government/uploads/system/uploads/attachment_data/file/564656/TB_annual_report_2016.pdf (last accessed April 2018).

Public Health England (2010). The Health Protection (Notification) Regulations). The Stationery Office, London.

Royal College of Nursing (RCN) (2013). Standards for assessing, measuring and monitoring vital signs in infants, children and young people. RCN Publications, London.

Royal College of Physicians (2015). Why Asthma Kills. Available at: https://www.rcplondon.ac.uk/projects/national-review-asthma-deaths (last accessed April 2018).

Smyth, A.R. (2013). Management of lung infection in children. In: Mighten, J. (ed.). *Children's Respiratory Nursing*. Wiley, Chichester.

Tate, P. (2010). *The Doctor's Communication Handbook*, 6th edn. Radcliffe Publishing, Oxford.

UK Immunisation Schedule (2016). Available at: https://www.gov.uk/government/publications/the-complete-routine-immunisation-schedule (last accessed 17 April 2018).

World Health Organization (WHO) (2014). Revised WHO classification and treatment of childhood pneumonia at health facilities. Evidence summaries. Available at: http://apps.who.int/iris/bitstream/10665/137319/1/9789241507813_eng.pdf?ua=1 (accessed October 2016).

Chapter 11

Disorders of the endocrine system

Julia Petty

Aim

The aim of this chapter is to offer a brief overview of the anatomy and physiology of the endocrine system. Altered pathophysiology is outlined and how this can impact on a person's development, health and wellbeing.

Learning outcomes

On completion of this chapter, the reader will be able to:

- List the organs and hormones of the endocrine system.
- Describe the key functions of the endocrine system.
- Discuss the normal and abnormal pathophysiological changes that may occur in the endocrine system.
- Outline the diagnosis and assessment of a range of endocrine disorders.
- Outline the care of children and/or young people who have endocrine disorders.

Keywords

- endocrine system
- endocrine glands
- hormones
- endocrine disorders
- hormone replacement
- lifelong effects

Fundamentals of Children's Applied Pathophysiology: An Essential Guide for Nursing and Healthcare Students, First Edition.
Edited by Elizabeth Gormley-Fleming and Ian Peate.
© 2019 John Wiley & Sons Ltd. Published 2019 by John Wiley & Sons Ltd.
Companion website: www.wileyfundamentalseries.com/childpathophysiology

Disorders of the endocrine system

Test your prior knowledge

1. Outline the role and functions of the endocrine system.
2. Identify each endocrine gland and the associated hormones along with their functions.
3. For each endocrine gland, identify the disorders that can occur.
4. Describe the pathophysiology of each disorder identified.
5. Outline how endocrine disorders are diagnosed.
6. Identify the signs and symptoms of key endocrine disorders.
7. Discuss the treatment and care of children and/or young people with a range of endocrine disorders.
8. Discuss how disorders of the endocrine system can impact on the child or young person's health and wellbeing.
9. Identify the long-term emotional effects of having an endocrine disorder.
10. Describe the role of the healthcare professional when providing care to a child with a disorder of the endocrine system.

Introduction

The endocrine system is a complex system that controls many vital functions of the body (Hinson, Raven & Chew, 2010; Jameson & De Groot, 2010). This chapter offers an outline of the endocrine system, the glands and hormones that make up this system and the associated pathophysiology when there is disease, injury or malfunction, for whatever reason. A number of endocrine-related conditions and their allied diagnosis, treatments and care are discussed.

Endocrine anatomy and function

The endocrine and nervous systems are responsible for the transmission of vital messages and the regulation of bodily functions. Whereas the nervous system works by transmission of electrical impulses, the endocrine system comprises a collection of ductless, highly vascular *glands* (Fig. 11.1) that secrete a range of different types of hormone directly into the blood stream. Hormones are then transported to distant target organs or tissues (Molina, 2013) where they take effect. Endocrine glands are controlled directly by stimulation from the nervous system, and by chemical receptors in the blood and hormones produced by other glands (Waugh & Grant, 2010). By regulating the functions of organs in the body, these glands help to maintain the body's homeostasis. Growth and development, sexual development and control of many internal body functions, such as glucose and mineral regulation, and the stress response, are among the many essential physiological processes regulated by the actions of hormones (Rogers, 2012; Petty, 2015). The anatomy of the endocrine system can be seen in Fig. 11.1.

The integrity and health of the endocrine system are essential to maintaining healthy body weight, growth, and physical and emotional development. Damage or disease to the endocrine system therefore can lead to significant consequences for the child or young person.

A summary of the endocrine organs, their functions and associated disorders can be seen in Table 11.1.

Disorders of the endocrine system Chapter 11

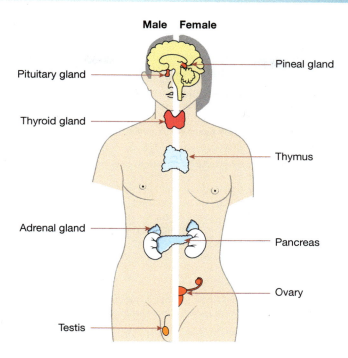

Figure 11.1 The endocrine system. *Source:* http://commons.wikimedia.org/wiki/File:Illu_endocrine_system.jpg

Endocrine disorders

Referring to the systems in Table 11.1, this chapter will now discuss each associated disorder in turn, outlining the pathophysiology, diagnosis and presenting signs along with a brief overview of care and management. For all conditions involving the endocrine system, referral to a paediatric endocrinology team and/or other health professionals, as appropriate, is necessary, for ongoing follow-up and management.

Disorders of the hypothalamus and pituitary gland
Hypothalamic disease

This is a disorder of the hypothalamus caused by damage from malnutrition, including anorexia and other eating disorders, genetic disorders, radiation, surgery, head trauma, lesion, tumour or other physical injury. Damage to the hypothalamus may impact any of the hormones outlined in Table 11.1 and the related endocrine systems. As many of these hypothalamic hormones act on the pituitary gland, hypothalamic disease in turn affects it's function as well as the target organs controlled by the pituitary, including the adrenal glands, ovaries and testes, and the thyroid gland.

Damage to the hypothalamus may cause disruptions in body temperature regulation, growth, weight, sodium and water balance, milk production, emotions, and sleep cycles. Hypopituitarism, neurogenic diabetes insipidus, hypothyroidism and problems with development of puberty are examples of conditions caused by hypothalamic disease. The signs and symptoms exhibited by these conditions, and the associated care will be covered in the sections that follow.

Table 11.1 Overview of the endocrine system, its associated functions and disorders. (For full details of endocrine system function and specific hormones as relevant to children, see Petty, 2015)

Endocrine organ	Function	Associated disorders
Hypothalamus	Serves as a central endocrine control centre by communication with the pituitary gland and has many different functions such as growth, thermoregulation, control of hunger and thirst, sexual development and regulation of stress defences	Hypothalamic disease, which in turn can cause the disorders below
Pituitary gland	Controlled by the releasing and inhibiting hormones from the hypothalamus, many endocrine functions are regulated by this gland. The hormones either released or inhibited are: anti-diuretic hormone (ADH) and oxytocin from the posterior pituitary gland (PG) and growth hormone (somatotropin), thyroid-stimulating hormone (TSH), adreno-cortico trophic hormone (ACTH) follicle-stimulating hormone, luteinising hormone, prolactin, melanocyte-stimulating hormone, beta-endorphin from the anterior PG	• Hypopituitarism • Pituitary dwarfism/poor somatic growth • Gigantism • Diabetes insipidus • Pituitary tumours, such as: 　• craniopharyngioma 　• prolactinoma 　• pituitary adenoma
Pineal gland	Produces the hormone melatonin that helps to regulate the human sleep–wake cycle known as the circadian rhythm	• Pineal disease/dysfunction, e.g., disruption to the sleep–wake cycle (circadian rhythms)
Thyroid gland	Releases thyroxine that regulates metabolism, stimulates body oxygen and energy consumption, plays a part in growth by promoting protein synthesis and influences the activity of the nervous system. Calcitonin lowers calcium levels of calcium	• Hypothyroidism • Hyperthyroidism ('Graves')
Parathyroid gland	Releases parathyroid hormone that raises blood calcium level and decreases phosphate level by increasing the rate of calcium absorption from the intestine into the blood	• Hypoparathyroidism • Hyperparathyroidism
Thymus gland	Releases thymosin and other related hormones that play an integral role in the maturation of T cells as part of the immune system	• Thymus disease/dysfunction, e.g., interference with normal immune response
Adrenal gland	Produces mineralocorticoids that stimulate sodium reabsorption in the kidneys increasing blood levels of sodium and water, corticosteroids that stimulate gluconeogenesis and fat breakdown in adipose tissue so increasing glucose availability in the blood, promote metabolism and resistance to stress and gonadocorticoids, which influence masculinisation (virilisation) in both males and females. Adrenaline and noradrenaline from the adrenal medulla are an integral part of the body's flight–fight responses to stress	• Adrenal insufficiency: Addison's disease. • Cushing disease • Congenital adrenal hyperplasia
Pancreas	Produces and releases insulin which results in targets cells taking up free glucose so lowering blood levels. Conversely, glucagon is also released that targets the liver to break down glycogen into glucose which increases blood glucose levels	• Diabetes mellitus • Hyperinsulinemia/nesidioblastosis
Testes and ovaries	Release sex hormones testosterone or oestrogen from either the testes or ovaries	• Disorders of sex development (DSD) or ambiguous genitalia • Gonadotropin deficiency – failure to initiate or complete puberty • Precocious puberty • Ovarian disease

ACTH, adrenocorticotrophic hormone; ADH, anti-diuretic hormone; DSD, disorder of sex development; PG, pineal gland; TSH, thyroid-stimulating hormone.

Hypopituitarism

As for hypothalamic disease, because of the widespread functions of the pituitary gland (Dorton, 2000), there are many diseases associated with hypopituitarism. The term refers to an inability of the pituitary gland to provide sufficient hormones due to inadequate production or an insufficient supply of hypothalamic-releasing hormones. When pituitary hormone production is impaired, target gland hormone production is reduced because of a lack of trophic stimulus. Normally, sub-physiologic target hormone levels stimulate the pituitary gland to increase trophic hormone production; however, in hypopituitarism, the pituitary gland response is absent, suboptimal, or inappropriate. This results in progressive secondary failure of the target glands (Kim, 2015). It is usually a mixture of several hormonal deficiencies and can be chronic and lifelong, unless successful surgery or medical treatment of the underlying disorder can restore pituitary function (Schneider et al., 2007).

Children with hypopituitarism typically present with low target hormone levels accompanied by low or inappropriately normal levels of the corresponding trophic hormone (Coremblum, 2016). Thus, pituitary function is assessed by the target gland function, not by measuring the pituitary hormone as an isolated event. Symptoms depend on the degree and type of hormone depletion, the rapidity of onset and the specific condition that manifests as a result of reduced pituitary function.

Specific conditions caused by hypopituitarism are now described, namely: growth disorder, diabetes insipidus, and tumours of the pituitary gland.

Growth disorders

Growth disorders can be due to a number of constitutional and genetic causes such as achondroplasia, hypothyroidism, Cushing syndrome, Silver-Russell syndrome, nutritional short stature, intrauterine growth restriction and bone disorders. The causation relevant to this chapter is short stature due to hormone deficiency in hypopituitarism. This type of growth disorder is characterised by growth that is very slow or delayed early in childhood before the ossification of bone cartilages (Dattani & Preece, 2004) and is caused by insufficient secretion of pituitary growth hormone.

The condition begins in childhood, and poor growth and/or shortness becomes more evident during puberty. It usually starts to show from late in the first year until mid-teens. The most obvious sign is a noticeable slowing of growth. Children may also possess signs of low blood sugar or obesity but they display average body proportions and average intelligence (Human Growth Foundation, 2015).

Through the use of injections of synthetic human growth hormone (HGH) over a period of several years, these children can achieve average height.

Conversely, acromegaly is due to an over-production of growth hormone during childhood characterised by excessive growth and height well above the average. Rarely, it affects children. If it develops in a child, usually between the ages of 15 and 17 years, it causes the condition known as gigantism and promotes growth of bones in the body.

Diabetes insipidus

Diabetes insipidus (DI) can be classified according to the primary cause. Neurogenic or cranial DI is of interest for this chapter, caused by a reduced amount of anti-diuretic hormone (ADH) being produced and released by the pituitary gland. Other forms of DI are nephrogenic DI, which originates in the kidney where the renal tubules are unresponsive to ADH, and idiopathic DI where the cells in the hypothalamus become damaged by an autoimmune response and stop producing ADH.

ADH, also called arginine vasopressin, is a hormone that constantly regulates and balances the amount of water in the blood. Osmoreceptors in the hypothalamus cells detect changes in the osmotic pressure in blood capillaries. A nerve message is sent to the pituitary to release ADH, which then travels in the blood to the kidneys. ADH increases the permeability of the distal tubule and collecting duct, so more water is reabsorbed. This causes the urine to be more concentrated. Osmoreceptors also regulate the body's sense of thirst. However, if less ADH is released, an increased volume of dilute urine will be passed (Roth & Kemp, 2015) and the child will become more thirsty leading to neurogenic DI. Signs and symptoms therefore include excessive thirst and excessive urination (Khardori & Ulla, 2012). Signs of dehydration may ensue if this condition continues without recognition or diagnosis. Neurogenic DI may just be a problem on its own but it can also occur with other problems because the production of other hormones that are released by the pituitary gland is also affected. For an example of the presenting signs of diabetes insipidus, refer to Case Study 1 at the end of this chapter.

For neurogenic DI, the treatment of choice is the synthetic ADH analogue desmopressin (1-deamino-8-D-arginine vasopressin [DDAVP]) (Mishra & Chandrashekhar, 2011). Parents must be educated regarding water replacement in infants and young children who cannot express thirst or access fluids without assistance. Gastrointestinal illnesses that cause decreased intake, increased stool losses, or both, must receive early and serious attention to prevent life-threatening electrolyte and fluid balance abnormalities (Roth & Kemp, 2015).

Medication Alert

Hormone drug therapy is often lifelong and there are risks associated with sudden cessation so education is essential for the child or young person and their family.

For endocrine conditions that require hormone replacement, for example, diabetes insipidus, hypothyroidism and diabetes mellitus, drug therapy is long term or lifelong. Therefore education of the child and family is paramount in order to teach them about the importance of continuing regular and timely administration of the hormone, the correct administration for self-care and how this is incorporated into their lifestyle and daily routine. It is essential to make them aware not to miss doses and prevent sudden cessation of the hormone, particularly in those associated with a risk of sudden withdrawal such as steroids. Education is a vital part of the role of the specialist endocrine and/or community children's multidisciplinary team in conjunction with the child, young person, family and/or carers.

Investigations: Assessing endocrine function

There are several ways to measure endocrine function and hormone levels (Matfin, 2009).

Measuring the effect of the hormone on body function: For example, blood glucose is measured to indirectly measure insulin availability.

Laboratory testing: The role of accurate and reliable laboratory testing is particularly important when investigating a potential endocrine disorder. Measuring hormones can be challenging as most circulate at very low concentrations, typically in the pico- (10–12) or nanomolar (10–9) range, and sensitivity and specificity can be affected by many variables (Wallace, 2011). Because hormones circulate in low quantities in blood, accurate measurement of these substances requires sensitive assays, usually in the form of a competitive immunoassay. A common method is radioimmunoassay that uses an antibody directed against the hormone and a radio-labelled form of the hormone (Barth, 2014). These are designed for detecting and quantifying substances such as peptides, proteins, antibodies and hormones. The use of radioactive tags permits detection of low concentrations of hormone. The labelled hormone competes with unlabelled hormone for antibody-binding sites. A standard range is used for comparison to calculate the concentration of hormone in blood samples. One example is IRMA (immunoradiometric assay). In recent years, non-radioactive tags, such as ELISA methods, have also been developed for hormone measurement. Blood tests can also test for the trophic hormone that stimulates the target organ, for example, TSH and actual thyroxine levels can both be measured (Elmlinger, 2011).

Urine testing: Hormone metabolites can be measured by urine testing usually preferred on a 24-hour collection basis.

Stimulation and suppression tests: Dynamic tests of endocrine function. A trophic or stimulating hormone is given to test the capacity of a gland in the case of hypofunction. Conversely, in hyperfunction when a gland is not responding to the normal negative feedback mechanisms and continues to release a hormone, a suppression agent can be given to confirm this situation.

Imaging: This is useful in diagnosing and follow-up. Isotopic imaging includes radioactive scanning of the thyroid gland, for example. Non-isotopic methods include magnetic resonance imaging (MRI) and computed tomography (CT), which are useful to visualize the hypothalamus/pituitary and adrenal/abdominal organs, respectively. Ultrasound also produces clear imaging of certain glands, such as the thyroid, as well as the neighbouring structures.

Tumours of the pituitary gland

Tumours can also be a cause of pituitary dysfunction. They are usually benign and can cause problems either due to local effects of the tumour, or because of excessive hormone production or inadequate hormone production by the remaining, unaffected pituitary gland. Pituitary tumours include:

- Craniopharyngioma: a benign tumour that develops near the pituitary gland. This tumour most commonly affects children 5–10 years of age.
- Pituitary adenoma: a small, benign tumour, usually less than 1 cm in size, which is made of abnormal cells that produce ACTH. This stimulates the adrenal glands, which then release cortisol. The abnormal cells in the adenoma are not downregulated by feedback from the high levels of cortisol. Excluding cases caused by steroid medication, the majority of cases of Cushing syndrome in children are caused by a pituitary adenoma.
- Prolactinoma: a non-cancerous swelling that produces excess prolactin.
- Others: Growth hormone (GH)-secreting, thyroid-stimulating hormone-secreting, and luteinising hormone/follicle-stimulating hormone (LH/FSH)-secreting tumours, named according to the hormone that is produced in excess (Keil & Stratakis, 2008).

Tumours can potentially cause symptoms in the following ways:

- by increasing intracranial pressure on the brain;
- by disrupting the function of the pituitary gland and the related hormones;
- by damaging the optic nerve.

In craniopharyngioma, increased pressure on the brain causes headache, nausea, vomiting and difficulty with balance. Damage to the pituitary gland causes hormone imbalances that can lead to various problems with the associated functions of those hormones, such as DI and stunted growth. When the optic nerve is damaged by the tumour, visual problems can develop. These defects are often permanent and may get worse after surgery to remove the tumour. Children will show evidence of decreased hormone production at the time of diagnosis. Investigations for diagnosis include:

- endocrine hormone evaluations to look for any imbalances (see Investigations box: Assessing endocrine function);
- CT scan or MRI scan of the brain;
- neurological examination.

In pituitary adenoma, the onset of the signs of Cushing disease may be insidious. Growth failure or deceleration associated with weight gain is a hallmark of Cushing syndrome in children. Other signs and symptoms often seen in children and adolescents with this condition include facial plethora, increased fine downy hair on the face, body and extremities, a temporal fat pad, round face, and diabetes. In prolactinoma, this can cause various symptoms including reduced fertility, breast changes, and headaches. In children there may be reduced growth or delayed puberty.

The management of the condition depends on the tumour. Traditionally, surgery has been the main treatment for craniopharyngioma but radiation treatment instead of surgery may be the best choice for some patients. In tumours that cannot be removed completely with surgery, radiation therapy is usually necessary. A biopsy may not be necessary if treatment with radiation alone is planned. In general, the prognosis for patients with craniopharyngioma is good, with an 80–90% chance of permanent cure if the tumour can be completely removed with surgery or treated with high doses of radiation. Recurrences may occur within the first 2 years after surgery. The prognosis for an individual child depends on whether the tumour is completely removed and the neurological deficits and hormonal imbalances caused by the tumour and the treatment. A significant percentage of patients have long-term hormonal, visual, and neurological problems following the treatment of craniopharyngioma. In patients where the tumour is not completely removed, the condition may recur (Maity *et al.*, 2008).

For a pituitary adenoma, the first-line treatment in childhood is surgical in the form of an adenomectomy or radiation for children in whom surgical intervention has failed (Keil & Stratakis, 2008). Prolactinomas can be treated successfully usually with medication using dopamine agonists to shrink the mass (Colao & Loche, 2009).

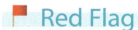
Red Flag

Multi-system effects and symptoms of endocrine disorders

The healthcare professional must be aware that there are many multi-system manifestations of endocrine disorders in children and young people, because of the widespread and diverse effects of this system and the associated hormones. Any unexplained or persistent signs and symptoms could potentially be due to an undiagnosed endocrine disorder. Some examples are:

Neurological (Jeesuk, 2014; Yu, 2014): headache, altered consciousness levels, abnormal muscle tone, strength and gait, movement problems and developmental delay.

Skin (Quatrano & Loechner, 2012): hypothyroidism – hair loss, the skin is cold and pale, with myxedematous changes, mainly in the hands and in the periorbital region. The striking features of Cushing syndrome are centripetal obesity, moon facies, supraclavicular fat pads, and abdominal striae. In Addison disease, the skin is hyperpigmented, mostly on the face, neck and back of the hands.

Pulmonary (Milla & Zirbes, 2012): acute and chronic pulmonary infections are the most common respiratory abnormalities in diabetes mellitus, hypo- and hyperthyroidism may alter lung function and affect the central respiratory drive.

Complications of hypoparathyroidism are due to hypocalcaemia. Laryngospasm can lead to stridor and airway obstruction.

In addition, it is reported that the incidence of endocrine disorders may increase in children with disabilities (Zacharin, 2013), and in those who have undergone previous childhood treatment in the form of chemotherapy and/or radiotherapy for cancer (Nandagopal et al., 2008).

Medication Alert

The methods of administering hormones.
Hormones can be administered by a range of different routes, depending on the actual type of hormone, age of the child or sometimes, their preference or choice. Oral preparations can be given for drugs such as steroids or thyroxine, subcutaneous in the case of insulin or growth hormone, intramuscularly (e.g., testosterone), intranasal (for vasopressin), and via skin patch for female sex hormones, to give some selected examples. Dosage can be based on the child's weight or in the case of diabetes, according to the measured levels of blood sugar, i.e., monitoring may influence dosage on a sliding scale basis.

For any drug route, it is essential to observe for potential side effects and to teach the child or young person what to watch out for.

Disorders of the pineal gland

The pineal gland is the centre for production of the hormone melatonin, which is implicated in a wide range of human activities. It regulates daily body rhythms, most notably the day/night cycle (circadian rhythms). Melatonin is released in the dark, during sleep. Benign pineal cysts are a common finding in children and do not usually cause any serious consequences (Lacroix-Boudhrioua et al., 2011). Generally, pineal dysfunction is rare.

Disruption of the circadian system can occur as a result of external factors such as crossing meridian time zones (jet lag), but it can also be related to a genetic predisposition or abnormalities that affect the functioning of the retinohypothalamic system, the production of melatonin, physical damage or tumours of the pineal gland. Sleep problems can manifest in children with these conditions but these are, of course, also a common finding in children (Carr et al., 2007); it is reported that problems of sleep initiation and maintenance occur in 15–25% of children and adolescents (Cummings, 2012). Studies of the benefits of melatonin for sleep disorders have been published for children and adolescents with chronic insomnia, attention deficit hyperactivity disorder, neurological injury, visual problems and for children with autism. These studies demonstrate short-term benefit with minimal side effects although data concerning the safety and efficacy of long-term melatonin use is limited (Buck, 2003; Phillips & Appleton, 2004).

Disorders of the thyroid gland

The pituitary gland secretes a hormone called thyroid-stimulating hormone (TSH), which tightly controls the amount of thyroid hormone produced. The system is designed as a feedback loop where the pituitary senses how much thyroid hormone is being released by the thyroid and adjusts the amount by making more or less TSH. An elevated TSH with a low or low-normal thyroid hormone level is called hypothyroidism, and a low or suppressed TSH with an elevated thyroid hormone level is called hyperthyroidism.

Hypothyroidism

Congenital hypothyroidism (CH) can be defined as a lack of thyroid hormones present from birth, which, unless detected and treated early, is associated with irreversible neurological problems and poor growth (BSPED, 2013). Hypothalamic or pituitary dysfunction accounts also for some cases of hypothyroidism (Willacy, 2011). Pituitary hypothyroidism usually occurs with other disorders of pituitary dysfunction, for example, lack of growth. Some infants may develop a lack of thyroid hormones after birth and this may represent primary hypothyroidism rather than CH. Children with primary hypothyroidism do not experience the irreversible neurological problems that are seen with untreated CH. There may be thyroid aplasia, hypoplasia or ectopic thyroid tissue. It is not inherited, so the chances of another sibling being affected are low. There may also be disorders of thyroid hormone metabolism, such as TSH unresponsiveness and defects in thyroglobulin. This is usually inherited and therefore there is a risk that further children may also be affected.

Transient hypothyroidism may also occur, although rarely in children, and is usually related to either maternal medications, for example, carbimazole, or to maternal antibodies. In maternal thyroid disease, IgG auto-antibodies can cross the placenta and block thyroid function in utero; this improves after delivery.

A number of genetic defects have been associated with CH (Wassner & Brown, 2013).

Infants are usually clinically normal at birth due to the presence of maternal thyroid hormones. Symptoms that develop in due course include feeding difficulties, drowsiness, lethargy, constipation and clinical signs include large fontanelles, myxoedema with coarse features, large head, oedema of the genitalia and extremities, nasal obstruction, macroglossia, low temperature (often <35 °C) with cold and mottled skin on the extremities, prolonged jaundice, umbilical hernia, hypotonia, cardiomegaly, bradycardia, failure of fusion of distal femoral epiphyses. The growing child may exhibit short stature, hypertelorism, depressed bridge of nose, narrow palpebral fissures and oedema of the eyelids. A goitre (enlarged thyroid gland) may also be present.

A blood test can diagnose hypothyroidism or may also rule it out if symptoms suggest that it could be a possible diagnosis. One or both of the following may be measured in a blood sample: thyroid-stimulating hormone (TSH) and thyroxine (T4). If the level of thyroxine in the blood is low, then the pituitary releases more TSH. Therefore, a high level of TSH means that the thyroid gland is underactive and is making too little thyroxine. A low level of T4 confirms hypothyroidism.

For an example of the presenting signs of hypothyroidism, refer to Case Study 2 at the end of this chapter.

In congenital hypothyroidism, treatment with thyroxine replacement should be initiated as soon as the diagnosis is suggested, immediately after obtaining blood for confirmatory tests. Delaying treatment after 6 weeks of life is associated with a substantial risk of delayed cognitive development. Newborns with elevated TSH should be treated with thyroid hormone replacement until they are aged 2 years to eliminate any possibility of permanent cognitive deficits caused by hypothyroidism. Once treatment is initiated for congenital hypothyroidism, serum total T4 and TSH concentrations should be assessed monthly until the total or free T4 levels normalize, then every 3 months until the patient is aged 3 years. Thereafter, total T4 and TSH should be measured every 6 months (Sinha & Kemp, 2014). Therapeutic goals are normalization of thyroid function test results and elimination of all signs and symptoms of hypothyroidism (Monzani et al., 2012).

Hyperthyroidism

Hyperthyroidism means a raised level of thyroid hormone. Thyrotoxicosis is an alternative term, and the two terms mean much the same.

There are various causes, which include the following: Graves' disease, an autoimmune disease, which is the most common cause; and autoimmune thyroiditis (Cappa, Bizzarri & Crea, 2011). Hyperthyroidism is most common in women aged 20–50 years but can affect children and young people; there is often a family history of the condition as well as other autoimmune diseases, such as diabetes, rheumatoid arthritis and myasthenia gravis.

Symptoms of hyperthyroidism include: being restless, nervous, emotional, irritable, sleeping poorly, tremor, weight loss, palpitations, sweating, diarrhoea or increased frequency of bowel movements, shortness of breath, skin problems, such as hair thinning and itch, menstrual changes, tiredness and muscle weakness. In Graves' disease, the thyroid gland usually enlarges causing a goitre in the neck. The eyes may also be affected in some cases and are pushed forwards looking more prominent (proptosis) causing discomfort and watering eyes. Problems with eye muscles may also occur and lead to double vision. For an example of presenting vital signs in a 12-year-old child with hyperthyroidism, see the following Vital signs box.

Vital sign	Observation	Normal
Temperature	37.8 °C	36.5–37.5 °C
Pulse	140 beats per minute	60–100
Respiration	25 breaths per minute	15–20
Blood pressure	130/85 mmHg	100–120 mmHg (systolic)
PEWS	3	0–1
Other	Low thyroid-stimulating hormone (TSH) and high T4 (thyroxine), calcium low	

As for hypothyroidism, a blood test can diagnose hyperthyroidism and again, a normal blood test will also rule it out if symptoms suggest that it may be a possible diagnosis. If the level of thyroxine in the blood is high, then the pituitary releases less TSH. Therefore, a low level of TSH means that the thyroid gland is overactive and is making too much thyroxine. A high level of T4 confirms hyperthyroidism. Sometimes the results of the tests are borderline and so the tests may be repeated a few weeks later, as borderline tests can be due to another illness.

Treatment options to reduce the thyroxine level include: medication, such as carbimazole, radio-iodine and surgery. Beta-blockers can ease some symptoms. Long-term follow-up is important, even after successful treatment. With treatment, the outlook is good, and if this is successful, most of the symptoms and risks of complications will go. The main aim of treatment is to reduce thyroxine levels to normal. Other problems, such as a large goitre or associated eye problems, may also need treatment.

It can be difficult to judge the correct dose of carbimazole, or just the right amount of radio-iodine in each case. Too much treatment may make T4 levels drop too low and insufficient treatment means levels remain higher than normal. Regular blood tests are needed to check T4. One option is to take a high dose of carbimazole each day or to receive a one-off high dose of radio-iodine. This stops the thyroid gland making any thyroxine. The child or young person needs to take a daily dose of thyroxine to keep their blood level within the normal range.

Some young people are given a beta-blocker drug (e.g., propranolol, and atenolol) for a few weeks while the level of thyroxine is reduced gradually by one of the treatments mentioned earlier. Beta-blockers can help to reduce symptoms of tremor, palpitations, sweating, agitation and anxiety. Surgery involves removing part of the thyroid gland; however, if too much thyroid tissue is removed then thyroxine medication may be required to keep the T4 level normal. Regular follow-up is recommended, even after successful treatment is completed. It is very important to have a regular blood test to check T4 levels as some people can become hyperthyroid again in the future. Others who have been treated successfully later develop an underactive thyroid. If this occurs, it can usually be treated easily with thyroxine tablets.

Red Flag

Long-term effects need to be prevented by early referral and treatment
The healthcare professional must be aware that there are potential permanent and long-term effects of hormone deficiency on the developing brain and nervous system. To avoid any damage in the long term, it is vital that identification, diagnosis and treatment is undertaken as early as possible. A key example of this is congenital hypothyroidism, which is screened for using the 5-day bloodspot test. If a high-risk sample is identified, urgent referral and further investigation is required in order to confirm diagnosis or not. If positive, the baby must be started on thyroxine therapy. This highlights the need for accurate and timely screening (Wassner & Brown, 2013).

Parathyroid disorders

As seen in Table 11.1, parathyroid hormone (PTH) is secreted by the four parathyroid glands, located in the neck behind the thyroid gland. It regulates serum calcium and phosphate levels and also plays a part in bone metabolism.

Hyperparathyroidism

Hyperparathyroidism results when there is excessive secretion of parathyroid hormone (PTH). High levels of PTH cause serum calcium levels to increase and serum phosphate levels to fall. In primary hyperparathyroidism (PHPT), excess PTH is produced by one or more of the parathyroid glands. The most common cause is a single parathyroid gland adenoma; other causes are hyperplasia or parathyroid carcinoma (rare). Secondary hyperparathyroidism is rare and can be as a result of kidney failure or vitamin D deficiency.

Diagnosis is made after hypercalcaemia is found. Clinical features are due to excessive calcium resorption from bone and may include osteopenia, presenting as bone pain and pathological fractures, muscle weakness, proximal myopathy, fatigue, excessive renal calcium excretion and renal calculi.

Appropriate management of PHPT in children and adolescents requires distinction between familial hypocalciuric hypercalcemia, which generally requires no specific treatment, and other forms of PHPT that are best treated by parathyroidectomy (Roizen & Levine, 2012). Medical management has not been satisfactory because no agents are available that can produce either sustained blockage of PTH release by parathyroid glands or sustained blockage of hypercalcemia. Subtotal or total parathyroidectomy is the most common choice for adults or children.

Hypoparathyroidism

Hypoparathyroidism occurs when too little parathyroid hormone is released by the parathyroid glands, or the parathyroid hormone that is released does not function properly. The most common cause is accidental injury to the glands during surgery or radiation but there may also be an autoimmune cause of cell destruction, as has been mentioned for previous conditions. The resulting low level of active parathyroid hormone causes the calcium level in the blood to fall and the phosphate level to rise. Either of these situations leads to low levels of calcium in the blood, which can cause a number of different symptoms, such as muscle cramps, pain and twitching. Hypoparathyroidism can be successfully treated with calcium and vitamin D supplements but regular blood test monitoring is also needed.

Disorders of the thymus gland

The thymus gland, despite containing glandular tissue and producing several hormones, is associated with both the immune system and the endocrine system. It plays a vital role in the development of T lymphocytes (Sauce & Appay, 2011). Thymus disorders include thymoma (cancer of the thymus), congenital athyma (absence of thymus), and DiGeorge syndrome. The latter condition will be discussed under this subsection.

DiGeorge syndrome

DiGeorge syndrome, or congenital thymic hypoplasia, is a rare condition in which a missing portion of chromosome 22 causes a child to be born without a thymus or with one that is underdeveloped. Some children will also present with hypoparathyroidism.

The child will be vulnerable to infection and may also have heart defects, a cleft palate, abnormal facial features and/or abnormally low calcium leading to problems with bone and muscle, such as hypotonia, scoliosis, clumsiness, leg pain, arthritis and muscle weakness. Most children nowadays, however, survive into adulthood and the number of T cells usually increases through childhood. Survivors are likely to have learning disabilities and other physical developmental issues, with the potential for slow speech development and poor concentration/attention deficit hyperactivity disorder (ADHD). Definitive diagnosis is made via chromosome testing using fluorescent in situ hybridization (FISH), which shows the deletion 22q11. There is no cure for DiGeorge syndrome and the child requires referral to a multidisciplinary team, as required, for physiotherapy, speech therapy, and cardiac surgical teams if heart surgery is necessary. Regular monitoring includes blood tests for hormone and calcium levels, signs of infection, kidney, heart scans and developmental, hearing and eye examinations.

Disorders of the adrenal glands

The adrenal glands produce a range of hormones with various effects so adrenal dysfunction can impact many different functions. The two conditions covered in this subsection are adrenal insufficiency, known as Addison's disease, and congenital adrenal hyperplasia (CAH).

Adrenal insufficiency: Addison's disease

Adrenal insufficiency leads to a reduction in adrenal hormone release, i.e., glucocorticoids and/or mineralocorticoids. Primary insufficiency is an inability of the adrenal glands to produce enough steroid hormones. Addison's disease is the name given to the autoimmune cause. Secondary insufficiency is where there is inadequate pituitary or hypothalamic stimulation of the adrenal glands. Adrenal insufficiency is rare in children.

Symptoms can include fatigue and weakness, anorexia, nausea, vomiting, weight loss, cramps, dizziness and confusion (Arlt & Allolio, 2003). Over time, the problems may worsen leading to exhaustion, and darkened skin and lips may be noted. Any child with Addison's disease and their family must be aware of a potential risk of sudden worsened symptoms, known as an adrenal crisis, where the cortisol levels fall significantly. This is an emergency situation requiring urgent treatment because the body requires cortisol on a constant basis to be able to regulate or modulate many of the changes that occur in the body in response to stress, including glucose levels, fat, protein and carbohydrate metabolism. Addison's is treated with hormone replacement, which is given on a lifelong basis (BSPED, 2011a).

Congenital adrenal hyperplasia

The term congenital adrenal hyperplasia (CAH) encompasses a set of autosomal recessive disorders where there is a deficiency of specific enzymes such as 21-hydroxylase, which is responsible for the synthesis of cortisol and aldosterone (Knowles *et al.*, 2011). The clinical manifestations of each form of congenital adrenal hyperplasia are related to the degree of cortisol deficiency and/or the degree of aldosterone deficiency (Speiser *et al.*, 2011). Overall, the condition is associated with a decrease in the blood levels of cortisol and aldosterone and an increase in the level of androgens in both sexes. The resulting deficiencies make the child unable to regulate the stress response and renders them vulnerable to salt loss from the body, both with life-threatening potential.

Females with severe forms of adrenal hyperplasia due to deficiencies of 21-hydroxylase have ambiguous genitalia at birth due to excess adrenal androgen (male sex hormones) production in utero. This is often called classic virilising adrenal hyperplasia. Mild forms of 21-hydroxylase deficiency in females are identified later in childhood because of precocious pubic hair, clitoromegaly, or both, often accompanied by accelerated growth and skeletal maturation due to excess postnatal exposure to adrenal androgens. This is called simple virilising adrenal hyperplasia.

21-Hydroxylase deficiency in males is generally not identified in the neonatal period because the genitalia are normal. If the defect is severe and results in salt wasting, these male neonates present at age 1–4 weeks with failure to thrive, recurrent vomiting, dehydration, hypotension, hyponatremia, hyperkalaemia, and shock (classic salt-wasting adrenal hyperplasia). Patients with less severe deficiencies of 21-hydroxylase present later in childhood because of the early development of pubic hair, phallic enlargement, or both, accompanied by accelerated linear growth and advancement of skeletal maturation (simple virilising adrenal hyperplasia) (Speiser & White, 2003). For an example of presenting vital signs in a 5-month-old child with congenital adrenal hyperplasia, see the following Vital signs box.

Vital sign	Observation	Normal
Temperature	36.8 °C	36.5–37.5 °C
Pulse	180 beats per minute	110–160
Respiration	65 breaths per minute	30–40
Blood pressure	60/40 mmHg	70–90 mmHg
PEWS	4	0–1
CRT	4 seconds	<3 seconds
Other	Blood sodium low	

Children with CAH are usually cared for by a multidisciplinary team including endocrinologists and genitourinary system specialists. Initially, they must be stabilised with intravenous fluids to restore their electrolyte levels followed by cortisol and/or aldosterone replacement therapy. Regular blood tests to monitor hormone levels are necessary so the most effective dose can be prescribed and adjustments made if needed (BSPED, 2011b). Children with CAH will need to take hormone replacement every day for the rest of their lives. As for Addison's disease, the child should be observed closely for adrenal crisis, especially if s/he becomes very stressed or unwell, either emotionally or physically, and is unable to increase the production of cortisol in their system to help the body cope. Long-term follow-up and monitoring is essential. Many children have short stature as they grow older and may benefit from growth hormone therapy.

Females with CAH may require surgery to correct virilised genitals; this is carried out by surgeons specialised in disorders of sex development. If precocious puberty (puberty starting before the expected age) occurs, further hormone replacement may be required. Males usually have normal fertility levels but females may have problems conceiving and may require additional help to have children. As CAH is an inherited disorder, genetic counselling may be helpful for the family.

Red Flag

Endocrine reasons for childhood obesity
In the light of recent public health concerns about the increasing level of childhood obesity, the potential for endocrine causes needs consideration. Such causes may be as follows (Crocker & Yanovski, 2009):

- Some classic endocrine disorders are associated with weight gain, such as hypothyroidism, growth hormone deficiency and Cushing syndrome.
- Obesity may arise after injury to, or congenital malformation of, the hypothalamus.
- Leptin, a hormone produced by adipose tissue, may be disrupted.

While obesity is not a disease, the long-term effects are well documented and so endocrine reasons need to be ruled out.

Medication Alert

Careful titration of hormones is essential.
For certain hormones, such as steroids, insulin and other hormone replacements, it is very important to adhere to careful titration in relation to dosage. Generally speaking, hormones should never be stopped suddenly; this is particularly vital with hormones such as cortisol, because the body's natural steroid manufacture and release is either absent or will cease during hormone replacement. The dose should be reviewed as the child or young person gets older and bigger, or in other situations that might necessitate dose changes. Follow-up and hormone therapy review is an essential part of ongoing consultations with the endocrine and/or community paediatric multidisciplinary team.

Disorders of the pancreas

The pancreas is not strictly an endocrine gland but because it produces and secretes the hormones insulin and glucagon, it is included in this chapter. The two conditions caused by abnormal insulin metabolism are: diabetes mellitus and congenital hyperinsulinaemia.

Diabetes mellitus

Diabetes mellitus is a disease caused by deficiency or diminished effectiveness of endogenous insulin. There are several types of diabetes in children and young people. Type 1 diabetes mellitus results from the body's failure to produce sufficient insulin (Dunger & Todd, 2008; NICE, 2010, 2015) as a result of an autoimmune response of the body, which damages the beta cells of the pancreas. Type 2 results from resistance to insulin (Beckwith, 2010; Reinehr, 2005) and arises due to lifestyle risk factors, such as obesity and poor diet. Gestational diabetes occurs in pregnant women who have high blood glucose levels during pregnancy. Maturity-onset diabetes of the young (MODY) involves beta-cell function and impaired insulin secretion, usually manifesting as mild hyperglycaemia at a young age (Vivian, 2006). MODY is caused by a mutation in a single gene; if a parent has this gene mutation, any child has a chance of inheriting the condition from them. Secondary diabetes accounts for a small incidence of diabetes mellitus and can be due to pancreatic disease and endocrine conditions, such as Cushing syndrome, acromegaly, thyrotoxicosis, and glucagonoma, for example.

Diabetes mellitus is characterised by hyperglycaemia, deranged metabolism and chronic complications. The presentation includes key signs, such as polyuria, polydipsia, lethargy, weight loss, dehydration and ketonuria. Diabetes can be diagnosed on the basis of one abnormal plasma glucose (random ≥11.1 mmol/L or fasting ≥7 mmol/L) (NICE, 2015) in the presence of diabetic symptoms such as thirst, increased urination, recurrent infections, weight loss, drowsiness and in the worst case scenario, coma. Diabetic ketoacidosis (DKA) is caused by a critical relative or absolute deficit of insulin, resulting in intracellular starvation of insulin-dependent tissues (muscle, liver, adipose), stimulating the release of the counter-regulatory hormones glucagon, catecholamine, cortisol, and growth hormone (Rosenbloom, 2010). An acidosis caused by high levels of blood ketones ensues. The severity of DKA is determined by the degree of acidosis. For an example of presenting vital signs in an 8-year-old child with moderate to severe DKA, see the Vital signs box below.

Referral to a specialized paediatric diabetes team is required for ongoing management. The main goal of diabetes management is to restore blood glucose levels and carbohydrate metabolism to a normal state. To achieve this, children with type 1 diabetes and an absolute deficiency of insulin require insulin replacement therapy, which is given through injections or an insulin pump. Children with type 2 may be controlled initially by lifestyle modifications, such as increased physical activity and dietary changes with lower caloric intake; weight loss reduces the rate of progression to more serious diabetes (Flint & Arsanian, 2011). Insulin may be required if such modifications are not successful. Ketoacidosis is an emergency situation leading to cerebral oedema and coma, if rapid

Vital sign	Observation	Normal
Temperature	36.8 °C	36.5–37.5 °C
Pulse	140 beats per minute	80–120
Respiration	40 breaths per minute	20–15
Blood pressure	85/45 mmHg	90–110 mmHg (systolic)
Blood gas	pH 7.15, bicarbonate 10 mml/L (metabolic acidosis)	
PEWS	4	0–1
CRT	4 seconds	<3 seconds
Other	Ketonaemia, glucosuria, and ketonuria Glasgow Coma Score 12 Oxygen saturation 91%	

insulin administration and/or resuscitation measures are not implemented (WHO, 2006). It is essential to follow recent, evidence-based guidelines in the care of diabetes as for any other clinical disorder; in this case, see those produced by BSPED (2015). Finally, the use of glucagon must be considered in the emergency care of severe hypoglycaemia, when a child's blood glucose levels are poorly stabilised and fluctuate between high and low.

Hyperinsulinaemia

Congenital hyperinsulinism (CHI) is a rare disease of the pancreas, often termed nesidioblastosis (McKenna, 2000), which describes the neodifferentiation of islets of Langerhans leading to inappropriate and unregulated insulin secretion from the pancreatic beta cells. High levels of insulin lead to hypoglycaemia. Some cases have a genetic cause while others have secondary, more transient causes, such as intrauterine growth restriction and infants from diabetic mothers.

A child usually starts to show symptoms within the first few days of life, sometimes later. Symptoms of hypoglycaemia include hypotonia, jitteriness, poor feeding and lethargy, all of which are due to the low blood glucose levels. Seizures can also occur, again due to low blood glucose levels. If the child's blood glucose level is not corrected, it can lead to loss of consciousness and potential brain injury. Children with suspected CHI should be transferred to a specialist centre with the expertise to carry out the detailed repeated blood glucose monitoring needed to deliver treatment.

The initial task is to stabilise the child, usually with intravenous glucose or a high carbohydrate feed. Once a child is stable, the team will confirm or rule out a diagnosis of CHI. This is usually done through detailed blood and urine tests taken while a child's blood glucose level is low, i.e., 'diagnostic fast'. Once CHI is confirmed, positron emission tomography (PET) scanning can identify the area of the pancreas from which excessive insulin is being produced. Medical management aims to keep a child's blood glucose level stable in a normal range. This can be managed by regular high carbohydrate feeds alongside medication to reduce insulin secretion. Diazoxide, chlorothiazide, glucagon and octreotide are options. Surgical treatment may also be an option if medical management does not stabilise the blood glucose levels. The area of the pancreas containing the defective beta cells is removed and this can offer a cure for CHI. Surgery to remove all or most of the pancreas is only an option for diffuse disease if medical management fails, but has a greater risk of long-term effects, such as diabetes or pancreatic insufficiency.

Disorders of the gonads

Two conditions will be discussed under this final system in the chapter: disorders of sex development (formerly known as intersex conditions), and problems with the onset of puberty.

Disorders of sex development (DSD)

When a baby cannot be identified immediately at birth as male or female, it is often referred to as having ambiguous genitalia. The more recent term is DSD, which is used to describe this finding caused by conditions such as congenital adrenal hyperplasia (CAH; see earlier section) (Knowles *et al*., 2011; Speiser *et al*., 2011), ovotesticular DSD (formerly termed hermaphroditism), and mixed gonadal dysgenesis (MGD).

A newborn with DSD may show a male appearance but with associated abnormalities of genitalia, severe hypospadias *with* bifid scrotum, undescended testis/testes *with* hypospadias, and bilateral non-palpable testes in a full-term apparently male infant. There may also be a baby with a female appearance but again, with associated abnormalities such as clitoral hypertrophy of any degree, non-palpable gonads and a vulva with single opening (BSPED, 2009; Hutcheson & Snyder, 2012).

The possibility of DSDs requires immediate referral to an experienced multidisciplinary team accompanied by kind, sensitive and clear explanation to parents. Naming and registration of such babies should be delayed for as long as possible (Hughes et al., 2006). It is essential to follow clear and comprehensive guidelines for management, such as that detailed in Ahmed *et al.* (2015). These state that the rationale for investigating a newborn or an adolescent with a suspected DSD includes the need to determine the sex of rearing, anticipate and treat early medical problems, explain the aetiology to the child, young person and parents, and to develop a management plan that leads to an optimal long-term outcome. A diagnosis confirmed by biochemical and genetic methods is often required. The approach to reaching a diagnosis needs to be explained to parents and the most important goals of the initial period of assessment should be to support the child and the parents.

Sex assignment and corrective surgery are necessary to enable a child to lead a 'normal' life as a boy or a girl. Depending on the decision, treatment may include hormone replacement therapy. As the child grows up and enters puberty, there is a chance that they will identify with a sex other than the one they were assigned. In this case, a gender transition may be necessary. In such cases, it may be preferred to wait until the child is an adolescent before beginning the hormone therapy process involved in a transition. Any hormone therapy needed for this condition must be distinguished from that given for gender dysphoria as the latter is not an endocrine disorder. A detailed discussion of DSD is beyond the remit of this chapter.

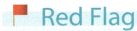

Red Flag

The emotional and psychological effects of endocrine disorders.
The health professional should be aware that lifelong endocrine conditions can potentially have significant emotional and psychological effects as a child grows and develops through puberty and into adolescence. This is particularly important in young people with disorders of sex development, such as those born with ambiguous genitalia, delayed or precocious puberty, and individuals who have gender dysphoria. Children and young people with the latter condition may be receiving hormones to develop the traits of the sex with which they identify or drugs to suppress puberty. A sensitive approach to counselling, support and consistent advice for the child, young person and family is essential (BSPED, 2009).

Medication Alert

Drugs may be required that suppress hormone action or counteract their effects.
In some instances, it may be necessary to suppress or counteract the release or action of a hormone. For example, in hyperthyroidism, anti-thyroid medication is given to inhibit the production of thyroid hormones. In precocious puberty, a gonadotrophic-releasing hormone analogue may be given to block the brain receptors for the release of luteinizing hormone, which acts on the gonads to release sex hormones at puberty onset. In disorders of sex development, the decision to bring a child up as male or female may necessitate sex hormone suppression as may be the case in gender dysphoria. Some drugs may also be required to counteract a hormone's action in the case of an emergency, for example, if a diabetic person becomes hypoglycemic, the hormone glucagon can be administered as it works in opposition to insulin.

Disorders of the endocrine system   Chapter 11

Delayed or precocious puberty

Generally, puberty begins at any point between the ages of 8 and 13 in girls, and 9 and 14 in boys. However, there are wide variations in age of onset that are still the norm (Nakamoto, 2000). That said, there are *some* cases when early puberty or delayed puberty could be a sign of an underlying condition that may need to be treated (Cesario & Hughes, 2007; Kaplowitz, 2010).

Precocious puberty: It is not always clear what causes early puberty and it may not have an obvious cause, particularly in girls. In boys it is less common and so is more likely to be linked to an underlying problem. In any sex, it can be caused by damage to hypothalamic–pituitary function as a result of a tumour, infection, surgery or radiotherapy, ovarian dysfunction (Zacharin, 2010), thyroid dysfunction, or due to a genetic disorder, such as McCune-Albright syndrome.

Delayed puberty refers to onset of puberty that is past the expected norms for age. In boys, there may be no sign of testicular development, and in girls, absence of breast development and onset of menstruation.

Conversely, delayed puberty tends to be common in boys and there may be no known cause. Documented causes include: chronic illness, such as cystic fibrosis, diabetes, coeliac disease or kidney disease, malnutrition, eating disorders, or a problem with endocrine control of the sex hormones because of damage to the ovaries, testes, thyroid gland, and/or the pituitary gland. Certain DSDs can also lead to delayed puberty, such as androgen insensitivity syndrome, or genetic conditions, such as Kallmann syndrome and Klinefelter syndrome.

Tests for either precocious or delayed puberty include blood tests to check sex hormone levels and possibly scanning to exclude tumours. Treating any underlying cause is a key aim. Precocious puberty can be managed by using medication to reduce hormone levels and delay sexual development for a few years. GnRH agonists are used in central precocious puberty, as well as for other aetiologies, including McCune–Albright syndrome (MAS) and testotoxicosis. These come in a number of depot preparations. They work by overstimulating the pituitary, causing desensitisation and thereby reducing release of LH and FSH. They are continued until the time for normal puberty arrives. Delayed puberty can be treated by using medication such as testosterone in boys or oestrogen in girls, to increase hormone levels and trigger the start of puberty (BSPED 2011c). Management with drugs, however, is only undertaken if it is thought that early or delayed puberty will cause emotional or physical problems.

Case Study 1   Pituitary insufficiency – diabetes insipidus

A 4-year-old boy is admitted with his mother to the children's emergency department with signs of dehydration. He has a history of excessive thirst, increased urine production and poor weight gain and growth. He is under the 10th centile for his weight and height, both of which have dropped a centile in the last year. He is subsequently admitted for further investigations with a provisional diagnosis of diabetes insipidus.

Chapter 11 — Disorders of the endocrine system

The following vital signs were noted and recorded:

Vital sign	Observation	Normal
Temperature	37.9 °C	36.5–37.5 °C
Pulse	165 beats per minute	95–150
Respiration	50 breaths per minute	25–35
Blood pressure	75/40 mmHg	80–100 mmHg
CRT	4 seconds	<3 seconds
PEWS		
Behaviour	2: Irritable	
Cardiovascular	2: Prolonged capillary refill time and tachycardia	
Respiratory	1: >10 above normal rate	
TOTAL SCORE	5	

The following parameters were also seen:

Test	Result	Guideline normal values
Urine output	6–7 mL/kg/hour	<4 mL/kg/hour
Urine: specific gravity	1.002	1.005–1.020
Urine osmolarity	300 mOsm/kg	500–800 mOsm/kg
Blood osmolarity	360 mOsm/kg	275–295 mOsm/kg
Blood sodium	147 mmol/L	135–145 mmol/L
Blood potassium	4 mmol/L	3.5–5 mmol/L
Blood creatinine	0.9 mg/dL	0.5–1.0 mg/dL
Blood urea	15 mg/dL	5–25 mg/dL

Reflect on this case and consider the following.

1. Why do the above signs and symptoms present in this condition?
2. What are the possible causes of this situation?
3. What are the goals and priorities of treatment?
4. What advice and education is required for the child and family in relation to the short- and long-term care?

Case Study 2   Hypothyroidism

A two-and-a-half-week-old baby presents with a low central temperature, cool and pale skin, and a low heart rate. There were concerns at birth that she was floppy, was slow to feed and wake for feeds, and then became constipated with reduced weight gain. The baby also has prolonged jaundice beyond 10 days and has a hoarse cry and large abdomen. The family have recently moved and so the results of the baby's blood spot screening have not been reported to the parents. These show a high risk of the baby having congenital hypothyroidism and referral to an endocrine team is needed. After referral, the baby and family are admitted for further investigations and confirmation of a diagnosis.

On admission to the endocrine ward, the following vital signs were noted and recorded:

Vital sign	Observation	Normal
Temperature	35 °C	36.5–37.5 °C
Pulse	85–90 beats per minute	100–190
Respiration	40–50 breaths per minute	30–40
Blood pressure	70/40 mmHg	70–90 mmHg (systolic)
O_2 saturation	94%	• 95%

Other tests were performed with the following results:

Test	Result	Guideline normal values
Thyroid-stimulating hormone (TSH)	35	<20 mU/L*
Thyroxine (T4)	5	9–25 mmol/L (free T4)
Calcium	1.6 mmol/L	1–1.3 mmol/L (ionized)

*UK NHS newborn bloodspot screening programme (2014)

Reflect on this case and consider the following.

1. Why does the infant present in this way?
2. What are the goals and priorities of treatment?
3. What are the potential short-term and long-term effects of this condition?
4. What advice and education is required for the child and the family?

Conclusion

This chapter has provided insight into the normal and abnormal anatomy and physiology of the endocrine system, as well as providing discussion on a number of pathological changes that may occur in this system in the child or young person. Emphasis has been placed on the provision of key information points in a clear format to assist the reader to understand the complex physical, emotional and lifelong issues encountered by children, young people and their families who are living with an endocrine disorder.

References

Ahmed, S.F., Achermann, J.C., Arlt, W., *et al.* (2011). UK guidance on the initial evaluation of an infant or an adolescent with a suspected disorder of sex development. *Clinical Endocrinology* 75(1), 12–26.

Arlt, W. & Allolio, B. (2003). Adrenal insufficiency. *Lancet* 361(9372), 1881–1893.

Barth, J.H. (2014). How are hormones measured? A journey into endocrinology. *The Endocrinologist* 111, 2–32.

Beckwith, S. (2010). Diagnosing type 2 diabetes in children and young people. *British Journal of School Nursing* 5(1), 15–19.

British Society for Paediatric Endocrinology and Diabetes (BSPED) (2009). Statement on the management of Gender Identity Disorder (GID) in children & adolescents. Available at: http://www.gires.org.uk/wp-content/uploads/2014/10/BSPEDStatementOnTheManagementOfGID.pdf (last accessed April 2018).

British Society for Paediatric Endocrinology and Diabetes (BSPED) (2011a). Steroid replacement in adrenal insufficiency. Available at: https://www.bsped.org.uk/clinical-resources/guidelines/ (last accessed April 2018).

British Society for Paediatric Endocrinology and Diabetes (BSPED) (2011b). Congenital adrenal hyperplasia.

British Society for Paediatric Endocrinology and Diabetes (BSPED) (2011c). Delayed puberty. Available at: https://www.bsped.org.uk/clinical-resources/guidelines/ (last accessed April 2018).

British Society for Paediatric Endocrinology and Diabetes (BSPED) (2013). Congenital hypothyroidism – Initial Clinical Referral Standards and Guidelines, and UK Newborn Screening Programme Centre. Available at: https://www.bsped.org.uk/clinical-resources/guidelines/ (last accessed April 2018).

British Society for Paediatric Endocrinology and Diabetes (BSPED) (2015). Recommended guideline for the management of children and young people under the age of 18 years with diabetic ketoacidosis. Available at: https://www.bsped.org.uk/clinical-resources/guidelines/ (last accessed April 2018).

Buck, M.L. (2003). The use of melatonin in children with sleep disturbances. *Pediatric Pharmacotherapy* 9, 1–4.

Cappa, M., Bizzarri, C. & Crea, F. (2010). Autoimmune thyroid diseases in children. *Journal of Thyroid Research* 2011, 675703.

Carr, R., Wasdell, M.B., Hamilton, D., *et al.* (2007). Long-term effectiveness outcome of melatonin therapy in children with treatment-resistant circadian rhythm sleep disorders. *Journal of Pineal Research* 43, 351–359.

Cesario, S.K. & Hughes, L.A. (2007). Precocious puberty: a comprehensive review of literature. *Journal of Obstetric, Gynecologic, & Neonatal Nursing* 36(3), 263–274.

Colao, A. & Loche, S. (2009). Prolactinomas in children and adolescents. *Pediatric Neuroendocrinology* 17, 146–159.

Corumblum, B. (2016). Hypopituitarism (Panhypopituitarism). Medscape. http://emedicine.medscape.com/article/122287-overview#a4 (last accessed April 2018).

Crocker, M.K. & Yanovski, J.A. (2009). Pediatric obesity: etiology and treatment. *Endocrinology and Metabolism Clinics of North America* 38(3), 525–548.

Cummings, C. & Canadian Paediatric Society, Community Paediatrics Committee. (2012). Melatonin for the management of sleep disorders in children and adolescents. *Paediatrics & Child Health* 17(6), 331–333.

Dattani, M. & Preece, M. (2004). Growth hormone deficiency and related disorders: insights into causation, diagnosis, and treatment. *Lancet* 363(12), 1977–1987.

Dorton, A.M. (2000). The pituitary gland: embryology, physiology and pathophysiology. *Neonatal Network* 19(2), 9–17.

Dunger, D.B. & Todd, J.A. (2008). Prevention of type 1 diabetes: what next? *Lancet* 372(9651), 1710–1711.

Elmlinger, M.W. (2011). Laboratory measurements of hormones and related biomarkers: technologies, quality management and validation. In: Ranke, M.B., Mullis, P.-E. (eds). *Diagnostics of Endocrine Function in Children and Adolescents*, 4th edn. Karger, Basel, pp. 1–31.

Hinson, J.P., Raven, P. & Chew, S.L. (2010). *The Endocrine System: Systems of the Body Series*, 2nd edn. Churchill Livingstone, Edinburgh.

Hughes, I.A., Houk, C., Ahmed, S.F., Lee, P.A. & LWPES1/ESPE2 Consensus Group. (2006). Consensus statement on management of intersex disorders. *Archives of Disease in Childhood* 91(7), 554–563.

Human Growth Foundation (2015). Disorders of short stature. Available at: http://hgfound.org/resources/disorders-of-short-stature/ (last accessed April 2018).

Hutcheson, J. & Snyder, H.M. (2012). Ambiguous genitalia and intersexuality, Medscape. Available at: http://emedicine.medscape.com/article/1015520-overview (last accessed April 2018).

Jameson, J.L. & De Groot, L.J. (2010) *Endocrinology: Adult and Pediatric*, 6th edn. Saunders, Philadelphia.

Jeesuk, Y. (2014). Endocrine disorders and the neurologic manifestations. *Annals of Pediatric Endocrinology & Metabolism* 19(4), 184–190.

Kaplowitz, P. (2010). Precocious Puberty, *Medscape*. http://emedicine.medscape.com/article/924002-overview (last accessed April 2018).

Keil, M.F. & Stratakis, C.A. (2008). Pituitary tumors in childhood: an update in their diagnosis, treatment and molecular genetics. *Expert Review of Neurotherapeutics* 8(4), 563–574.

Khardori, R. & Ulla, J. (2012). Diabetes Insipidus. *Medscape*. http://emedicine.medscape.com/article/117648-overview (last accessed April 2018).

Kim, S.Y. (2015). Diagnosis and treatment of hypopituitarism. *Endocrinology and Metabolism* 30(4), 443–455.

Knowles, R.L., Oerton, J.M., Khalid, J.M., et al.; British Society for Paediatric Endocrinology and Diabetes Clinical Genetics Group (2011). Clinical outcome of congenital adrenal hyperplasia (CAH) one year following diagnosis: a UK-wide study. *Archives of Disease in Childhood* 96, A27.

Lacroix-Boudhrioua, V., Linglart, A., Ancel, P.Y., et al. (2011). Pineal cysts in children. *Insights into Imaging* 2(6), 671–678.

Maity, A., Pruitt, A.A., Judy, K.D., Phillips, P.C. & Lustig, R. (2008). Cancer of the central nervous system. In: Abeloff, M.D., Armitage, J.O., Niederhuber, J.E., Kastan, M.B. & McKenna, W.G. (eds). *Abeloff's Clinical Oncology*, 4th edn. Elsevier Churchill Livingstone, Philadelphia, Chap. 70.

Matfin, G. (2009). Mechanisms of hormonal control. In: Pooler, C. (ed.). *Pathophysiology: Concepts of Altered Health States*. Lippincott Williams & Wilkins, New York, Chap. 40.

McKenna, L.L. (2000). Pancreatic disorders in the newborn. *Neonatal Network* 19(4), 13–20.

Milla, C.E. & Zirbes, J. (2012). Pulmonary complications of endocrine and metabolic disorders. *Paediatric Respiratory Reviews* 13(1), 23–28.

Mishra, G. & Chandrashekhar, S.R. (2011). Management of diabetes insipidus in children. *Indian Journal of Endocrinology and Metabolism* 15(Suppl 3), S180–S187.

Molina, P. (2013). *Endocrine Physiology*, 4th edn. McGraw-Hill Medical, New York.

Monzani, A., Prodam, F., Rapa, A., et al. (2012). Natural history of subclinical hypothyroidism in children and adolescents and potential effects of replacement therapy: a review. *European Journal of Endocrinology* EJE-12.

Nakamoto, J.M. (2000). Myths and variations in normal pubertal development. *Western Journal of Medicine* 172(3), 182–185.

Nandagopal, R., Laverdière, C., Mulrooney, D., Hudson, M.M. & Meacham, L. (2008). Endocrine late effects of childhood cancer therapy: a report from the Children's Oncology Group. *Hormone Research in Paediatrics* 69(2), 65–74.

National Institute for Health and Care Excellence (NICE) (2010). Clinical Knowledge Summary. Diabetes – type 1. Available at: http://cks.nice.org.uk/diabetes-type-1 (last accessed April 2018).

National Institute for Health and Care Excellence (NICE) (2015; updated 2016). Diabetes (type 1 and type 2) in children and young people: diagnosis and management. NICE guideline [NG18]. Available at: https://www.nice.org.uk/guidance/ng18 (last accessed April 2018).

Petty, J. (2015). Endocrine disorders. In: Peate, I. & Gormley-Fleming, E. (eds). *Fundamentals of Children's Anatomy and Physiology*. Wiley, Oxford, Chap. 10.

Phillips, L. & Appleton, R.E. (2004). Systematic review of melatonin treatment in children with neurodevelopmental disabilities and sleep impairment. *Developmental Medicine & Child Neurology* 46(11), 771–775.

Quatrano, N.A. & Loechner, K.J. (2012). Dermatologic manifestations of endocrine disorders. *Current Opinion in Pediatrics* 24(4), 487–493.

Reinehr, T. (2005). Clinical presentation of type 2 diabetes mellitus in children and adolescents. *International Journal of Obesity* 29, S105–S110.

Rogers, K. (2012). *The Endocrine System*. Britannia Educational Publishers, New York.

Roizen, J. & Levine, M.A. (2012). Primary hyperparathyroidism in children and adolescents. *Journal of the Chinese Medical Association* 75(9), 425–434.

Rosenbloom, A.L. (2010). The management of diabetic ketoacidosis in children. *Diabetes Therapy* 1(2), 103–120.

Roth, K.S. & Kemp, S. (2015). Pediatric Diabetes Insipidus. *Medscape*. http://emedicine.medscape.com/article/919886-overview (last accessed April 2018).

Sauce, D. & Appay, V. (2011). Altered thymic activity in early life: how does it affect the immune system in young adults? *Current Opinion in Immunology* 23(4), 543–548.

Schneider, H.J., Aimaretti, G., Kreitschmann-Andermahr, I., *et al.* (2007). Hypopituitarism. *Lancet* 369(9571), 1461–1470.

Sinha, S. & Kemp, S. (2014). Pediatric Hypothyroidsim. Medscape. http://reference.medscape.com/article/922777-overview (last accessed April 2018).

Speiser, P.W., Azziz, R., Baskin, L.S., *et al.* (2011). Congenital adrenal hyperplasia due to steroid 21-hydroxylase deficiency: an Endocrine Society clinical practice guideline. *Archives of Disease in Childhood* 96, A27.

Speiser, P.W. & White, P.C. (2003). Congenital adrenal hyperplasia. *New England Journal of Medicine* 349(8), 776–788.

Vivian, M. (2006). Type 2 diabetes in children and adolescents – the next epidemic? *Current Medical Research and Opinion* 22, 297–306.

Wallace, M. (2011). Part one: Principles of international endocrine practice. 1.7: Measurement of hormones. In: Wass, J.A.H., Stewart, P.M., Amiel, S.A. & Davies, M.E. (eds). *Oxford Textbook of Endocrinology and Diabetes*, 2nd edn. Oxford University Press, Oxford.

Wassner, A.J. & Brown, R.S. (2013). Hypothyroidism in the newborn period. *Current Opinion in Endocrinology, Diabetes, and Obesity* 20(5), 449.

Waugh, A. & Grant, A. (2010). *Ross and Wilson Anatomy and Physiology in Health and Illness*, 11th edn. Churchill Livingstone, Edinburgh.

Willacy, H. (2011). *Childhood and Congenital Hypothyroidism*. Document ID: 1164 Version: 22 © EMIS. Available at: www.patient.co.uk/doctor/childhood-and-congenital-hypothyroidism (last accessed April 2018).

World Health Organization (WHO) (2006). Definition and diagnosis of diabetes mellitus and intermediate hyperglycaemia. WHO, Geneva.

Yu, J. (2014). Endocrine disorders and the neurologic manifestations. *Annals of Pediatric Endocrinology & Metabolism* 19(4), 184–190.

Zacharin, M. (2010). Disorders of ovarian function in childhood and adolescence: evolving needs of the growing child. An endocrine perspective. *BJOG* 117, 156–162.

Zacharin, M. (2013). Endocrine problems in children and adolescents who have disabilities. *Hormone Research in Paediatrics* 80(4), 221–228.

Chapter 12

Disorders of the digestive system

Ann L. Bevan

Aim

This chapter explores the role of the digestive system as it removes nutrients from the food that a child eats to enable growth and development, and the changes that can occur when pathology is disturbed.

Learning outcomes

On completion of this chapter, the reader will be able to:

- Describe the general function of the gastrointestinal system.
- Discuss the pathological processes of disorders of the gastrointestinal system.
- Identify structural defects in the newborn.
- Identify signs and symptoms indicating gastrointestinal disorders.
- Be familiar with the management of disorders in infants, children and young people.

Keywords

- oesophagus
- motility
- inflammation
- obstruction
- structural defects
- malabsorption

Fundamentals of Children's Applied Pathophysiology: An Essential Guide for Nursing and Healthcare Students, First Edition.
Edited by Elizabeth Gormley-Fleming and Ian Peate.
© 2019 John Wiley & Sons Ltd. Published 2019 by John Wiley & Sons Ltd.
Companion website: www.wileyfundamentalseries.com/childpathophysiology

Chapter 12

Disorders of the digestive system

Test your prior knowledge

1. What structures and organs make up the gastrointestinal system?
2. What function does the gastro-oesophageal sphincter have?
3. What is meconium and when would you expect to see it?
4. At what stage of embryonic/foetal development is the palate and mouth formed
5. What is the function of bile and where is it produced?
6. What function do intestinal villi play in digestion and absorption?
7. Label the diagram:

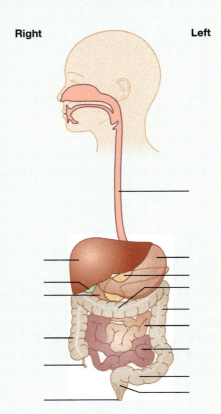

How can having a problem with the digestive system impact on a person's physical and psychological wellbeing?

8. How does food move through the gastrointestinal system from the mouth to the anus?
9. Where is the appendix located?
10. Why do infants regurgitate milk and when does it become of concern?

Introduction

The gastrointestinal system includes the mouth, pharynx, oesophagus, stomach and intestines, ending at the anus; in total it measures approximately 10 metres in length. Supporting structures include accessory organs necessary for digestion, such as salivary glands, liver, pancreas and gallbladders. The function of the gastrointestinal tract is to digest and absorb nutrients and then eliminate waste products.

Disorders of the digestive system　　Chapter 12

In this chapter some of the most common gastrointestinal disorders in infants, children and young people will be presented. Nursing care of the infant, child or young person and management of these disorders will be considered within the context of a family-centred approach to care. The chapter is organised under the main headings of motility disorders, inflammatory conditions, obstructive disorders, malabsorption disorders, structural defects, and hernias.

Motility disorders

Motility disorders include all those affecting the normal movement of matter through the GI system. Any condition that slows or speeds the movement of matter through the GI system alters the absorption rate of fluids and nutrients. Symptoms may include diarrhoea and vomiting, resulting in fluid and electrolyte disturbances.

Gastroenteritis (diarrhoea)

Gastroenteritis is an acute or chronic inflammation of the stomach and intestines often accompanied by vomiting and diarrhoea. It can affect any part of the gastrointestinal tract and may be caused by a viral, bacterial or parasitic infection. This condition is common in children under 5 years who on average experience two episodes per year with rotavirus being the most common cause in this age group (Ball, Bindler & Cowen, 2015). Frequent episodes of diarrhoea, especially if accompanied by vomiting, can lead to severe dehydration in infants and young children putting them at risk for hypovolemic shock if fluid and electrolytes are not replaced. This may necessitate a hospital admission for intravenous fluids.

Diarrhoea can be acute or chronic. Acute diarrhoea is defined as a sudden increase in frequency and change in consistency of stools often caused by an infection. This is usually self-limiting and may or may not be severe enough to cause dehydration. Chronic diarrhoea occurs over more than 14 days and is often caused by chronic conditions, such as inflammatory bowel disease (IBD), malabsorption syndromes, food allergies or non-specific causes. Causes of acute and chronic diarrhoea are presented in Table 12.1.

Diarrhoea can be mild, moderate, or severe. This is determined by the number of stools and how liquid they are. In addition, the severity of other accompanying symptoms, such as irritability, anorexia, nausea and vomiting and electrolyte imbalance, determine the severity and subsequent treatment.

Diagnosis is based on history, physical examination, and laboratory results. A thorough history should include questions about recent travel, day-care attendance and recent medications or dietary changes. Questions should also be asked about the frequency and character of stools, urinary output and intake of food and fluids, and the presence of fever

Table 12.1　Possible causes of acute and chronic diarrhoea

Acute diarrhoea	Chronic diarrhoea
• Bacterial, viral and parasitic infections • Associated conditions, such as upper respiratory tract infections, urinary tract infections and otitis media • Dietary cause, such as overfeeding, incorrect formula reconstitution, or excess sugar • Medications: iron, antibiotics • Ingestion of a toxin, such as lead or organic phosphates • Irritable bowel syndrome, Hirschsprung disease • Colon disease: necrotising enterocolitis, colitis	• Malabsorption causes: coeliac disease, short-bowel syndrome, lactose intolerance, pancreatic or enzyme deficiency • Allergies • Immunodeficiency conditions • Inflammatory bowel diseases: ulcerative colitis, Crohn disease • Endocrine causes: hyperthyroidism, adrenal hyperplasia, Addison disease • Motility disorders: Hirschsprung disease, intestinal obstruction • Parasitic infestations • Abdominal tumours

or vomiting. Physical examination gives an indication of the severity of the dehydration. Laboratory evaluation of blood and urine gives an indication of electrolyte imbalance, and stools can be examined for the presence of infectious organisms, viruses, parasites, ova, fat and undigested sugars.

Medical management depends on the severity of the diarrhoea and dehydration. Rehydration with an intravenous solution chosen to correct the specific dehydration will be used in those children with severe diarrhoea and accompanying dehydration. Clear oral fluids or breast milk will be introduced as soon as possible and then progression to normal diet. If the diarrhoea is caused by bacteria or parasites, antibiotics may be prescribed.

Medication Alert

Because of the risk of masking the signs and symptoms of more serious illnesses, anti-emetics and anti-diarrhoeal medications are not generally used in children.

Constipation

Constipation is a common problem in childhood; depending on the criteria used to diagnose the condition, the prevalence may be as high as 30%, and in one-third of those the condition becomes chronic (NICE, 2010).

The cause of constipation may be dietary, an underlying disease or as a result of psychological factors, or it may be idiopathic and therefore have no known cause. It may also be as a result of defects in filling or emptying of the rectum, such as in Hirschsprung disease, stricture or stenosis. Constipation in infancy is uncommon and most often associated with changes of diet, such as from breastfeeding to cow's milk due to the protein content. The most common time for the condition is during toddler and childhood years when withholding of stool may be the cause because of the unpleasant sensations associated with defecating. In the older child it is more commonly associated with lack of fibre in the diet and a sedentary lifestyle. Children and young people with physical disabilities and associated impaired mobility are more prone to constipation.

Signs and symptoms may include: abdominal pain, abdominal distension, hard painful stools, a decrease in stool frequency, excessive flatulence, lack of appetite, general malaise, constipation with faecal soiling (encopresis), and irritability. Diagnosis is made on a thorough history of stool frequency and consistency, and a physical examination. Early diagnosis and treatment of an acute episode of constipation is important in order to prevent the condition becoming chronic. Early identification of constipation and effective treatment can improve outcomes for children and young people (NICE, 2010).

The first line of treatment for constipation that has no underlying pathological cause is dietary management. However, for children with impacted faeces an enema and/or laxatives will be administered, accompanied by both behavioural interventions and dietary modification to ensure a balanced diet and adequate fluid intake. The goals for management are to restore and maintain regular toileting routines and evacuation of stool. Nursing care focuses on teaching patents about normal bowel patterns in children and the appearance of a normal stool. Families need reassurance that establishing normal patterns can take time and they need to be persistent and consistent, and provide the child with positive reinforcement.

Vomiting

Vomiting is one of the most common symptoms in childhood. In infants it is normal to regurgitate small amounts of milk, called posseting, but in childhood it is often due to gastroenteritis. It may also be associated with other conditions, see Table 12.2 for some of

Table 12.2 Possible causes of vomiting

Newborns and infants	Older children and adolescents
• Overfeeding • Gastro-oesophageal reflux • Pyloric stenosis • Whooping cough • Small bowel obstruction • Constipation • Systemic infection	• Gastroenteritis • Migraine • Raised intracranial pressure • Toxic ingestion or medication • Pregnancy • Stress

the causes. The history of vomiting and associated symptoms may help to identify the cause. Vomiting in childhood is usually self-limiting with no treatment required; however, complications can occur and these may include: dehydration, electrolyte imbalances, aspiration or malnutrition.

The vomiting reflex is under the central nervous system control, specifically the medulla. Nausea, meaning the desire to vomit, is a sensation that may be induced by a number of causes including inner ear, visceral or emotional stimuli. It may lead to retching due to contraction of the abdominal muscles.

A thorough history should be taken to ascertain the underlying cause alongside a physical examination to identify any abdominal pain or dehydration. The type of vomitus and its relation to meals or specific foods, behaviour and any accompanying pain need to be ascertained. It is also important to assess for the presence of constipation, diarrhoea or jaundice. Other causes, such as urinary infections, brain tumour, and any anatomic abnormalities, need to be ruled out with diagnostic tests, such as blood and urine analysis, X-ray, and brain scan. If a cyclic vomiting pattern is present, it may indicate an eating disorder such as bulimia, and therefore a psychiatric assessment may be needed.

If the vomiting persists for more than 24 hours, parenteral fluids may need to be considered in order to correct or prevent dehydration. Anti-emetic drugs are usually only administered in cases of extensive post-operative vomiting, chemotherapy-induced vomiting, or for travel sickness. Nursing care is determined by the cause of the vomiting but in general includes observing the type of vomit, placing the infant or child who is vomiting in a position to prevent aspiration, cleaning the mouth after vomiting to prevent the acid damaging teeth, assessing for dehydration, carrying out routine observations and encouraging small amounts of fluid regularly when tolerated. Once vomiting has ceased, fluids and small amounts of diet can be encouraged.

Gastro-oesophageal reflux

Gastro-oesophageal reflux (GOR) refers to the return of gastric contents into the oesophagus, and is a common symptom affecting 40% of infants and young children (NICE, 2015a). The cause of GOR is a poorly functioning gastro-oesophageal sphincter, which normally prevents stomach contents from regurgitating back into the oesophagus. Some positing of milk is considered normal in newborns following a feed; however, regurgitation that continues or increases requires further investigation. Infants with reflux are at risk of aspiration and apnoea, particularly if lying down.

GOR usually begins before the infant is 8 weeks old and may occur several times a day, but this lessens in frequency over time. It is important to reassure parents that in well infants, with no symptoms other than effortless regurgitation, 90% of cases usually resolve before they are 1 year old and do not require further investigation (NICE, 2015a). There is an increased prevalence of GOR in premature infants, children or young people with obesity, hiatus hernia, diaphragmatic hernia or oesophageal atresia repair, and children with a neuro-disability.

Table 12.3 Possible complications of gastro-oesophageal reflux (GOR)

- Reflux oesophagitis due to acid irritation of the membranes
- Recurrent aspiration pneumonia due to the risk of aspiration
- Frequent otitis media
- Dental erosion in a child or young person with neuro-disability, in particular cerebral palsy

Source: NICE 2015a.

Other symptoms include heartburn, regurgitation, epigastric and retrosternal pain, and weight loss, and most sufferers are irritable. Infants with GOR, particularly premature infants, are at risk for aspiration and apnoea. Diagnosis is made on the symptoms and an upper GI contrast study for those with persistent or recurring symptoms. In infants with unexplained bile-stained vomiting, an upper GI contrast study will be done urgently in order to rule out more serious disorders, such as intestinal obstruction (NICE, 2015a).

Treatment depends on the severity and cause of GOR. Initially in infants, feeding with thickened feeds and upright positioning may be enough for milder cases. Feeding smaller amounts more often may help to reduce abdominal distension and associated reflux. Frequent winding throughout a feed also helps to prevent the build-up of abdominal wind associated with feeding. Depending on the healthcare provider, pharmacological treatment may be administered; this would depend on the cause of the problem and the severity. In some cases where there is failure to thrive or persistent weight loss enteral tube feeding may be considered. Surgery for GOR is only performed when medical therapy has failed and complications develop (see Table 12.3).

Nursing management focuses on ensuring the infant or child receives adequate nutrition. Daily weights and plotting infant or child weight and height on a percentile chart will monitor growth. Sandifer syndrome is the abnormal posturing that may occur in cases of severe acid reflux and may be mistakenly diagnosed as a seizure.

⚑ Red Flag

Infant positioning

Infants must always be put to sleep on their back in order to reduce the risk of sudden infant death syndrome (SIDS), and this is still the case if they have GOR. Infants can be fed in a more upright position to help prevent regurgitation.

(NHS, 2015; NICE, 2015a)

Hirschsprung disease (Fig. 12.1)

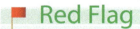

Hirschsprung disease (congenital aganglionic megacolon) is a congenital anomaly that causes inadequate motility due to the absence of parasympathetic ganglion cells in the affected areas of the intestine, mostly the recto-sigmoid region of the colon. This lack of motility leads to mechanical obstruction of the intestine and a distended sigmoid colon. The incidence is 1 in 5000 live births and is more common in males than females (Ball *et al.*, 2015); in many cases it has a familial pattern.

The age of onset will determine the clinical manifestations of the disease. In newborn infants there may be a failure to pass meconium in the first 48 hours, abdominal distension, feeding intolerance and bilious vomiting. In the older infant or child there may be a history of ribbon-like foul-smelling stools, visible peristalsis, easily palpable faecal mass, failure to thrive, chronic progressive constipation, which may be accompanied by episodes of faecal impaction.

Disorders of the digestive system Chapter 12

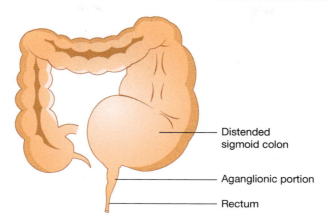

Figure 12.1 Distended sigmoid colon in Hirschsprung disease. *Source:* Hockenberry & Wilson 2015.

Diagnosis is made on the history and physical examination. An abdominal X-ray will show the distended colon and a lack of stool in the rectum. A rectal biopsy will be performed to confirm the absence of ganglion cells. Treatment is to remove the aganglionic portion of the bowel and a procedure consisting of pulling through the normal bowel to the end of the rectum to replace the removed portion. If the area of colon affected is too large for an immediate pull-through or it is inflamed, a temporary colostomy may be created and surgery performed later. Following the pull-through procedure incontinence and stricture may occur, requiring dilations or bowel retraining. Surgery is usually delayed in infants until they are 10 months old.

Nursing care is focused around observing for infection and ensuring adequate nutrition, maintaining hydration, pain management and providing support to the child and family. One very serious complication in infancy is enterocolitis, which can be fatal if not recognised early. Following a pull-through operation it is important to monitor the return of bowel function. If a colostomy is performed, post-operative stoma care and parent and child education in the care of a stoma will be needed.

Inflammatory conditions

Inflammatory disorders may be acute or chronic and be anywhere in the gastrointestinal tract. Causes may include injuries, foreign bodies, surgery, micro-organisms or chemicals. Included here are appendicitis and inflammatory bowel disease.

Appendicitis

Appendicitis is an inflammation of the vermiform appendix, which is a blind sac located near the end of the caecum. Appendicitis is the most common cause of acute abdominal surgery in children and can occur at any age although it is most often seen in children over 5 years with a peak incidence at 10 years (Ball *et al.*, 2015; Hockenberry & Wilson, 2015).

Appendicitis results from an obstruction in lumen of the appendix usually by a faecalith, which is a hardened faecal mass. It can also be caused by a parasitic infestation, stenosis lymphoid tissue or a tumour. The tissue becomes swollen due to the continuing production of mucus secretions causing build-up and pressure within the lumen, which results in compression of blood vessels. This compression can lead to ischaemia, tissue death and necrosis. The appendix may perforate or rupture allowing faecal matter and bacteria to be

Chapter 12 — Disorders of the digestive system

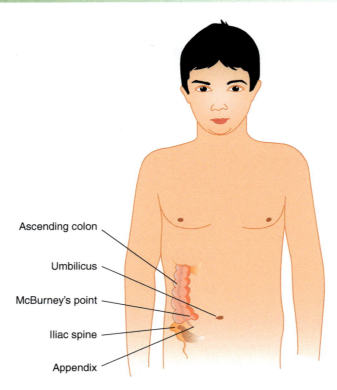

Figure 12.2 Common location of pain in children and adolescents with appendicitis. *Source:* Ball *et al.* 2015.

released into the peritoneal cavity. This then spreads rapidly throughout the abdomen causing peritonitis. Progressive peritoneal infection can lead to small bowel obstruction, septicaemia, electrolyte imbalance and hypovolaemic shock.

Early abdominal symptoms of appendicitis include tenderness, colicky cramping pain around the umbilicus, anorexia, nausea and fever. The pain experienced around the umbilicus is known as referred pain. Focal abdominal tenderness occurs at the site of McBurney's point, which is located two-thirds along the line between the umbilicus and the left antero-superior iliac spine (see Fig. 12.2). Rebound tenderness, guarding and rigidity may also be present.

⚑ Red Flag

Appendicitis pain

Any sudden relief of pain may indicate a ruptured appendix. The initial pain relief is due to the release of pressure.

(Ball *et al.*, 2015)

Diagnosis can be difficult as children often present with appendix symptoms when they have other conditions, such as Meckel diverticulum, gastroenteritis, pelvic inflammatory disease, mesenteric adenitis. Delaying treatment can result in the appendix rupturing. Blood analysis for white cell count and CT scan may assist with the diagnosis although this is mainly done on the symptoms and physical examination. The treatment is surgical removal of the inflamed appendix and the child can generally be discharged fairly quickly following surgery if they have an uncomplicated recovery.

Children with a ruptured appendix will need intravenous antibiotic therapy and fluids prior to surgery. Irrigation of the peritoneal cavity during surgery will be performed to remove any infected exudate and subsequent abdominal drainage may continue for a few days post-operatively. Oral fluids are slowly introduced and diet not commenced until bowel sounds are active due to the risk of a paralytic ileus.

Pain management is essential and should be assessed using a pain assessment tool; however, pain is to be expected following any abdominal surgery and the nurse should anticipate this and treat accordingly. A sudden admission for an acute condition is very worrying for both the child and parents and they will need to be reassured. Once bowel sounds have returned following surgery the child will be allowed home. On discharge parents will need to be educated on the signs of infection and when their child will be able to return to normal activities.

Inflammatory bowel disease (IBD)

Crohn's disease and ulcerative colitis are two distinct chronic disorders with similar aetiologies and clinical features, even though their histology differs. They both have a similar impact on the child and family. Onset is before age 20 years with the majority diagnosed around 12 years (Ball *et al.*, 2015).

Crohn's disease occurs commonly in the ileum, colon and rectum whereas ulcerative colitis is limited to the colon. The aetiology is unknown but they may be related to allergies, dietary factors, immune disorders, or infection. There may be a genetic association, which is more common in children with Crohn's disease. There is also a link between developing IBD and limited exposure to gastrointestinal pathogens in early childhood (Winter, 2010).

Although many symptoms are shared between Crohn's disease and ulcerative colitis there are differences illustrated in Table 12.4. Diagnosis of IBD may be made initially on history and blood testing; however, further tests, such as endoscopy, biopsy and radiological tests, are needed to confirm the diagnosis.

Management of the two conditions differs slightly although the aim is to induce and maintain remission and reduce the incidence of flare-ups while still promoting normal growth and development, control inflammation and reduce or eliminate symptoms (Winter, 2010). Treatment includes medical treatment with 5-aminosalicylates (5-ASAs) to support remission induction, corticosteroids are used in moderate to severe disease, but long-term use may cause side effects and they are therefore limited to short periods of treatment. Surgery is more of an option in ulcerative colitis because it is limited to the colon. Crohn's disease is more disabling and may result in more serious complications (Rodgers & Wilson, 2015). Long-term complications of IBD include the need for a permanent ileostomy or colostomy, and colorectal cancer.

Table 12.4 Clinical manifestations of inflammatory bowel diseases (IBD)

Characteristics	Ulcerative colitis	Crohn's disease
Rectal bleeding	Common	Uncommon
Diarrhoea	Often severe	Moderate to severe
Pain	Less frequent	Common
Anorexia	Mild or moderate	May be severe
Weight loss	Moderate	May be severe
Growth retardation	Usually mild	May be severe
Anal and perianal lesions	Rare	Common
Fistulas and strictures	Rare	Common
Rashes	Mild	Mild
Joint pain	Mild to moderate	Mild to moderate

Nutritional support is needed and a nutritionist will be involved in planning the dietary needs of the child. The emotional impact of the disease on the child and family requires support both during exacerbations when hospitalised and in the community, where the majority of management occurs. Frequent absences from school can affect a child's self-esteem and cause social isolation from their peers. Body image is a concern for children, particularly adolescents and with prolonged corticosteroid treatment delayed sexual maturation and growth retardation may result. In cases where an ostomy has been performed the child and family will need support and encouragement for the child to lead as normal a life as possible.

Obstructive disorders
Pyloric stenosis (Fig. 12.3)

Pyloric stenosis is a hypertophic obstruction caused by hyperplasia and hypertrophy of the circular pyloric muscle at the lower opening of the stomach. This thickened muscle results in narrowing of the pyloric canal leading to an outlet obstruction. It is more common in first-born babies, with boys being affected 4–6 times more frequently than girls. The condition is more common in Caucasians and more likely in full-term newborns (Rodgers & Wilson, 2015). The exact cause is unknown but there may be a family history of the disorder.

Manifestations include progressive vomiting, which may be projectile; this is non-bilious in the early stages but may become brown if gastritis develops. The thickened pylorus can be felt as an olive-like mass and may be palpable in the abdomen. Initially the infant appears well with only slight regurgitations after feeds, but as the obstruction becomes worse due to swelling causing increasing narrowing of the lumen, the vomiting becomes worse; this usually occurs at around 3 weeks. There may also be visible gastric peristalsis on the abdomen. The infant becomes increasingly irritable and fails to gain the expected weight. Diagnosis is confirmed by an ultrasound and upper GI radiography.

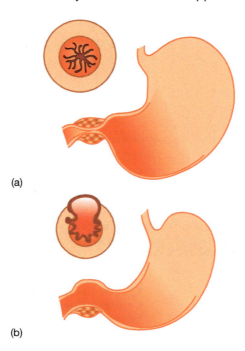

Figure 12.3 Hypertrophic pyloric stenosis. (a) Enlarged muscular tumour nearly obliterates pyloric canal. (b) Longitudinal surgical division of muscle down to submucosa establishes adequate passageway. *Source:* Hockenberry & Wilson 2015.

Pre-operatively, infants need intravenous fluids to correct any dehydration and electrolyte imbalance. A naso-gastric tube will be inserted to remove any remaining fluids prior to surgery. Treatment is a surgical pyloromyotomy, which consists of an incision in the pyloric muscle to expand the opening. Feeds are recommended according to the surgeon's protocol but usually commence 4–6 hours following surgery with clear fluids unless breastfeeding. Intravenous fluids may be necessary until adequate amounts of fluid are taken orally in order to maintain fluid and electrolyte balance. Some vomiting may still occur following surgery and parents need to be reassured that this is normal. Parents also need reassurance that the treatment is usually successful with no reoccurrence in the affected infant. It is unusual for subsequent infants to be affected with the condition.

Intussusception (Fig. 12.4)

Intussusception is a common cause of intestinal obstruction in infants and young children, usually before the age of 3 years but most commonly around age 6 months. It is more common in males than females. Generally the cause is unknown; however, it is common in children with cystic fibrosis. It may also follow a recent infection, or be caused by a polyp, lymphoma, or Meckel diverticulum.

Intussusception occurs when one portion of the bowel telescopes into a more distal portion of the bowel propelled by continuing peristalsis, the most common site being the ileocaecal valve. The mesentery is still attached to the telescoped portion of the bowel and is compressed causing lymphatic and venous obstruction. Mucus production is increased producing jelly-like stools. This results in oedema and pressure causing obstruction, which can also lead to ischaemia.

Manifestations include sudden onset of colicky pain, inconsolable crying, and drawing up of the knees to the chest in a previously healthy infant or child. This is usually accompanied by vomiting that contains bile or faecal material. Electrolyte imbalance and dehydration can develop. On palpation the abdomen is tender with a palpable sausage-shaped

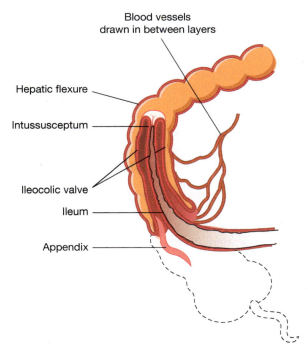

Figure 12.4 Ileocaecal valve (ileocolic) intussusception. *Source:* Hockenberry & Wilson 2015.

mass. Continuing symptoms may include fever, shallow respirations, rapid pulse and decreased blood pressure. If not treated, ischaemia can lead to necrosis, perforation and peritonitis.

Ten percent of children may have a spontaneous reduction of the vaginated bowel (Devitt & Thain, 2011). This may be indicated by the passage of a normal brown stool and will need reporting immediately as the course of treatment may be altered. Treatment consists of a hydrostatic reduction of air pressure or liquid contrast medium given rectally to reverse the telescopic segment of the bowel. Surgery consists of manual reduction only when the hydrostatic reduction fails. If this is unsuccessful or if the portion of effected bowel is gangrenous or strangulated then a resection is performed.

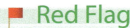
Red Flag

Nursing considerations

Because this is a potentially fatal condition nurses need to be alert to older children presenting with a more chronic picture of diarrhoea, anorexia, weight loss, periodic pain and vomiting.

Nursing management includes monitoring and correcting any imbalance in fluid and electrolytes by administering intravenous fluids. Post-operative care focuses on observing the child for infection, maintaining patency of the naso-gastric tube and controlling pain. The presence of bowel sounds is important prior to commencing any oral intake in order to prevent the development of a paralytic ileus. Clear fluids or breastfeeding may then be commenced and slowly increased according to the practitioner's protocol.

Malabsorption syndromes
Coeliac disease

Coeliac disease (gluten-sensitive enteropathy) is an immunologic disorder characterised by intolerance to dietary gluten, the protein present in wheat, rye, oats and barley. This protein causes damage to the villi in the small intestine leading to malabsorption of nutrients. The incidence is 1 in 100 people in the UK (NICE, 2015b) and is usually diagnosed between 6 to 18 months of age when these proteins are first introduced in the diet. It is more common among family members of the same family and in children with Down syndrome, Turner syndrome, type 1 diabetes, and autoimmune thyroid disease (NICE, 2015b).

Coeliac disease can present with a number of symptoms, both gastrointestinal and non-gastrointestinal (see Table 12.5). Diagnosis is confirmed through serological testing and intestinal biopsy of the upper GI tract to confirm changes in the villi.

If not detected and properly treated coeliac disease can cause serious malnourishment and debilitation. The complications of coeliac disease may include anaemia, small bowel ulcerations, bleeding disorders, malignancy (intestinal lymphoma), osteoporosis, vitamin D and iron deficiency, and lactose intolerance. Treatment is a lifelong elimination of gluten from the diet and dietary supplements such as calcium and vitamin D. It is important for the family to access a dietician to provide information and ongoing support. Many of the problems with the disease are due to poor compliance with a gluten-free diet.

Disorders of the digestive system — Chapter 12

Table 12.5 Symptoms of coeliac disease

Gastrointestinal symptoms	Non-gastrointestinal symptoms
• Indigestion • Diarrhoea • Abdominal pain • Bloating • Distension • Constipation	• Fatigue • Dermatitis • Herpetiformis • Anaemia • Osteoporosis • Reproductive problems • Neuropathy • Ataxia • Delayed puberty • Growth delay • Weight loss or static weight

Source: NICE 2015b.

Nursing care priorities focus mostly around helping the child and family adhere to a dietary regime and providing them with information about the disease. It is difficult for a child to understand that they need to stick to the restricted diet when they have no symptoms. This may lead to exacerbation of symptoms due to non-compliance with the dietary requirements.

Structural defects
Tracheoesophageal fistula (TOF) and oesophageal atresia (OA)

Tracheoesophageal fistula (TOF) and oesophageal atresia (OA) are congenital malformations of the oesophagus. In TOF the oesophagus fails to develop in the foetal stage as one continuous passage and either results in a blind end known as oesophageal atresia or connects to the trachea via a fistula. See Fig. 12.5 for the most common formations. The most common manifestation is when the oesophagus ends in a blind end and the distal section attached to the stomach inserts into the trachea (example (c) in Fig. 12.5) (Rodgers & Wilson, 2015).

The incidence is slightly higher in males than females and these infants usually have lower birth weights with a higher incidence of pre-term births than average (Rodgers & Wilson, 2015). Associated anomalies may include gastrointestinal abnormalities

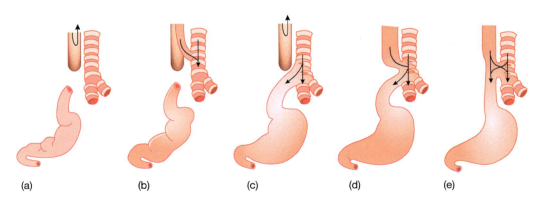

Figure 12.5 (a)-(e) Five most common types of oesophageal atresia and tracheoesophageal fistula. (See text for discussion) *Source:* Hockenberry & Wilson 2015.

including imperforate anus, urinary tract anomalies, vertebral defects, and cardiac defects.

Newborns with the defect will present with frothy saliva and drooling from the mouth and nose and choking and coughing with associated respiratory distress. This may be mild or more serious depending on the type of defect present. On feeding the infant may begin coughing and gagging despite swallowing normally and fluid will return through the nose and mouth. Due to milk aspiration apnoea and cyanosis may result. In mild cases diagnosis may not occur until later in life when the child has experienced chronic respiratory problems and oesophageal reflux. A distended stomach may also be evident due to inspiratory air entering the stomach via a fistula. The type of defect is confirmed by the presenting signs and symptoms and also by radiographic studies.

The priority for treatment is to maintain a patent airway, necessitating nil by mouth to prevent aspiration and intravenous solutions to maintain fluid and electrolyte balance. Accumulated secretions will be removed by suction, and if there is an oesophageal pouch a permanent sump pump may also be inserted. A naso-gastric tube may be inserted into type E (see Fig. 12.5) or a gastrostomy tube to remove air from the stomach. Surgical correction of the malformation will be performed in one or two stages. Success is dependent on the type of defect and an early diagnosis.

Prior to surgery these infants should be nursed with the head of the bed slightly elevated in order to reduce aspiration. Airway, respirations, oxygen saturation and colour should be continuously monitored for any deterioration. Suction equipment should be at hand and no oral fluids should be given. Infants should not be given a pacifier pre-surgery as this increases the production of secretions. Following surgery nurses need to monitor the secretions from the low-suction naso-gastric tube by recording the character and amount removed. Respiratory function needs to be closely monitored and nurses should be alert to any signs of infection. Gastrostomy feeds may be given until the surgical site is healed or begin oral feeds with sterile water and then increase to feeding as per practitioner protocol. Sucking on a pacifier post-surgery prevents oral aversion. Parents need reassurance and should be encouraged to participate in the care of their infant.

Cleft lip and palate (Fig. 12.6)

Cleft lip with or without cleft palate is one of the most common birth defects (Wilson & Wilson, 2015). Globally, approximately one in 700 babies are born each year with a cleft, which equates to 1000 babies each year in the UK (Cleft Lip & Palate Association [CLAPA], 2016). The cause may be due to environmental or genetic factors. There is an increased incidence in families with a history of cleft lip and palate. Environmental factors or teratogens during the first trimester of pregnancy may include alcohol consumption, ingestion of some medications, such as anticonvulsants, retinoids, steroids, or illegal drugs such as cocaine, and smoking. However, folic acid supplements during pregnancy are known to have a protective action against the condition.

The variations seen in the defect are due to the different stages in palatine development (see Fig. 12.7). Interruption in any of these stages can result in the defect. A cleft lip and palate may occur together or alone and may be bilateral or unilateral. It may involve both the soft and hard palates and depending on severity may extend up into the floor of the nasal cavity. It is usually diagnosed at birth; however, a cleft palate without involvement of the lip may not be diagnosed immediately.

Treatment consists of surgical repair to the lip (cheiloplasty) and palate (palatoplasy). Cleft lip repair usually occurs when the infant is around 3 months old; further aesthetic surgery is sometimes needed when the child is older. Cleft palate repair usually occurs later between 6 and 12 months of age, again with the possibility of further surgery as the child grows and develops (CLAPA, 2016).

Disorders of the digestive system　　　　　　　　　　　　　　　　　　　　Chapter 12

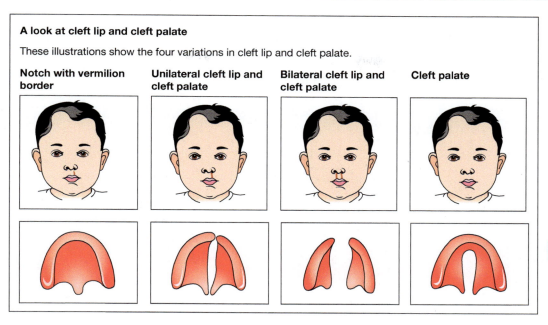

Figure 12.6 Cleft lip and cleft palate. *Source:* Devitt & Thain 2011.

For pre- and post-operative nursing care see Table 12.6. There are a number of specialist feeding devices available to assist with feeding prior to repair. Mothers need to be alerted to the fact that infants and children with a cleft palate are at increased risk of otitis media due to the altered position of the Eustachian tubes. On discharge, parents should be taught how to care for the suture line and monitor the child's feeding to maintain a healthy weight gain. These children are often followed into their teenage years and further surgery may be necessary.

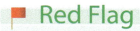 Red Flag

Nursing considerations

Following surgery nothing (such as tongue depressors, suction tubes, spoons or straws) should be inserted into the mouth in order to prevent compromising the suture line.

Hernias

A hernia is a protrusion of an organ or part of an organ through an abnormal opening in the muscle wall. The abnormal opening may be as a result of incomplete fetal closure or from a musculature weakness. The organ protrudes due to pressure, with the danger that it could lose function, or blood flow could be reduced ultimately causing ischaemia. Two common hernias that present in infancy and childhood are the umbilical hernia and inguinal hernia.

The umbilical hernia is common in infants and occurs when there is incomplete development of the umbilical ring. It may be associated with some congenital anomalies such as Down syndrome. Any abdominal pressure increases the size of the hernia, such as crying. The hernia usually resolves on its own by 3–5 years, but if it persists elective surgery may be needed. If the hernia becomes incarcerated and is not reducible manually then surgical intervention is indicated as there is a danger of ischaemia.

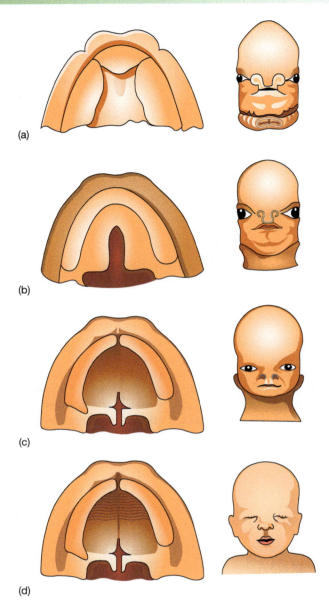

Figure 12.7 (a)-(d) Stages in palatine development. (See text for discussion). *Source:* Hockenberry & Wilson 2015.

Inguinal hernia is the most common and accounts for approximately 80% of all hernias in childhood (Hockenberry & Wilson, 2015). It is more common in black children and very low birthweight infants (Ball *et al.*, 2015). Inguinal hernia is caused by the persistence of the processus vaginalis, which is the tube preceding the testicle as it travels through the inguinal canal to reach the scrotum in boys, or the round ligament into the labia in girls. This occurs around 8 months' gestation. Normally the upper portion atrophies and the lower portion forms the tunica vaginalis which encloses the testicle within the scrotum. When the upper portion fails to atrophy abdominal fluid descends creating a bulge or mass (see Fig. 12.8).

Table 12.6 Pre- and post-operative nursing care of the infant with a cleft lip and/or palate

Pre-operative nursing care	Post-operative nursing care
Cleft lip • Provide parental emotional support • Feed the infant slowly to decrease aspiration risk • Small frequent feeds and wind frequently • Promote sucking between feeds to aid speech development • Position upright to feed to aid swallowing and prevent milk from entering the nasal cavity	Cleft lip • Maintain a patent airway and observe for respiratory distress • Maintain a patent airway and observe for respiratory distress • Restrict hand to mouth movement in order to protect the suture line • Clean the wound following a feed • Keep the infant calm as crying stresses the suture line • Use a syringe and soft tube to feed at the side of the mouth initially to protect the suture line • Monitor pain and administer analgesia • No soothers until the wound is healed
Cleft palate • Give a small amount of water after feeds to clean the palate • Wean onto a cup prior to surgery • Observe for fluids entering the nasal cavity and compromising respiration • Feed sitting up to aid swallowing and prevent aspiration	Cleft palate • Maintain a patent airway and observe for respiratory distress • Provide a clear drink following feeds to clean the suture line • Use a cup to feed • Start with clear fluids and increase up to soft foods • Monitor pain and administer analgesia • No soothers • Provide soft toys to prevent injury

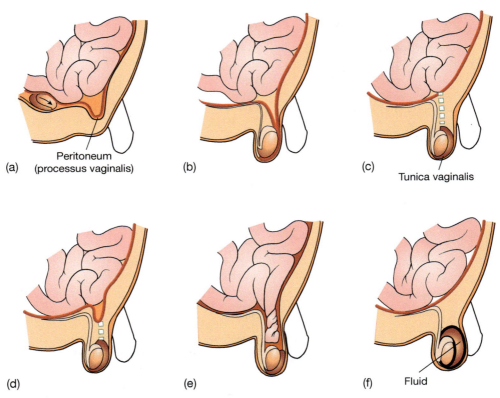

Figure 12.8 Development of inguinal hernias. (a) and (b), prenatal migration of processus vaginalis (c), Normal. (d), partially obliterated processus vaginalis. (e), Hernia, (f), Hydrocele. *Source:* Hockenberry & Wilson 2015.

This defect may cause no symptoms and usually presents as a painless inguinal swelling. It can be reduced with gentle pressure and diminishes in size with rest. It becomes more prominent when the infant cries or when the child coughs, strains or is active. It becomes a problem if the herniated loop of intestine becomes compressed or partially obstructed. Symptoms then may include redness, oedema, tenderness, anorexia or abdominal swelling. Occasionally strangulation occurs when there is a loss of blood supply, which can lead to necrosis. The treatment is surgical repair, usually elective unless strangulated, in which case it is a surgical emergency. Nursing management consists of early recognition of the hernia and post-operative care of the wound. This includes monitoring for normal bowel function and pain control (Table 12.7).

Table 12.7 Causes of potential alteration in post-operative vital signs

Potential alteration	Potential causes
Heart rate	
Increase:	Pyrexia Pain Haemorrhage leading to decreased profusion and shock Respiratory distress – early Medication
Decrease:	Hypoxia Respiratory distress – late stage Raised intracranial pressure Medication
Respiratory rate	
Increase:	Respiratory distress Pain Hypothermia Pyrexia Increase in circulating fluid volume – fluid overload
Decrease:	Medication including anaesthetic agents Pain
Blood pressure	
Increase:	Excessive intravascular volume Raised intracranial pressure Pain CO_2 retention Medication
Decrease:	Medication especially opioids Anaesthetic agents – vasodilators
Temperature	
Increase:	Sepsis Shock – late sign Malignant hyperthermia Environmental factors – room, heating blankets
Decrease:	Anaesthetic agents – vasodilators Medication – muscle relaxants Cold intravenous fluids and/or blood Environmental factors – room too cold

Source: Hockenberry & Wilson 2015.

Disorders of the digestive system Chapter 12

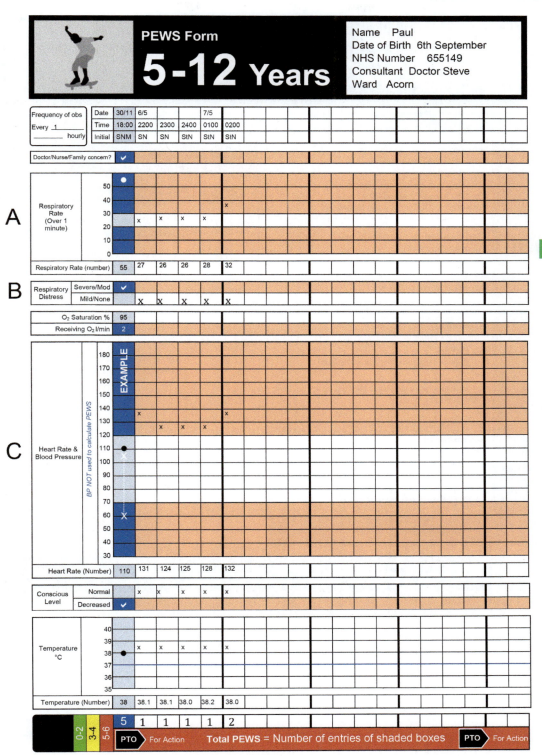

Figure 12.9   PEWS chart for Paul in Case Study 1.

Chapter 12 — Disorders of the digestive system

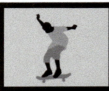

PEWS Form
5-12 Years

Name Paul
Date of Birth 6th September
NHS Number 655149
Consultant Dr Steve
Ward Acorn

PEWS Escalation Aid

S — Situation:
I am (name), a nurse on ward (X)
I am calling about (child X)
I am calling because I am concerned that…
(e.g. BP is low/high, pulse is XXX
temperature is XX, Early Warning Score is XX)

B — Background:
Child (X) was admitted on (XX date) with
(e.g. respiratory infection)
They have had (X operation/procedure/investigation)
Child (X)'s condition has changed in the last (XX mins)
Their last set of obs were (XXX)
The child's normal condition is…
(e.g. alert/drowsy/confused, pain free)

A — Assessment:
I think the problem is (XXX)
and I have…
(e.g. given O2 /analgesia, stopped the infusion)
OR
I am not sure what the problem is but child (X)
is deteriorating
OR
I don't know what's wrong but I am really worried

R — Recommendation:
I need you to…
Come to see the child in the next (XX mins)
AND
Is there anything I need to do in the meantime?
(e.g. stop the fluid/repeat the obs)

Download SBAR prompt cards and pads at
www.institute.nhs.uk/SBAR

Remember: If you feel you need more help at any time, call for help – regardless of PEW Score

Score	Action
0 1	Continue monitoring
2	Nurse in charge MUST review
3	Nurse in charge & Doctor MUST review
4	Nurse in charge & Doctor MUST review & inform Consultant
5 6	Nurse in charge & Consultant MUST review

Record Call When PEWS 3 Or More

Date	Time	PEWS	Print Name (nurse)
01/01/12	09:00	5	SN Morton

Record Time of Review, Who by & Plan

Time	Plan	Print Name
09:15	ED consultant called Anaesthetic review	Sister JACKS

Download documents to use or edit at
www.institute.nhs.uk/PEWScharts

NHS Institute for Innovation and Improvement

© NHS Institute for Innovation and Improvement 2012

Figure 12.9 (continued).

Paediatric early warning system – related to a case study

Case Study 1

At 10 p.m. on a Friday evening, 7-year-old Paul's mother brings him into the accident and emergency department with severe abdominal cramping pain. This pain started suddenly the evening before and has slowly worsened over that period. Paul has a fever of 38.5 °C and is now unable to keep any food or fluids down. He also has diarrhoea. On palpation he has rebound tenderness in the lower right abdominal quadrant. The pain is worse on palpation and he is most comfortable with his knees drawn up to his chest. He is diagnosed with acute appendicitis and scheduled for an appendectomy. Paul returned to the ward following the surgery with a dry dressing, an intravenous infusion and pain medication.

This is the first time Paul has been in hospital and his parents are worried how he will cope with the experience and the pain following surgery. They are concerned about how quickly he became ill and wonder if they could have done something to prevent it.

- What would you say to these parents?
- How would you prepare Paul for surgery?

Observations are recorded on a PEWS chart (see Fig. 12.9).
What actions might the nurse take based on the score on this chart?

Case Study 2

Logan, a 6-week-old baby, is brought to the hospital by his parents with a history of worsening vomiting and failure to gain expected weight. On examination Logan has been vomiting since 3 weeks of age and is hungry and irritable. He has mild dehydration and visible gastric peristalsis. An olive-shaped mass is palpable in the epigastrium right of the umbilicus. Logan's mother describes his vomiting as forceful.

A diagnosis of pyloric stenosis is made and Logan is made nil by mouth in preparation for a pyloromyotomy surgical procedure. Intravenous fluids and electrolytes are commenced to correct any dehydration and restore the electrolyte balance.

Logan's parents are very upset as this is their first child and they are worried that this could happen again in future children.

- What information would you give Logan's parents about this condition?
- What post-operative care would you provide to Logan?

References

Ball, J., Bindler, R. & Cowen, K. (2015). *Caring for Children: Principles of Pediatric Nursing*, 6th edn. Pearson, New Jersey.

Cleft Lip & Palate Association (CLAPA) (2016). What is cleft lip and palate? Available at: https://www.clapa.com/what-is-cleft-lip-palate/ (accessed 25 April 2016).

Devitt, P. & Thain, J. (2011). *Children's and Young People's Nursing Made Incredibly Easy*. Lippincott Williams & Wilkins, London.

Hockenberry, M.J. & Wilson, D. (eds) (2015). *Wong's Nursing Care of Infants and Children*, 10th edn. Elsevier Mosby, Canada.

National Health Service (NHS) (2015). Sudden infant death syndrome (SIDS). Available at: http://www.nhs.uk/Conditions/Sudden-infant-death-syndrome/Pages/Introduction.aspx (last accessed April 2018).

National Institute for Health and Care Excellence (NICE) (2010). Constipation in children and young people: diagnosis and management. NICE guideline [CG99]. Available at: http://www.nice.org.uk/guidance/CG99/chapter/Introduction (last accessed April 2018).

National Institute for Health and Care Excellence (NICE) (2015a). Gastro-oesophageal reflux disease in children and young people: diagnosis and management. NICE guideline [NG1]. Available at: https://www.nice.org.uk/guidance/NG1/chapter/1-recommendations#/diagnosing-and-investigating-gord (last accessed April 2018).

National Institute for Health and Care Excellence (NICE) (2015b). September Coeliac disease: recognition, assessment and management. NICE guideline [NG20]. Available at: https://www.nice.org.uk/guidance/ng20/chapter/Update-information (last accessed April 2018).

Rodgers, C.C. & Wilson, D. (2015). The child with gastrointestinal dysfunction. In: Hockenberry, M.J. & Wilson, D. (eds). *Wong's Nursing Care of Infants and Children*, 10th edn. Elsevier Mosby, Canada.

Winter, J.M. (2010). Caring for children with gastrointestinal problems. In: Glasper, A. & Richardson, J. (eds). *A Textbook of Children's and Young People's Nursing*, 2nd edn. Churchill Livingstone Elsevier, London.

Chapter 13

Disorders of the renal system

Cathy Poole

Aim

The aim of this chapter is to help the reader develop an understanding of diseases of the renal system and the care required to help children and young people.

Learning outcomes

On completion of this chapter, the reader will be able to:

- Distinguish between upper renal tract and lower renal tract disorders.
- Identify a selection of renal anomalies identified during routine antenatal ultrasound scanning.
- Describe a renal disorder-focused nursing assessment.
- Describe some of the more common medical and surgical renal disorders.
- Discuss some specific renal medical and renal surgical nursing care.

Keywords

- upper renal tract
- lower renal tract
- congenital anomalies
- fluid overload
- preservation of kidney and bladder function
- renal investigations

Fundamentals of Children's Applied Pathophysiology: An Essential Guide for Nursing and Healthcare Students, First Edition.
Edited by Elizabeth Gormley-Fleming and Ian Peate.
© 2019 John Wiley & Sons Ltd. Published 2019 by John Wiley & Sons Ltd.
Companion website: www.wileyfundamentalseries.com/childpathophysiology

Test your prior knowledge

1. What does the urinary system consist of?
2. List the functions of the kidney
3. At what point during pregnancy is a detailed ultrasound scan done of the unborn fetus?
4. Name two renal anomalies which can be diagnosed by fetal ultrasound scanning.
5. Describe the nursing care of a child with nephrotic syndrome.
6. Describe the physiology of periorbital oedema associated with heavy proteinuria.
7. What can cause haematuria in children?
8. What is a pyeloplasty and why is it performed?
9. What is hypospadias?
10. Why is hand hygiene so important when visiting community farms?

Introduction

Some disorders of the renal system are common, such as urinary tract infections, while others are less so, bladder exstrophy, for example. This chapter will discuss the most common disorders seen in the general children's nursing environment and will also introduce you to some of the more complex and rarer disorders. When referring to renal disorders the reader should consider the urinary tract as a whole, kidneys, ureters, bladder, and the urethra (Fig. 13.1). Disorders of the urinary system are often referred to as either upper or lower urinary tract disorders (Peate & Gormley-Fleming, 2015). This chapter is divided into disorders of the upper urinary tract and disorders of the lower urinary tract. In addition to this, management of disorders of the urinary system can be either medical or surgical, and in some cases a combination of both. The nursing care of the infant, child or young person with a medical or surgical disorder of the entire urinary system will be outlined.

Prior to the advent of antenatal ultrasound screening few congenital malformations of the renal system were diagnosed until they caused symptoms in infancy, childhood, or later in adult life. The importance of early diagnosis is well recognised and a section in this chapter will be dedicated to renal anomalies that can be detected during the antenatal

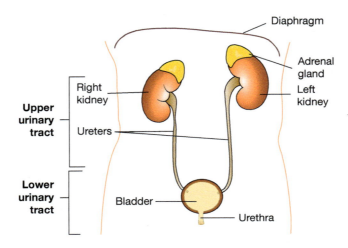

Figure 13.1   Upper and lower urinary tract.

Antenatal detection of renal anomalies

Early identification of renal system anomalies is important as they may be associated with abnormal renal development and function. They may also predispose to postnatal infection and involve urinary tract obstruction, which may require surgical intervention (Lissauer & Clayden, 2007). Early detection, therefore, has the potential for early intervention and affords the opportunity to reduce, minimise or even prevent progressive renal system damage. However, a concern with this early detection is that very minor anomalies are also detected, the most common being renal pelvic dilatation (RPD). RPD rarely requires intervention, but does require follow-up during the antenatal period and potentially further investigations postnatally depending on the degree of dilatation. This can consequently lead to unnecessary anxiety for the parents. It is estimated that antenatal anomalies of the urinary system are identified in 1 in 200–400 births (Lissauer & Clayden, 2007). Table 13.1 provides an insight into these anomalies.

In summary, kidney and urinary tract anomalies are the most common antenatal abnormality detected. The use of antenatal ultrasound scanning is recommended during all pregnancies to aid early diagnosis of urinary tract abnormalities, thus establishing plans for postnatal care to optimise the outcome and reduce or delay the progress of renal function deterioration.

Table 13.1 Antenatal urinary tract abnormalities

Antenatal anomaly detected	Brief description of anomaly
Renal agenesis (Potter syndrome)	Absence of both kidneys, associated with reduced volume of amniotic fluid (oligohydramniosis), lung hypoplasia, low-set ears, beaked nose, downward eye slants, and limb abnormalities. Incompatible with life. Affects 1 in 4000 pregnancies.
Solitary kidney	Solitary kidney is a condition in which children have a single kidney instead of two kidneys.
Horseshoe kidney	During embryonic development the kidneys fuse together to form a horseshoe-shape. Reported to affect about 1 in 600 children.
Duplex kidney	Children with a duplex kidney (also called a duplicated collecting system) have two ureters coming from a single kidney. Duplex kidneys can occur in one (unilateral) or both (bilateral) kidneys (Fig. 13.2).
Ectopic kidney (or renal ectopia)	An ectopic kidney does not grow in the proper location. It occurs in about 1 in 900 births. Infants, children and young people with an ectopic kidney usually have no symptoms, but sometimes it may cause urinary problems, e.g., urine blockage, infection, or urinary stones.
Hydronephrosis	One or both kidneys are stretched and swollen (dilated). It is quite common, affecting about 1 in 100 pregnancies. Most cases are not serious.
Multicystic dysplastic kidney (MCDK)	The kidneys have bundles of cysts in them, which are like sacs filled with liquid. MCDK can be unilateral or bilateral. The cysts can be very large initially; however, over time they become smaller and the kidney gradually shrinks.
Posterior urethral valves (PUV)	Affects only boys as only boys have a posterior urethra. PUV are extra flaps of tissue in the urethra. Babies with PUV may not be able to micturate normally, during fetal development and after they are born.

Source: Adapted from Lissauer & Clayden 2007, and infoKID; www.infokid.org.uk/ (accessed 6 December 2016).

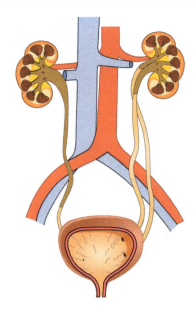

Figure 13.2 Duplex left kidney.

Assessment of the renal system

Nursing assessment is a key component of nursing practice, which forms the foundation for planning and provision of patient- and family-centred care. The Nursing and Midwifery Council (NMC) (2015) states that nurses must 'make sure that people's physical, social and psychological needs are assessed and responded to'. It is therefore really important when undertaking a holistic nursing assessment that criteria relating to the renal system are taken into account (see Table 13.2).

Medication Alert

A review of patients with reduced renal function identified a link with the use of supplements, and it listed 15 herbs and supplements reported to have caused kidney problems, including chromium, creatine, liquorice, willow bark, vitamin C and yohimbe (Gabardi, Munz & Ulbricht, 2007). Families should always be advised to discuss the use of such treatments with their doctors or pharmacists as these may also interfere with the pharmacodynamics of prescribed treatments.

Commonly, infants, children and young people who present with symptoms of a urinary tract disorder will be required to undergo further tests to confirm the diagnosis. These tests may include the following;

- blood tests to assess renal function
- renal ultrasound, which provides a non-invasive assessment of urinary tract anatomy
- CT (computed tomography) scan – this type of X-ray uses a computer to produce detailed images of many structures inside the body, including the internal organs, blood vessels and bones
- DMSA (dimercaptosuccinic acid) scan – a type of radioisotope scan that shows which areas of the kidneys are working normally and which areas have been damaged (usually following kidney infections)
- intravenous urogram to show detailed anatomy of the renal calyces or ureter

Disorders of the renal system Chapter 13

Table 13.2 Assessment of the renal system

Urinary symptoms: enuresis (bed wetting), new-onset incontinence, frequency, urgency, quantity, dysuria and its timing during voiding (at beginning or end, throughout), change in colour and odour of urine, haematuria, presence of stones or sediment in the urine, toilet-training problems, reduced urine output.

Hydration status, including blood pressure, fluid balance, and weight, ankle and eye oedema (periorbital oedema).

Growth and feeding, diet or fluid restrictions, sudden weight loss.

Urine output (neonates 1–3 mL [kg/h]; children <2 yrs 2–3 mL [kg/h]; >2 yrs 0.5–1 mL [kg/h]).

Urinalysis (pH, ketones, protein, blood, leukocytes, nitrite, glucose, specific gravity). Proteinuria and haematuria are early signs of disorders of the renal system.

Review blood chemistry results, urea, creatinine, electrolytes, albumin and haemoglobin, and estimated GRF (glomerular filtration rate).

Skin condition: temperature, turgor and moisture, colour, evidence of any rashes, enlarged painful nodes (axilla, groin).

Inexplicable crying, holding genitalia, discolouration of external genitalia, pain or swelling of the testicles, penile discharge, itching or swelling of the genitalia, urethral or vaginal discharge.

Location of pain, flank, suprapubic, genital, groin or low back pain.

Medication: prescribed, over-the-counter or herbal remedies and supplements.

Source: Adapted from The Royal Children's Hospital Melbourne 2014.

- micturating cystourethrogram (MCUG) uses X-rays that show the bladder and urethra while the child is passing urine. It identifies whether or not the urine goes from the bladder back up to the kidneys instead of out through the urethra, known as vesicoureteric reflux (VUR)
- MAG3 scan – MAG is an abbreviation for a chemical called mercaptoacetyltriglycine (MAG3 or MAG III), which is injected to perform this test. It shows how well each kidney is working, how well urine is draining from the kidneys, and can help to identify if there is any blockage that affects the flow of urine from kidneys
- kidney biopsy – this involves the removal of small samples of kidney tissue, which are then examined under high-powered microscopes to find out more about the kidneys.

For a successful outcome to these specialist investigations, the child and family need full preparation, explanation and, where required, provide informed consent. *The Great Ormond Street Hospital Manual of Children's Nursing Practices*, Chap. 14 (Macqueen, Bruce & Gibson, 2012), provides a comprehensive account of the nursing implications for these investigations as does infoKID, a web resource for parents and carers of children with renal disorders (www.infokid.org.uk).

In summary, while this section has focused on renal-specific assessment skills, these should form part of the full holistic assessment of all infants, children and young people for whom you care.

Medical disorders of the upper urinary tract
Proteinuria

Proteinuria is leakage of protein from the blood into the urine. Normally, significant amounts of protein do not pass into urine when the blood is filtered in the glomeruli, because protein molecules are too large to pass through the tiny holes (fenestrae) in the kidney filters. However, the glomeruli can be damaged in renal disease, which allows protein to pass into the urine. Most proteinuria is identified by urinalysis using a dipstick. It is quite normal for small amounts of protein to be detected in urine during febrile illnesses or after excessive exercise and this would not require further investigation. Additional investigations would, however, be required if proteinuria continues as there are several causes, and the management would be determined dependent upon the diagnosis (Table 13.3).

Table 13.3 Some causes of proteinuria

Nephrotic syndrome
Glomerulonephritis
Renal dysplasia
Vesicouretric reflux (VUR)
Vasculitis
Orthostatic proteinuria
Acute kidney injury (AKI)
Renal tubular diseases – very rare in children, Fanconi syndrome, for example
Hypertension
Diabetes – rare in children very common in adults, known as diabetic nephropathy

Source: Adapted from infoKID; www.infokid.org.uk/ (accessed 6 December 2016).

Nephrotic syndrome

Nephrotic syndrome can occur at any age and it affects more boys than girls. It often starts when a child is between 2 and 5 years old. There is a congenital form of nephrotic syndrome, Finnish type which appears during the first year of life; however, it is very rare. There are different types of nephrotic syndrome which are classified according to whether steroid drugs treat and resolve the symptoms, or what the causes of the symptoms are. Sometimes it is not possible to know what type of nephrotic syndrome children have until they have tried a course of steroid treatment.

Children with nephrotic syndrome present with classical clinical signs:

- periorbital oedema, especially first thing in the morning after waking
- generalised oedema, scrotal, vulval, leg and ankle
- breathlessness due to pleural effusions and abdominal distension from ascites.

The amount of protein in the urine can be so large that the urine appears 'frothy' and is so full of albumin that it looks like the white of an egg. For 85–90% of children, the proteinuria resolves with corticosteroid therapy, the so-called steroid-sensitive nephrotic syndrome. Complications, for example, hypovolemia, thrombosis and infection, require close monitoring and the nursing team should be mindful of the following assessment needs:

- temperature min. every 4 hours
- pulse min. every 4 hours
- respirations min. every 4 hours
- blood pressure min. every 4 hours
- weight – this is commonly done twice a day.

It may be necessary to undertake vital signs more frequently depending on the child's clinical status.

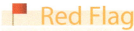

Red Flag

Nursing consideration

Careful hydration assessment is needed for children with nephrotic syndrome as they often have generalised oedema giving the impression of being hypervolemic when in reality they are much more likely to be hypovolemic. Large losses of plasma proteins (proteinuria) impact on osmotic and colloid osmotic pressure, which causes intravascular fluid to move from the intravascular space into the interstitial space.

In summary, the majority of children who have nephrotic syndrome respond to steroid therapy, and while they may have relapses, they usually grow out of it. For further detail on some general renal nursing principles, please see the section on this later in the chapter.

Disorders of the renal system   Chapter 13

Glomerulonephritis

Glomerulonephritis is a type of kidney disease that involves the glomeruli, which sit in the Bowman's capsule in the nephron (Fig. 13.3). During glomerulonephritis, the glomeruli become inflamed, which impacts on the kidney's ability to filter urine normally. There are many causes of glomerulonephritis, for example:

- acute glomerulonephritis is a common condition in children following a streptococcal infection, often referred to as post-streptococcal glomerulonephritis (PSGN);
- systemic immune disease, such as systemic lupus erythematosus (SLE or lupus) – very rare in children;
- other systemic diseases which are also rare in children: polyarteritis nodosa and Wegener vasculitis, which are inflammatory diseases of the arteries, and Henoch–Schönlein purpura;
- Alport syndrome, which is an inherited disease.

Children who present with glomerulonephritis can have a wide variety of signs and symptoms. The most common are listed in Table 13.4.

Diagnosis is made on the history and physical examination, supported by a variety of tests, which may include the following;

- Urinalysis – laboratory examination of urine to assess for infection, and to accurately measure the amount of protein in the urine. In the case of haematuria, to count the number and types of blood cells.
- Blood tests, as well as a full blood count and urea and electrolytes tests, will be undertaken to look for antibodies and measure complement levels, which will provide information linked to infections. An estimation of the eGFR (estimated glomerular filtration rate) will also be performed.
- Renal ultrasound scan to look at the shape and size of the kidneys.
- Chest X-ray, especially if the child presents with breathing problems.

The management and nursing care of children with glomerulonephritis is very much dependent upon the presenting symptoms and the underlying cause. Some children may

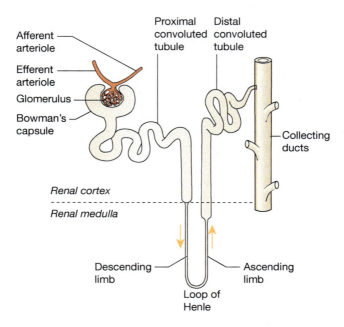

Figure 13.3   The nephron. *Source:* Peate & Gormley-Fleming 2015.

Table 13.4 Possible signs and symptoms of glomerulonephritis

Haematuria and proteinuria	Urine looks dark brown in colour
Fluid overloaded	Hypertensive
	Increase in body weight
	Oedema
	Headaches
	Seizures
	Reduced urine output (oliguria)
	Increased respiratory rate
Changes in physical appearance	Pale skin colour
	Skin rash, especially over the buttocks and legs
	Lethargic
Other	Sore throat
	Decreased appetite

Source: Adapted from Children's Hospital of Philadelphia n.d. (accessed 6 December 2016).

need to have some dietary restrictions, for example, a no added salt diet, or a fluid restriction. Others may need to take medication, for example, antibiotics, antihypertensives and diuretics. On rare occasions children may be prescribed immunosuppressive drugs, and in even rarer cases may require dialysis.

In summary, there are several causes of glomerulonephritis, the most common of which is associated with a streptococcal infection of the throat. For the majority of children the disease is mild, responds well to treatment and does not cause any long-term renal disease.

Henoch–Schönlein purpura

Henoch–Schönlein purpura (HSP) is a condition that can affect people of all ages; however, it is most often seen in children between the ages of 3 and 10 years, and is twice as common in boys. It is more common during the winter months and is frequently preceded by an upper respiratory tract infection.

Children with HSP often present with a fever, and have a rash that is characteristically symmetrically distributed over the buttocks, feet and ankles, backs of legs, lower back and arms. Children with HSP also commonly complain of pain in their joints and abdominal colic-like pain. Intussusception (see Chapter 14) can occur. Although renal involvement is common, it is not usually the first symptom (Lissaur & Clayden, 2007).

Most children with HSP do not need special treatment, and many will be monitored as outpatients. The mainstay of treatment is symptom management, i.e., analgesia for joint pain. After several days or a few weeks, the majority of children begin to feel better and the rash and other symptoms disappear. HSP sometimes comes back, usually within a few months, and may need further treatment. A few children have long-term problems, especially when their kidneys are affected. They will need to be monitored and may need specialist paediatric nephrology follow-up.

Medication Alert

Non-steroidal anti-inflammatory drugs (NSAIDs), for example, ibuprofen (e.g., Brufen®) are known to cause kidney damage and should be avoided as an analgesic in children with renal disease.

Haematuria

Haematuria indicates the presence of red blood cells in the urine. Urine does not normally contain red blood cells because these are too large to pass through the tiny holes (fenestrae) in the kidney filters. However, the glomeruli can be damaged in renal disease, which allows blood to pass into the urine. Microscopic haematuria means that the blood can only be detected during microscopy. Gross haematuria means the urine appears red in colour. Microscopic haematuria in healthy children does not usually need to be investigated unless it is present in at least three urine tests over several months. However, if a child has other symptoms, for example, hypertension or proteinuria, further investigations are warranted.

Haematuria is a common finding in children and has many causes, which include the following:

- abnormal structures in the urinary tract (renal cysts)
- inherited diseases (Alport syndrome)
- mineral imbalances in the urine (hypercalciuria causing renal stones – calculi)
- glomerulonephritis
- idiopathic, where no cause of haematuria is found.

In summary, care and management of children with haematuria may be minimal to complex depending on the underlying cause.

Chronic kidney disease

Chronic kidney disease (CKD) is characterised by permanent deterioration of renal function that gradually progresses to end-stage renal disease (ESRD). Congenital disorders, including congenital anomalies of the kidney and urinary tract, are responsible for about 66% of all cases of CKD in children in developed countries. All data on CKD in adults and children is reported to the UK Renal Registry by the specialist renal units across the UK and Ireland. An annual report is published by the UK Renal Registry, a section being dedicated to an analysis of CKD data in children. The last UK Renal Registry (2015) reported that a total of 917 children and young people under 18 years with established renal failure (ERF) were receiving treatment at paediatric nephrology centres in 2014. This clearly demonstrates that CKD is very rare in children and out of these, 79.3% had a functioning kidney transplant, 11.2% were receiving haemodialysis, and 9.5% were receiving peritoneal dialysis (UK Renal Registry, 2015). There are a variety of causes of CKD (Table 13.5), the most common primary renal diagnosis being renal dysplasia with reflux.

Understanding normal renal function (Peate & Gormley-Fleming, 2015) will enable you to appreciate the physiological consequences of CKD (Table 13.6), and to recognise the need for multidisciplinary specialist paediatric nephrology services. CKD is classified into

Table 13.5 Causes of CKD in children

Renal dysplasia with reflux
Obstructive uropathy
Glomerular disease
Congenital nephrotic syndrome
Tubulo-interstitial disease
Renovascular disease
Polycystic kidney disease
Metabolic
Malignancy and associated disease

Source: UK Renal Registry 2015.

Table 13.6 Consequences of CKD

Functions of the kidney	Clinical consequence of CKD
Fluid balance	Reduced/no urine output (oliguria/anuria) leading to fluid overload, peripheral oedema, pulmonary oedema, shortness of breath.
Removal of waste	Uraemia which causes nausea, vomiting and loss of appetite. Persistent itchy skin (pruritus) due to uraemia.
Renin and angiotensin secretion	Reduced blood supply (hypoperfusion) to damaged nephrons causes increased secretion of renin, angiotensin and aldosterone causing hypertension.
Erythropoietin (EPO) secretion	Reduced production of EPO and the circulation of toxic waste substances cause renal anaemia. Anorexia and lethargy, failure to thrive.
Vitamin D synthesis	Without vitamin D synthesis phosphate is retained and calcium levels drop (hypocalcaemia), which results in secondary hyperparathyroidism. If left untreated bones become painful, brittle and are prone to fracture (rickets, renal bone disease). Red eyes of uraemia, due to high plasma phosphate levels.
Acid–base balance	Reduction in the secretion of hydrogen ions culminates in metabolic acidosis.
Electrolyte balance	Hyperkalaemia causing heart arrhythmia. Kidneys normally excrete 90% of daily potassium intake.

Table 13.7 Stages of CKD and GFR

Stage	GFR	Kidney function	What this means
1	90 or higher	Normal, but other signs of kidney disease	Normally no symptoms
2	60–89	Mildly reduced	Normally no symptoms
3a	45–59	Moderately reduced	Normally no symptoms
3b	30–44	Moderately reduced	Children may start to have symptoms of CKD
4	15–29	Severely reduced	Many children have more symptoms of CKD. Start to plan for treatment options for next stage
5	Less than 15	Very severely reduced and cannot support the body	This is also called end-stage renal failure (ESRF) or established renal failure. Children are started on treatments, including dialysis and kidney transplantation

Source: infoKid; www.infokid.org.uk/ (accessed 6 December 2016).

five stages (Table 13.6), which are defined by the GFR. The GFR measures the volume in millilitres (mL) filtered by the kidneys each minute (min), which is an indication of kidney function. This is adjusted for children against a standard adult body size, which has a surface area of 1.73 square metres (m^2).

Table 13.7 describes the stages of CKD and GFR.

Unfortunately there is no cure for CKD. Treatment options include the following:

- Peritoneal dialysis (PD) (Fig. 13.4)
    - A treatment that uses the peritoneal membrane as a filter to remove waste and fluid. The peritoneal cavity is filled with dialysate fluid, which sits in the cavity for several hours allowing the peritoneum to filter the blood. The dialysate fluid is then drained out into a waste bag and fresh dialysate is replaced into the peritoneal cavity. PD is done at home either several times a day or overnight.

Disorders of the renal system Chapter 13

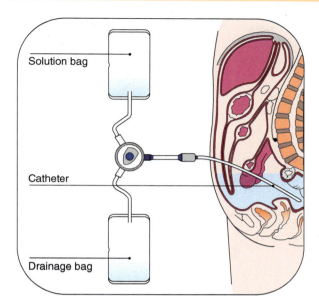

Figure 13.4   Peritoneal dialysis.

- Haemodialysis (HD) (Fig. 13.5)
    - Blood is pumped out of the body and into a haemodialysis filter (dialyser), often referred to as an 'artificial kidney', either by a central venous catheter or via an arteriovenous fistula; the blood is then returned to the body. This filter removes waste products and excess water. Each dialysis session takes 3–4 hours, and is done three or more times a week. It is commonly done in a specialist children's haemodialysis unit; however, some older children are able to do haemodialysis at home.
- Renal transplantation (Fig. 13.6)
    - This treatment is considered the best for children as it allows them to return to a much more normal way of life without the constraints of dialysis.
        - Types of transplantation:
            - Deceased donor transplant or a cadaveric transplant, where the deceased person has consented to organ donation.
            - Living donor is a living person (an adult) who agrees to give one of his or her two healthy kidneys to a recipient. The living donor is usually related to the child.
            - Altruistic donation, in this situation the donor does not usually know the recipient. An altruistic donor is a living donor.
- Supportive treatment
    - Unfortunately, in some cases the right option for the child and family is the decision not to have dialysis or a transplant. The child and family will be offered supportive treatment with the aim being to treat and control the symptoms of CKD focusing on family-centered care, which includes medical, psychological and practical support.

In summary, CKD is rare in children. It has many causes, the most common of which is associated with structural congenital malformations, which require the support of a specialist paediatric renal team to provide holistic family-centred care. There is no cure for CKD; however, with dialysis and transplantation many children with CKD now find themselves being transferred to adult renal units in their late teens.

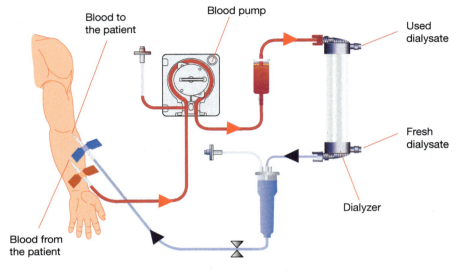

Figure 13.5 Haemodialysis.

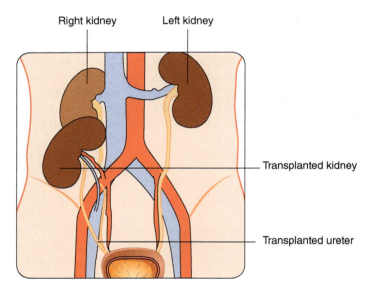

Figure 13.6 Renal transplantation.

Acute kidney injury

Acute kidney injury (AKI) can be defined as 'an abrupt decline in renal function resulting in loss of water, electrolyte and acid–base regulation, with collection of nitrogenous waste material in the body'. This produces disturbance of water, electrolyte, acid–base balance, and nitrogenous waste products and blood pressure. In order to understand the consequences of AKI you need to fully understand normal renal function as described by Peate & Gormley-Fleming (2015).

Like CKD, AKI is classified into stages (Table 13.8). AKI is much more common in children than CKD, and there are many causes. These are classified as follows:

- Pre-renal – the most common, resulting from compromised renal perfusion
  - Hypovolaemia from haemorrhage, dehydration, hypoxia, reduced cardiac output, vasodilation (warm shock), sepsis.
- Intrarenal or intrinsic – as a result of damage to the nephrons (acute tubular necrosis [ATN])
  - Acute glomerulonephritis, uric acid nephropathy (tumour lysis syndrome), renal vein thrombosis, haemolytic uraemic syndrome, pyelonephritis.
- Postrenal – due to urinary tract obstruction (congenital or acquired)
  - Posterior urethral valves, neurogenic bladder, phimosis, renal stone, blood clot, blocked urinary catheter.

Table 13.8 Classification of AKI

Stage	Serum creatinine	Urine output
1	eGFR < 75 mL/min/1.73 m^2 or decrease in eGFR by 25% or increase creatinine 1.5–2 × baseline	<0.5 mL/kg/h for 6 hours
2	eGFR < 50 mL/min/1.73 m^2 or decrease in eGFR by 50% or increase creatinine 2–3 × baseline	<0.5 mL/kg/h for 12 hours
3	eGFR < 35 mL/min/1.73 m^2 or decrease in eGFR by 75% or increase creatinine > 3 × baseline or requirement for renal replacement therapy	<0.3 mL/kg/h for 24 hours Or anuria for 12 hours

Source: Nottingham Children's Hospital 2014.

Red Flag

Nursing consideration
When caring for children with a urinary catheter, if the hourly urine output drops, never assume that this is an absolute finding until you have considered the patency of the catheter. You may need to discuss the need to undertake a catheter flush to ascertain the patency of the catheter.

Medication Alert

Several drugs are known to cause AKI, for example;
- prostaglandin synthetase inhibitors (ibuprofen)
- angiotensin-converting enzymes (ACE) inhibitors (lisinipril, enalapril)
- angiotensin receptor blockers (losartan)
- diuretics
- calcineurin inhibitors (cyclosporine A, tacrolimus)

During your nursing assessment take particular note of the medication that child has been prescribed or which has been bought over the counter.

Depending on the extent of the AKI and the involvement of other organs, children may be nursed either in paediatric intensive care units, on paediatric high-dependency units, or in paediatric renal units. Nursing care of these children focuses on an ABC approach where life-threatening features must be addressed in the first instance, for example:

- hydration, oxygenation, electrolyte derangements
- oedema
- blood pressure
- close monitoring
    - weight
    - 1 hourly input–output
    - 1 hourly PEWS, for example
    - 6-hourly BMs.

While dialysis can and does sometimes play a part in the overall management of children with AKI, it is an invasive treatment that is not without significant risks. Therefore careful consideration of the following will be taken when deciding whether or not to commence specialist dialysis therapies:

- clinical status
    - hyperkalaemia > 6.5 mmol/L
    - urea > 40 mmol/L (>30 mmol/L in neonates)
    - severe hypo-/hypernatraemia or acidosis
    - uraemia with bleeding and/or encephalopathy
    - anticipation of prolonged oliguria (i.e., haemolytic uraemic syndrome)
    - intoxications
    - inborn errors of metabolism (IEM)
    - need for nutritional support
- degree of fluid overload
- involvement of multiple organ systems
- metabolic/electrolyte imbalance.

In summary, the definitions and characterisation of AKI in children have advanced significantly over the past two decades. It is common in critically ill children and is associated with increased morbidity and mortality. When it is associated with sepsis, multiple organ involvement and fluid overload, it carries heightened risk. Treatment of AKI is problematic, but the use of renal replacement therapies in AKI and multiple organ system failure continue to grow in use and potential benefit (Fortenberry, Paden & Goldstein, 2013).

Haemolytic uraemic syndrome

Haemolytic uraemic syndrome (HUS) is a rare severe, life-threatening condition that can lead to acute kidney injury in children. However, more than 85% of children with the most common form of HUS recover complete kidney function. It is more common during the summer months and may occur in outbreaks. Outbreaks have been reported in nursery schools, following farm visits, and from fast-food restaurants as a result of inadequately cooked beef burgers.

There are several known and some unknown causes of HUS. The most common cause in children occurs following an infection with the *Escherichia coli* (*E. coli*) O157:H7 or other Shiga toxin-producing *E. coli*, which may be found in contaminated food, such as dairy products and meat. The toxins produced by these bacteria damage the small blood vessels in the kidney and they also cause haemolysis (breakdown of red blood cells). HUS can also develop as a result of taking certain medications or may result from a cancer present in the body, although these causes are less common. Some rare cases of HUS are familial, known as atypical HUS, which suggests a genetic link.

The children often present with the following common symptoms which can last for over 2 weeks:

- bloody or watery diarrhoea
- vomiting
- severe dehydration from the diarrhoea and vomiting
- acute abdominal pain – sometimes leading to severe bowel or colon problems
- fever
- irritability
- fatigue and pale skin – due to severe reduction in red blood cell count as a result of haemolysis
- small bruises in mouth – as a result of alteration in normal clotting from the bacterial toxins.

As the kidneys become involved, symptoms of AKI develop, for example, hypertension, raised urea, creatinine and potassium levels, and reduced urine output leading to fluid overload (oedema). Diagnosis is made using a combination of tests:

- blood samples for urea and electrolytes and full blood count and clotting screen
- stool culture
- abdominal X-ray
- urinalysis to assess for haematuria and proteinuria.

Management for children with HUS focuses on close monitoring, correction and management of hydration, management of blood pressure, prevention of infection, correction of anaemia through blood transfusions, correction of electrolyte imbalance, provision of adequate nutrition, and potentially haemodialysis. Due to the acute nature of this illness children will require treatment by paediatric nephrologists in specialist renal units and may be cared for in paediatric intensive care units depending on the severity of their illness.

In summary, HUS is a life-threatening illness that requires specialist nursing care and management. Thankfully the majority of children make a full recovery with no lasting chronic renal damage. Prevention is always better than cure so it is always worth reminding families to pay particular attention to the following:

- Good hand hygiene with soap and water – hand gels/wipes do not remove *E.coli* 0157 (infoKID)
  - pay attention to strict hygiene when visiting community farms, parks or camping sites.
- Cook all meats thoroughly especially meats cooked on barbeques, and wash salads thoroughly; pay particular attention to food storage and preparation recommendations.

Wilms' tumour

Every year in the UK around 90 children are diagnosed with renal tumours, 90% of these cases are Wilms' tumour (also known as nephroblastoma). Wilms' tumour mainly affects children less than 5 years of age with peak incidence between 1 and 3 years. Wilms' tumours can be unilateral or bilateral, and girls are twice as likely to be diagnosed with bilateral tumours (Children with Cancer UK, 2016).

The most common symptom of a renal tumour is a swelling in the abdomen, which is usually painless. Sometimes the child may have haematuria and be hypertensive. They may also present with a fever, diarrhoea and vomiting, weight loss or loss of appetite.

Table 13.9 Staging Wilms' tumour

Stage 1 – the tumour is only affecting the kidney and has not begun to spread. It can be completely removed with surgery.
Stage 2 – the tumour has begun to spread beyond the kidney to nearby structures, but it is still possible to remove it completely with surgery.
Stage 3 – the tumour has spread beyond the kidney, either because it has burst before or during the operation, or because it has spread to the lymph glands, or because it has not been completely removed by surgery.
Stage 4 – the tumour has spread (metastasized) to other parts of the body, such as the lungs or liver.
Stage 5 – there are tumours in both kidneys (bilateral Wilms' tumour).

Source: Children with Cancer UK 2016; http://www.childrenwithcancer.org.uk/wilms-tumour.

A variety of tests and investigations will be undertaken, which will include the following:

- urine and blood samples to check kidney function
- an abdominal ultrasound scan and CT
- scans of the chest and liver may be undertaken to check for any spread of the disease
- a biopsy of the tumour will be performed to assist in determining the type and stage (Table 13.9) of the tumour. This will help the paediatric oncologists to decide on the most suitable treatment.

Treatment for Wilms' tumour depends on a number of things, for example, the histology as well as the staging. Nephrectomy or partial nephrectomy may be performed either at diagnosis or following a course of chemotherapy to shrink the tumour, or occasionally radiotherapy may be used to shrink the tumour. Depending on the stage of the tumour, radiotherapy may also be required. For children with bilateral Wilms', the surgical goal is to remove as much of the tumour as possible, while leaving as much healthy kidney as possible (Children with Cancer UK, 2016).

All children with cancer must be cared for in specialist paediatric oncology centres. The majority of children with Wilms' tumour can be cured, with 90% of patients surviving to 5 years (Children with Cancer UK, 2016).

General medical renal nursing principles

A holistic family-centred approach is needed for children with renal medical disorders. However, there are some elements of nursing care provided to infants and children which have renal significance as detailed in the following.

1. Risk of hypertension – ensure the correct size BP cuff is used and that the size used is documented in the child's care plan; give antihypertensives as prescribed.
2. Risk of fluid overload due to reduced urine output – weigh twice a day, monitor and record input and output. Administer intravenous fluids as prescribed. Adhere to prescribed fluid restrictions – look out for 'hidden fluids' in foods, e.g. custard. Be alert for signs of dehydration as renal function recovers, obtain urine samples for urinalysis or laboratory assessment.
3. Risk of infection due to disease state – record vital signs, and document accurately; may require isolation nursing.
4. Potential to be prescribed several different medications, i.e. diuretics, antibiotics, antihypertensives and corticosteroids – ensure administration times and methods are adhered to and be alert for any medication complications.
5. May need dietary supplements and or dietary restrictions – liaise with the dietitian if renal-specific diets are required, for example, low sodium, low potassium, reduced

protein and/or high calorie. Stress the importance of adhering to the special diet with the child and family.
6. Risk of skin damage due to oedema and or reduced nutritional state – provide meticulous skin use local tissue viability assessment scale.

Surgical disorders of the upper urinary tract
Hydronephrosis

Hydronephrosis is a condition that can occur prenatally, where the baby's kidneys fill up with urine and become dilated. It affects the drainage of urine from the urinary system and in children who have mild or, sometimes, moderate hydronephrosis, kidney function is frequently unharmed. The likelihood of surgery depends on the cause and severity of the hydronephrosis. The hydronephrosis is monitored using ultrasound scans and sometimes other radioisotope scans. The overall treatment for children with hydronephrosis really depends on what is causing it.

- If the cause is related to vesicoureteric reflux (VUR), the child will probably be treated using antibiotics.
- If the cause is due to a blockage of the urinary system, the child may need an operation called a pyeloplasty to remove it.
- If the cause is a due to multicystic kidney disease, the affected kidney will shrivel up and disappear and therefore does not need to be removed. Occasionally, if the hydronephrosis is severe and causing other symptoms, for example, high blood pressure, it may be need to be removed (nephrectomy).

Ureteropelvic junction obstruction

The ureteropelvic junction (UPJ) is located where the pelvis of the kidney meets the ureter, a UPJ obstruction describes a blockage to this area. The obstruction hinders the flow of urine down to the bladder, causing the urine to back up in the kidney and dilate it (hydronephrosis) (Fig. 13.7). UPJ obstruction is the most common cause of paediatric hydronephrosis, the incidence being between 1 per 1000–2000 newborns (Children's Hospital of Philadelphia, n.d.).

If the hydronephrosis is severe and does cause a PUJ obstruction, surgery is required. The area of obstruction in the ureter is removed and the normal area is reconnected to the kidney. This procedure is called a pyeloplasty, which is often performed through small incisions, known as minimally invasive surgery (keyhole surgery). The main advantages of keyhole surgery are smaller, less visible incisions, less post-operative pain, and a much faster post-operative recovery period. A drainage tube (stent) may be left in place to allow urine to flow across the surgical area to promote healing. The primary aim of this surgery is to improve the drainage, which reduces the hydronephrosis and prevents further renal damage.

Nursing management focuses on ensuring the infant or child receives safe pre- and post-operative care with a specific focus on prevention of infection, adherence to fasting times, maintenance of hydration and reintroduction of oral fluids/food. It is particularly important to monitor urine output and take note of when urine is first passed post-surgery.

Nephrectomy

Nephrectomy is a surgical procedure to remove all or part of a kidney:

- complete (radical) nephrectomy – the entire kidney is removed;
- partial nephrectomy – only diseased tissue is removed leaving healthy kidney tissue in place.

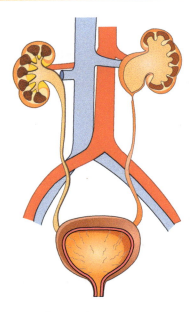

Figure 13.7 Ureteropelvic junction obstruction.

There are many reasons why kidneys may need to be removed, for example:

- cancer of the kidney, i.e., Wilms' tumour;
- kidney that has no remaining renal function and is causing symptoms of illness, i.e., pyelonephritis or hypertension;
- donor kidney for transplantation.

Most nephrectomies are performed using keyhole surgery (laparoscopically); however, occasionally traditional 'open' surgery may be needed if the kidney is very large or badly infected, for example. Whether the operation is done via a laparoscopic or open method, the surgeon ties off the blood vessels and removes the kidney through the incision.

The specific surgical nursing care for children who have had a nephrectomy focuses on the maintenance of a strict fluid balance with particular emphasis on the volume and colour of the child's urine. A wound drain may be in situ so careful monitoring of the volume drained off is important. The child may also have a urethral catheter in situ; this is usually removed 2 days after the operation and before the child is discharged home.

General surgical renal nursing principles

A holistic family-centred approach is essential for children with renal surgical disorders. However, there are some elements of nursing care for infants and children that have renal significance detailed as follows:

1. Risk of dehydration if surgery is delayed, which may compromise renal function; adhere to the preoperative evidence-based fasting recommendations (Smith *et al.*, 2011). Liaise with the theatre team if there is a delay.
2. Exclusion of a urinary tract infection (UTI) prior to surgery – obtain a clean-catch urine sample prior to surgery; perform a urinalysis and send a urine sample for microscopy and culture as requested.
3. Risk of UTI post-surgery – especially if a urinary catheter, nephrostomy tube or stent are in situ; adhere to local clinical guidelines on the management of these devices; monitor vital signs and obtain urine samples as requested.

Disorders of the renal system — Chapter 13

4. Risk of urinary retention post-surgery – document and report when urine is passed following return from theatre; monitor and document all urinary output.

Medical disorders of the lower urinary tract
Urinary tract infection

Urinary tract infection (UTI) is a common bacterial infection responsible for causing illness in infants and children worldwide. It has been estimated that UTIs are diagnosed in 1% of boys and 3–8% of girls (WHO, 2005). The diagnosis of UTI in infants and children can be problematic as the presenting symptoms and signs are often non-specific (Table 13.10). Confirmation of a UTI is dependent upon the collection of a clean uncontaminated urine sample, which can be particularly challenging from infants and young children.

The following methods of urine collection are recommended:

- a clean-catch urine sample
- if a clean-catch urine sample is not possible, the following can be used:
    - non-invasive urine collection pads; ensure you follow the manufacturer's instructions.
    - if it is not possible or practical, for example, when urine samples are needed as an emergency, to collect urine by non-invasive methods, catheter samples or suprapubic aspiration (SPA) under ultrasound guidance should be used (Marin et al., 2014).

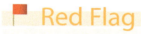

Red Flag

Nursing considerations

Cotton wool balls, gauze and sanitary towels should not be used to collect urine in infants and children as bactericidal agents incorporated in these materials may lead to false negative results.

Ideally, urine samples should be put under the microscope to identify organisms and cultured immediately. If this is not possible the urine sample must be refrigerated in order to prevent the overgrowth of bacteria. Treatment with antibiotics will depend upon the

Table 13.10 Symptoms and signs of UTI in infants and children

Age group	Most common	Symptoms and signs		Least common
Infants younger than 3 months	Fever Vomiting Lethargy Irritability	Poor feeding Failure to thrive		Abdominal pain Jaundice Haematuria Offensive urine
Infants and children, 3 months or older	**Pre-verbal**	Fever	Abdominal pain Loin tenderness Vomiting Poor feeding	Lethargy Irritability Haematuria Offensive urine Failure to thrive
	Verbal	Frequency Dysuria	Dysfunctional voiding Changes to continence Abdominal pain Loin tenderness	Fever Malaise Vomiting Haematuria Offensive urine Cloudy urine

Source: National Institute of Health and Care Excellence, Clinical guideline [CG54] 2007.

causative organism, and infants and children may need to undergo further investigations, for example:

- renal ultrasound scan
- DMSA scan
- micturating cystourethrogram.

In summary, UTIs are common in childhood. The nursing management and treatment of infants and children with UTIs are dependent upon the collection of a clean uncontaminated urine sample that is transported to the laboratory quickly to avoid the risk of false positive or false negative results. Parents are often skilled at catching urine samples as they have a vested interest to do so. It is important that parents are given good instruction on how to do this and reminded about the importance of administering the full prescribed course of antibiotics to their children.

Daytime wetting (enuresis)

According to ERIC (Enuresis Resource Information Centre) daytime wetting affects 1 in 75 children aged 5 and above. It is usual for younger children to have wetting accidents as part of the toilet-training process but as children get older, daytime wetting can be more difficult to manage at school or in social situations. It is known to be more common in girls and younger children, and for most children there is no serious underlying disorder.

There are several causes of daytime wetting. These include:

- UTI – can cause irritation of the bladder and urinary frequency. Sometimes the bladder does not empty completely, which perpetuates the problem;
- not consistently dry in the day following toilet training;
- constipation – due to the close proximity of the bowel to the bladder, a full bowel pressing on the bladder can prevent the bladder from emptying completely;
- stress and anxiety;
- overactive bladder (urge incontinence) – a form of urinary incontinence, which is the involuntary release of urine. Children with overactive bladders need to urinate frequently and, at times, urgently. As a consequence they may not make it to the toilet in time and urine leaks from the bladder.

The nursing assessment of these children is essential as it will form the basis of an appropriate management plan. The nursing management and care plan will commonly include:

- exclusion of or management of UTI;
- exclusion or management of constipation;
- ensure the child is drinking at least 6–8 cups of water a day;
- develop a regular toileting routine, sometimes with the help of a vibrating watch to remind them to go to the toilet;
- advise the child to take their time when going to the toilet.

Nursing tips for parents and children is to reinforce the fact that daytime wetting is not uncommon and can be treated but it may take some time and definitely requires commitment from the child and family in adhering to treatment plans. On rare occasions these young children may need to be referred to a nephrologist or urologist if conventional management has not been successful. In these cases further investigations may be needed, for example, urodynamic studies and the prescription of oxybutynin, an anticholinergic drug.

Nocturnal enuresis (bed wetting)

This is categorised into two types:

1. Primary nocturnal enuresis – involuntary urination during sleep by a child aged 5 years or older, who has never achieved consistent night-time dryness. It may be due to

excessive urine production at night, poor sleep arousal and/or reduced bladder capacity.
2. Secondary nocturnal enuresis – involuntary urination during sleep by a child who has previously been dry for at least 6 months.

Children with nocturnal enuresis may also have daytime urinary urgency, frequency or incontinence of urine. Children with a family history of nocturnal enuresis have a higher incidence of small bladder capacity and up to 23% of children who are wet at night are constipated and have associated daytime incontinence (ERIC).

A full nursing assessment is needed and should focus on, for example:

- the number of times a night and how many nights a week?
- the volume of urine in the bed
- whether there is any pattern to the bedwetting
- ask whether the child wakes up after wetting the bed
- establish what the daytime continence is like – children who are continent during the day will attain night-time continence
- identify if there are any other issues, for example, constipation or soiling, developmental delay, behavioural problems.

The nursing management and care for these children are very similar to that of the child with daytime enuresis. Other management strategies which can help are to encourage the child to empty their bladder before bed, and ensure there is access to the toilet at night. If they wake during the night it is a good idea to take them to the toilet before they settle back to sleep. The use of positive reward systems may be useful, for example, offering a reward for drinking the right quantities during the day, toilet before bed.

In summary, daytime bladder control always comes before night-time and children who are continent in the day will get dry during the night – it just might take a little longer.

Balanitis

This is inflammation of the glans penis and often the foreskin (NICE, 2015). It can be acute, chronic, or recurrent and can be caused by:

- trauma
- skin conditions
- exposure to irritants – soap and bubble bath, for example
- infection – *Candida* (thrush), streptococcal infection.

The nursing management includes identifying the cause through a full nursing history. Children, parents or carers should be advised to clean the penis with lukewarm water and dry gently. They should also be advised not to make any attempt to retract the foreskin to clean under it, if it is still fixed. Wherever possible soap, bubble bath, or baby wipes should not be used. If the child is still in nappies these should be changed frequently. If infection is the cause then appropriate topical antibiotic or antiviral creams will be prescribed, and in some cases of bacterial infection a course of oral antibiotics may be required.

Epididymitis

This is a very painful condition resulting from infection or inflammation of the epididymis (Fig. 13.8), which is the tube-shaped structure connected to the testicle (Bevan, 2015). It is caused by the spread of a bacterial infection from the urethra or the bladder. It often develops as a result of inflammation from direct trauma, torsion of the appendix epididymis (a small appendage on the top of the epididymis), or reflux of urine into the epididymis.

Boys typically complain of testicular pain, which increases in severity over time. The testicle becomes tender to touch, red and swollen. The boys may also complain of lower

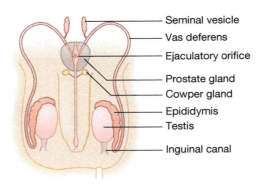

Figure 13.8 Male reproductive system. *Source:* Peate & Gormley-Fleming 2015. Reproduced with permission of Wiley.

abdominal pain, dysuria, discharge from the urethra, and they may have a fever. In the majority of cases rest and analgesia will resolve the pain. Occasionally antibiotics are required if the cause is bacterial or if the child has UTI.

Surgical disorders of the lower urinary tract

Hydrocele

This is a collection of fluid in the scrotum, surrounding the testicle, which can occur on one or both sides; despite this swelling, hydroceles are usually painless. Hydroceles occur more commonly in infants, especially premature infants, but can occur at any age. They are caused during embryonic development (Bevan, 2015).

There are several different types of hydroceles and treatment will vary according to the type. Some hydroceles disappear without treatment whereas others require surgical repair. A small incision is made in the groin (along a skin crease), the fluid is drained, and a portion of the hydrocele sac is removed.

Hypospadias

Hypospadias is a condition in which the meatus is not located at the tip of the penis, but somewhere on the underside of the glans or the shaft of the penis. Hypospadias is present in about 1 out of every 100 boys (Children's Hospital of Philadelphia, n.d.). Hypospadias is classified according to the location of the meatus on the penis. The opening can be located anywhere from just below the tip of the penis to the scrotum, and occasionally below the scrotum (Fig. 13.9).

Many different surgical approaches are used to correct hypospadias. The method chosen often depends on the surgeon's preference, and also on the position of the hypospadias. Surgical repair aims to correct the appearance of the meatal opening and overall appearance of the penis, as well as ensuring that it functions normally. During surgery a catheter (urethral stent) is stitched into the urethra to help maintain its shape and to prevent the risk of urinary obstruction as a result of post-operative inflammation. Some boys with severe hypospadias require extensive reconstructive surgery, which has to be done in stages.

🚩 Red Flag

Nursing consideration
It is important to advise parents of children with hypospadias that they should not be circumcised as the foreskin may be needed for the surgical repair.

Disorders of the renal system

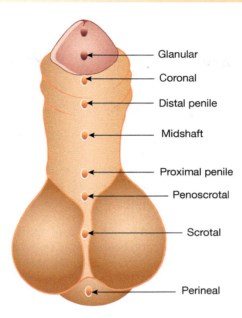

Figure 13.9 Classification of hypospadias.

The specific post-operative care for these boys is concerned with maintaining the stent in position to allow the urethra to heal. Dressings on the urethra need to be secure and the boys distracted from putting their hands down their nappies. The children are usually discharged with the dressing and stent in situ and parents are asked not to bathe the boys until the day they are brought back to the hospital when the dressing and stent will be removed. It is a good idea to ask the parents to give the children some analgesia on the morning they are due to have their dressing and stent removed.

Circumcision

Circumcision is a procedure that involves the removal of the foreskin of the penis. It can be performed for religious or medical reasons. The medical reasons for circumcision include the following:

- Non-retractable foreskin – in some boys, the foreskin can be retracted as early as infancy, in others not until 5 or 6 years of age. Once potty-trained, the uncircumcised boy should learn to retract his foreskin when he urinates and bathes and then pull it back forward again. If the foreskin cannot be pulled back this may increase a boy's chances of developing phimosis.
- Phimosis – is a constriction of the opening of the foreskin so that it cannot be drawn back over the glans of the penis. Phimosis is a normal occurrence in the newborn boy. Tight foreskins can sometimes cause bleeding and irritation, pain and stinging during micturition, and in some cases even cause an obstruction.
- Balanitis – inflammation of the head of the penis.
- Recurrent urinary tract infections.

Circumcision is usually carried out on a day-patient basis and is a reasonably simple procedure. The foreskin is removed just behind the head of the penis, and any bleeding is stopped using heat (cauterised). Dissolvable stitches are used to stitch the edges of skin and a dressing is applied. Children are usually discharged from hospital when they have passed urine. Parents should be advised to give regular analgesia and sometimes the wearing of loose pants and trousers is useful. They should be advised that it can take up to

6 weeks for the penis to heal completely, and that if there is any bleeding from the penis, or post-operative swelling has not resolved within 2 weeks, or if micturition is still painful after a couple of days, they should contact their GP or hospital.

Undescended testis (cryptorchidism)

Undescended testis is a common childhood condition of the lower urinary tract. For further information on this, please see Chapter 14.

Ureterovesical obstruction

The ureterovesical junction is where the ureter enters the bladder. Ureterovesical junction (UVJ) (Fig. 13.10) obstruction refers to a blockage in this area. The obstruction impedes the flow of urine down to the bladder, causing urine to back up into and dilate the ureters and kidney (megaureter and hydronephrosis).

UVJ obstruction generally occurs during fetal development. The obstruction is usually caused by narrowing of the connection between the ureter and the bladder. UVJ obstruction can also be due to scar tissue, infection or kidney stones. Radiological investigations, for example, renal ultrasound scan, MAG3 or MRI, may be undertaken to confirm the diagnosis.

The surgical correction of UVJ obstruction depends upon the cause and severity of obstruction. For example, in newborn babies with ureteral dilation (megaureter) or poor renal function, a temporary cutaneous distal ureterostomy may be recommended. During this procedure the ureter is brought to the abdominal surface and allows urine to drain into the nappy. This lets the affected kidney and ureter decompress and has the potential to preserve upper renal tract function, which is a key priority in this surgery. Sometime later the ureter will be reimplanted into the bladder. Sometimes ureteric reimplantation is the first procedure of choice. Reimplantation involves the removal of the ureter from the bladder; it is then reduced in size and reconnected (reimplanted) into the bladder.

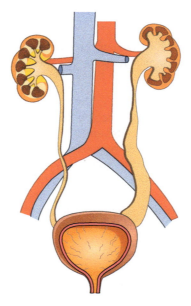

Figure 13.10   Ureterovesical junction obstruction.

Disorders of the renal system   Chapter 13

Vesicoureteric reflux

Vesicoureteric (or vesicoureteral) reflux (VUR) is quite a common condition, especially in babies and young children. When children with VUR micturate some urine refluxes back up the ureters towards the kidneys, it can be unilateral or bilateral. Children with VUR may be at greater risk of UTIs in their bladder (cystitis) or kidneys (pyelonephritis), and may need to take prophylactic antibiotics to prevent or treat infection (infoKID).

It is diagnosed by undertaking an MCUG, which grades the reflux from I to V (Fig. 13.11), by identifying the extent of reflux and whether it is unilateral or bilateral.

- Grades I and II are mild – children will be cared for as outpatients to monitor their renal function, and may be required to take prophylactic antibiotics.
- Grades III, IV and V are more serious – urine refluxes all the way to one or both kidneys, causing hydronephrosis and sometimes megaureter. In addition, the bladder may not empty completely. Children will be monitored closely by a paediatric nephrologist for signs of reflux nephropathy and will most likely be required to take prophylactic antibiotics. This higher grade often gets better over time. It was common for children with higher grades of VUR to have surgery to correct the reflex; however, nowadays surgery is only occasionally required. If the child gets recurrent UTIs this would be an indication for surgery.

There are two surgical approaches:

1. Endoscopic surgery – this is performed as a day case under general anaesthetic via cystoscopy. It allows the surgeon to visualise the ureteric orifice. A substance, called Deflux®, is injected into the area where the ureter enters the bladder, which helps to prevent urine from refluxing back into the ureter.
2. Ureteric reimplantation – as described earlier in the section on UVJ obstruction.

In summary, surgical correction for VUR is reserved for infants and children who have recurrent UTIs and whose upper renal tracts are at risk of renal damage (reflux nephropathy). The mainstay of treatment is prevention of UTIs through the use of prophylactic antibiotics.

Posterior urethral valves

Posterior urethral valves (PUV) (Fig. 13.12) are obstructive membranes that develop in the urethra close to the bladder during embryonic development. The abnormality affects only male infants and occurs in about 1 in 8000 births. This disorder is usually sporadic (occurs by chance). However, some cases have been seen in twins and siblings, suggesting a genetic link (Children's Hospital of Philadelphia, n.d.).

Treatment depends on the severity of the PUV, the child's age, and the degree of kidney involvement. The surgical goal is always to preserve both kidney and bladder functions (Children's Hospital of Philadelphia, n.d.).

Surgical correction can be undertaken in one of two ways:

1. Valve ablation: Once PUV are identified, they need to be surgically incised. During valve ablation, the urologist will insert a cystoscope, a small device with a light and a camera lens at the end. S/he will use this instrument to make incisions in the valves so they collapse and no longer obstruct the urethra.
2. Vesicostomy: In a situation where the baby is too small to undergo valve ablation or when a severe obstruction is noted, a vesicostomy may be recommended. A vesicostomy

Chapter 13　　　　　　　　　　　　　　　　　Disorders of the renal system

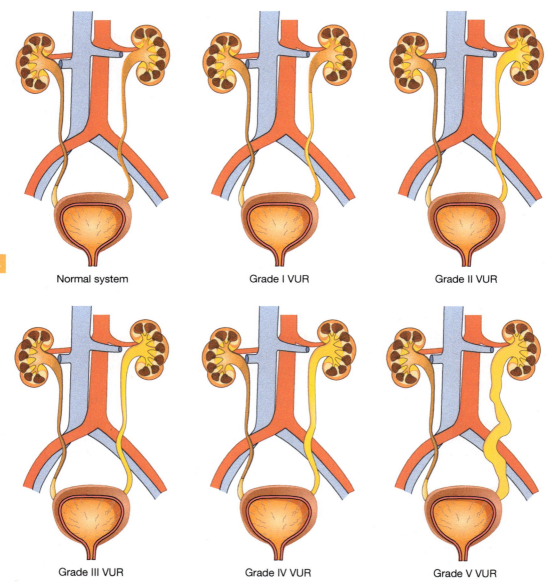

Figure 13.11　Stages of vesicoureteric reflux.

provides an opening to the bladder, so that urine drains freely from the lower abdominal opening. During surgery, a small part of the bladder wall is turned inside out and sewn to the abdomen. It looks like a small slit, surrounded by pink tissue. The vesicostomy is a temporary option and can be closed in the future.

The valves cause an obstruction to outflow of urine from the bladder, which leads to increasing dilatation of the bladder, ureters and kidneys, which in turn causes damage to the kidneys.

Disorders of the renal system Chapter 13

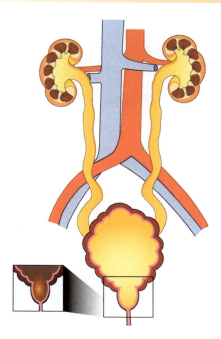

Figure 13.12 Posterior urethral valves.

Case Study 1

Emily, aged 4, is brought to the local emergency department by her dad with severe abdominal pain, bloody watery diarrhoea and vomiting; she is febrile with a temperature of 38.6 °C and is very pale and lethargic. Her dad reports that Emily began to feel unwell 2 days ago following a family trip to a local community farm where she and her older brother Josh had enjoyed petting some sheep and rabbits and bottle-fed a baby goat. Emily's parents are divorced and mum is away on a business trip and is not aware that Emily is unwell. Following a full nursing and medical assessment and a collection of investigations, it is confirmed that Emily has acute kidney injury due to haemolytic uraemic syndrome (HUS) and requires specialist paediatric nephrology care. This is not available locally but at a hospital some 50 miles away.

Emily has never been in hospital before and dad is really worried about how she will cope with this and how he will be able to look after both children and get to and from the specialist children's renal unit. Emily's dad calls his parents and breaks the frightening news to them. Emily's grandparents agree to come straight to the local hospital to collect Josh.

An ambulance is arranged to transfer Emily and her dad to the specialist children's renal unit. Emily's dad is very upset and is blaming himself for taking his children to the community farm; he is also concerned that Josh might develop the same illness.

- What information about HUS would you give to Emily and her dad?
- How will you prepare them for their transfer to the specialist children's renal unit?

While in the emergency department, Emily's observations are recorded on a PEWS chart (see Fig. 13.13).

- What actions would you take based on Emily's last score?
- How would you explain your actions to Emily and her dad?

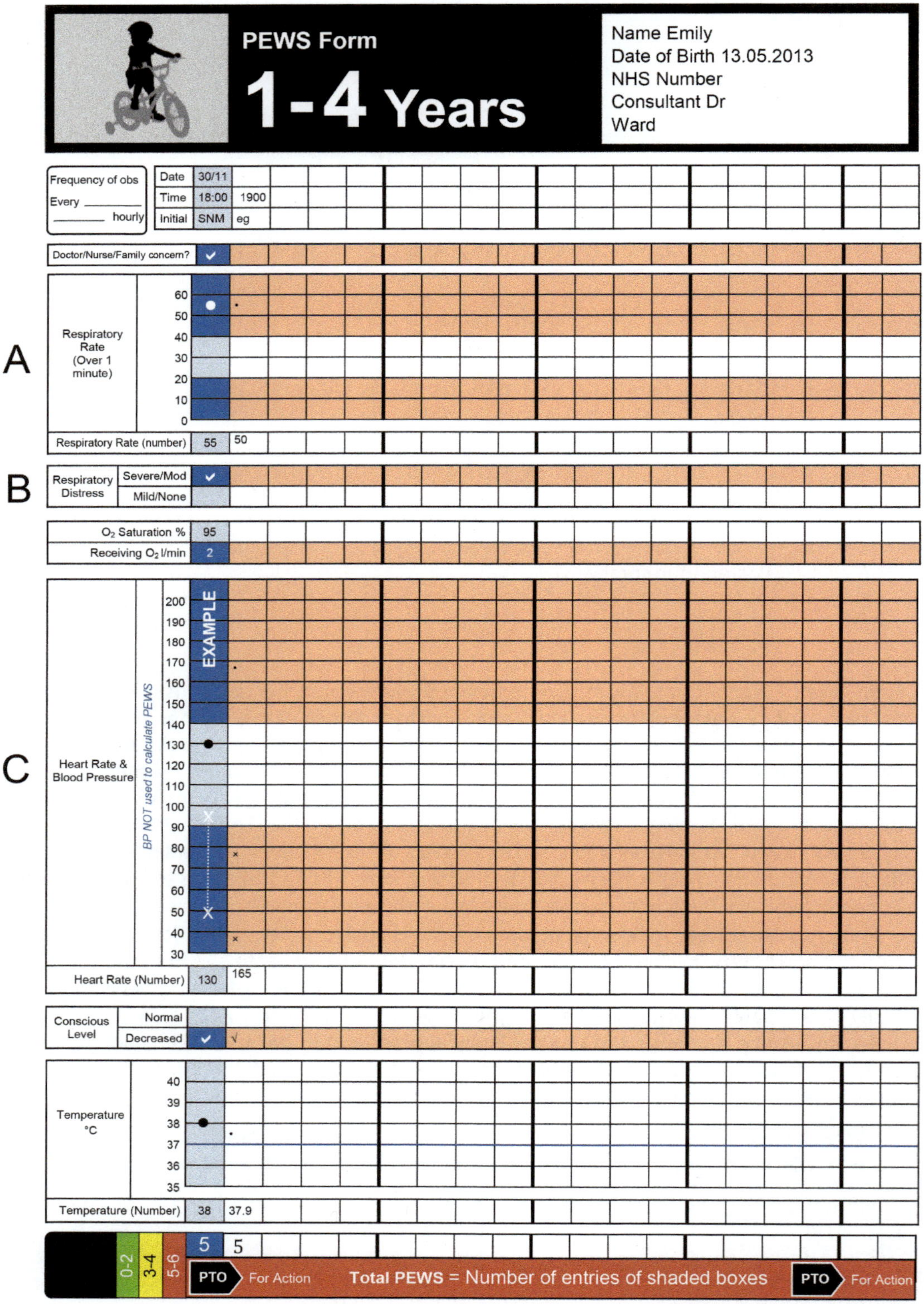

Figure 13.13 PEWS chart for Emily.

Disorders of the renal system — Chapter 13

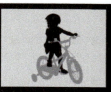

PEWS Form
1-4 Years

Name Emily
Date of Birth 13.05.2013
NHS Number
Consultant Dr
Ward

PEWS Escalation Aid

S — **Situation:**
I am (name), a nurse on ward (X)
I am calling about (child X)
I am calling because I am concerned that...
(e.g. BP is low/high, pulse is XXX
temperature is XX, Early Warning Score is XX)

B — **Background:**
Child (X) was admitted on (XX date) with
(e.g. respiratory infection)
They have had (X operation/procedure/investigation)
Child (X)'s condition has changed in the last (XX mins)
Their last set of obs were (XXX)
The child's normal condition is...
(e.g. alert/drowsy/confused, pain free)

A — **Assessment:**
I think the problem is (XXX)
and I have...
(e.g. given O2 /analgesia, stopped the infusion)
OR
I am not sure what the problem is but child (X)
is deteriorating
OR
I don't know what's wrong but I am really worried

R — **Recommendation:**
I need you to...
Come to see the child in the next (XX mins)
AND
Is there anything I need to do in the meantime?
(e.g. stop the fluid/repeat the obs)

Download SBAR prompt cards and pads at
www.institute.nhs.uk/SBAR

Remember: If you feel you need more help at any time, call for help – regardless of PEW Score

0 1	Continue monitoring	
2	Nurse in charge MUST review	
3	Nurse in charge & Doctor MUST review	
4	Nurse in charge & Doctor MUST review & inform Consultant	
5 6	Nurse in charge & Consultant MUST review	

307

Record Call When PEWS 3 Or More				Record Time of Review, Who by & Plan		
Date	Time	PEWS	Print Name (nurse)	Time	Plan	Print Name
01/01/12	09:00	5	SN ...	09:15	ED consultant called Anaesthetic review	Sister ...
30/11/2017	1900	5	SN ...	1905	Paed Registrar called to review. Consultant contacted.	Sr ...

NHS Institute for Innovation and Improvement

Download documents to use or edit at
www.institute.nhs.uk/PEWScharts

© NHS Institute for Innovation and Improvement 2012

Figure 13.13 (continued)

Case Study 2

Ben, aged 18 months, is admitted as a planned admission to the local children's hospital for surgical correction of his mid-shaft hypospadias. He is accompanied by his mum, Alice, who is 18 years old, and Ben's grandmother. Alice is going to be staying in hospital with Ben. His surgery is scheduled to take place at 4 p.m. that day, it is now 9 a.m.

- What advice would you give to Alice about Ben's fasting time prior to his surgery?
- What preoperative care and assessment would you provide?

Ben returns from theatre at 5.30 p.m. following his surgery. He has a dressing around his penis and a urethral stent in situ. He recovers well following his anaesthetic and asks for a drink almost as soon as he is back on the ward. He passes urine within 1 hour of returning to the ward. He is due to be discharged home the following day.

- What advice would you give to Alice regarding Ben's dressing and stent?
- What advice would you give regarding surgical follow-up?

Conclusion

The renal system consists of the upper and lower urinary tract: kidneys, ureters, bladder and urethra. Many renal system anomalies are detected during the antenatal period through detailed ultrasound scanning. Some renal diseases are treated medically, some surgically and some require a combination of both. It is essential the nursing care and management of infants and children with renal disorders are embedded in a family-centred approach, and that as a paediatric nurse, you are mindful of renal medical- and surgical-specific nurse assessment and care.

References

Bevan, A.L. (2015) cited in Peate, I. & Gormley-Fleming, E. (eds) (2015). *Fundamentals of Children's Anatomy and Physiology*. Wiley, Oxford.

Children's Hospital of Philadelphia (n.d.). Conditions and diseases. Available at: http://www.chop.edu/conditions-diseases (last accessed April 2018).

Children with Cancer UK (2016). Available at: http://www.childrenwithcancer.org.uk/wilms-tumour) (last accessed April 2018).

Fortenberry, J.D., Paden, M.L. & Goldstein, S.L. (2013). Acute kidney injury in children. An update on diagnosis and treatment. *Pediatric Clinics of North America* 60, 669–688.

Gabardi, S., Munz, K. & Ulbricht, C. (2007). A review of dietary supplement-induced renal dysfunction. *Clinical Journal of the American Society of Nephrology* 2, 757–765.

Lissauer, T. & Clayden, G. (2007). *Illustrated Textbook of Paediatrics*, 3rd edn. Mosby Elsevier, Philadelphia.

Macqueen, S., Bruce, E.A. & Gibson, F. (2012). *The Great Ormond Street Hospital Manual of Children's Nursing Practices*. Wiley, Chichester.

Marin, J.D., Shaikh, N., Docimo, S.G., et al. (2014). Suprapubic bladder aspiration. *New England Journal of Medicine* 371, e13.

National Institute for Health and Care Excellence (NICE) (2015). Balanitis. Clinical Knowledge Summary. NICE, London.

National Institute for Health and Care Excellence (NICE) (2007). Urinary tract infection in under 16s: diagnosis and management. Clinical guideline [CG54]. NICE, London.

Nottingham Children's Hospital (2014). Guideline for the assessment and management of acute kidney injury in children and young people. Nottingham University Hospitals NHS Trust, Nottingham.

Nursing and Midwifery Council (NMC) (2015). *The Code. Professional standards of practice and behaviour for nurses and midwives*. NMC, London.

Peate, I. & Gormley-Fleming, E. (2015). *Fundamentals of Children's Anatomy and Physiology*. Wiley, Oxford.

Smith, I., Kranke, P., Murat, I., *et al*. (2011). Perioperative fasting in adults and children: guidelines from the European Society of Anaesthesiology. *European Journal of Anaesthesiology* 28(8), 556–569.

The Royal Children's Hospital Melbourne (2014). Clinical Guidelines (Nursing). Available at: http://www.rch.org.au/rchcpg/hospital_clinical_guideline_index/nursing_assessment/#renal (last accessed April 2018).

UK Renal Registry (2015). The Eighteenth Annual Report of the Renal Association. *Nephron* 2016, 132(Suppl 1).

World Health Organization (2005). Urinary tract infections in infants and children in developing countries in the context of IMCI. WHO, Geneva. http://apps.who.int/iris/handle/10665/69160 (accessed April 2018).

Chapter 14

Disorders of the reproductive systems

Michele O'Grady

Aim

This chapter provides understanding and insight into disordered pathophysiology of male and female reproductive systems. Developing understanding and insight will help you to offer safer, high-quality and effective informed care.

Learning outcomes

On completion of this chapter, the reader will be able to:

- Describe common conditions in both boys and girls.
- Consider the psychological distress caused by reproductive ill health.
- Consider the role of the paediatric nurse in assessing reproductive health/ill health.
- Discuss consider common conditions related to both the male and female reproductive systems.

Keywords

- reproductive health
- male genitalia
- female genitalia
- female genital mutilation
- torsion
- psychological care
- sexually transmitted infection

Fundamentals of Children's Applied Pathophysiology: An Essential Guide for Nursing and Healthcare Students, First Edition.
Edited by Elizabeth Gormley-Fleming and Ian Peate.
© 2019 John Wiley & Sons Ltd. Published 2019 by John Wiley & Sons Ltd.
Companion website: www.wileyfundamentalseries.com/childpathophysiology

Test your prior knowledge

1. In male fetal development, when do testes descend down the inguinal canal into the scrotal sac?
2. Why are male gonads outside the body in the scrotal sac?
3. Spermatogenesis is the term for the production of what?
4. What is the age range of male puberty?
5. What does the male Tanner scale measure?
6. What shape are the ovaries?
7. What is the age range of female puberty?
8. What does the female Tanner scale measure?
9. At what age do the ovaries descend into the pelvis?
10. How many oogonia do females produce in their lifetime?

Introduction

There are a vast number of disorders of the reproductive systems of both boys and girls and it would be difficult to include all of them in a single chapter. However, common presentations have been chosen and an attempt made to select the common conditions that are likely to present throughout your career.

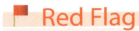
Red Flag

Throughout the chapter there will be conditions common in girls and to a lesser extent boys, which may be a symptom of sexual abuse, although this will be a rare cause of the complaint. It is essential whenever a gynaecological examination takes place that it is carried out by a professional trained to diagnose sexual abuse. History taking and systematic assessment are vitally important in conditions of the reproductive system in order to identify possible signs of abuse.

Why is dealing with the reproductive system more difficult than any other system in the body? The short answer is that adults are often embarrassed to talk about or even consider that their children are developing into sexual human beings. Alongside this, is the possibility that some reproductive health issues may affect future fertility, which is an emotional subject for parents (Wilson & Koo, 2010; Leser & Francis, 2014).

The use of language when dealing with children and young people can be challenging and depends on the conversations that parents may or may not have had with their children (Rogers et al., 2015). What children call their genitalia can be varied and in fact some girls do not have a name for their vagina, so taking a history can be tricky. Throughout the chapter, this issue will be highlighted with helpful tips to overcome language difficulties. However, you, as the practitioner, need to be comfortable discussing matters affecting reproductive health as children and young people will sense your discomfort, which will affect your therapeutic relationships.

The male reproductive system

One of the characteristics of the male reproductive organs is that the majority of the organs are outside the body. The reproductive system is closely linked with the neuroendocrine systems, which produce hormones that are required for development and sexual maturation.

Disorders of the reproductive systems Chapter 14

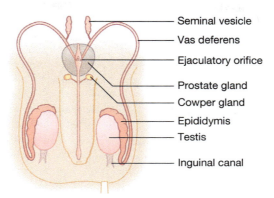

Figure 14.1 The male reproductive system. *Source:* Peate & Gormley-Fleming 2015. Reproduced with permission of Wiley.

The urinary system and the reproductive system are collocated. The testes are located in the scrotum outside the body because sperm production and storage need to be 3 degrees cooler than body temperature. For an in-depth examination of the anatomy and physiology, please see Peate and Gormley-Fleming (2015). See Fig. 14.1 for an overview of the male reproductive system (see also Chapter 13).

Male reproductive issues

There are a number of common male reproductive issues that boys may experience. The healthcare worker is likely to see many of these during their career. Common problems affecting the male reproductive tract are shown in Table 14.1.

It is possible and even highly likely that boys who have a problem with their genitalia may be embarrassed and reluctant to tell their parents or health professionals about their concern. In an ideal world, boys could choose if they want to be examined by a female or male nurse/doctor but often there is no option. Top tips for examination of boys' genitalia:

- Always take a detailed history first – it is important to use terminology that the child or young person is comfortable with, and not to portray any embarrassment.
- The nurse should carefully consider their choice of words.
- If examination is required, try to minimise the number of people and occasions involved. This may mean doctors and nurses doing a first examination jointly.

There are a number of conditions relating to male reproductive health, but this chapter will consider cryptorchidism, and testicular torsion, which is a surgical emergency.

Table 14.1 Some common male reproductive conditions

- Hydrocele
- Epididymitis
- Torsion of the testes
- Undescended testes
- Priapism
- Balanitis
- Inguinal hernia
- Hypospadias

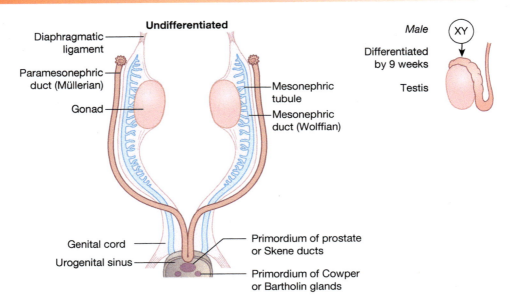

Figure 14.2 The development of the male reproductive tract. *Source:* Peate & Gormley-Fleming 2015. Reproduced with permission of Wiley.

Cryptorchidism (also known as undescended testes)

Cryptorchidism refers to the absence of one or both testes from the scrotum. It occurs in about 1% of infants over 3 months (Fawzy et al., 2015). The precise cause is still unclear, but it is considered to be a common condition. See Fig. 14.2 for a depiction of the development of the male reproductive tract.

Classification

Classification of undescended testes are based on testicular location, which may be either along the normal line of descent (abdomen, inguinal canal, external ring, pre-scrotal, upper scrotal) or in an ectopic position.
True undescended testes: The testes lie along the normal path of descent in the abdomen or inguinal region but do not reach the scrotum.
Ectopic testes: The testes lie outside the normal path, for example, the perineum or penile shaft.
Ascending testes: The testes have descended but are now lying outside the scrotum.
Causes: Not generally understood but there are some risk factors:

- father or sibling who has had undescended testes
- low birth weight
- small for gestational age
- preterm delivery
- another genital abnormality, e.g., hypospadias.

Diagnosis

- Wash hands and try to warm them prior to examination
- Examine the child lying down in a warm room, being careful to maintain privacy and dignity
- Visual inspection

Disorders of the reproductive systems   Chapter 14

- Palpation by a qualified practitioner, e.g., general practitioner (GP), surgeon
- Screening within 72 hours of birth (National Institute for Health and Care Excellence [NICE], 2006), at 6–8-week check-up and at 3 months if undescended testes discovered.

Treatment

Surgical intervention is the treatment option. The surgical procedure undertaken brings the testis into the scrotum and anchors it to the wall of the scrotal sac.

Potential complications

- Impaired fertility (Kolon *et al.*, 2014)
- Testicular cancer
- Testicular torsion
- Surgical complications, e.g., vascular damage

Psychological care

There are several factors that lead to parents' distress when treating this condition. Usually it is diagnosed in young babies and surgical intervention in a young baby is very traumatic for parents, carers and the whole family. Minimising distress is as important as treating the problem. Families require adequate explanations, detailed information and constant reassurance. Occasionally, an older child will present with one or both testes undescended. This can be very traumatic for all concerned and the outcome for future fertility may not be positive. For pre- and post-operative care, see Glasper and Richardson (2006).

Case Study

Testicular torsion

Carl is a 10-year-old boy who presents to the emergency department with a history of a sudden pain in his left testicle. His mum is concerned as he never complains of pain so she has brought him to hospital.

Carl is triaged by the nurse. He has a PEWS score of zero but he is complaining of moderate pain and is given analgesia of paracetamol 500 mg orally and ibuprofen 300 mg orally, having checked that he has no allergies and has not had any previous doses of these drugs today. As per protocol, an urgent call is made to the surgeons and they attend the department 10 minutes later.

Because of the severity of the pain, the surgeons advise mum that Carl needs to go to theatre for a surgical exploration of the testes to rule out testicular torsion and he might lose the testicle if untreated. Within minutes, the hospital porter arrives to take a tearful Carl and his mother to theatre.

The operation is a success, Carl had a testicular torsion, which was released and blood supply was restored to the testicle. Carl makes an unremarkable post-operative recovery with no complications and is discharged home that evening.

Investigations: Obtaining a urine sample

NICE (2007) recommends that a clean-catch specimen of urine is required from all children when ruling out a urinary tract infection, and a midstream specimen from older children.

Robinson *et al.* (2014) have argued that it is not necessary to wash a child's perineal area before a midstream specimen is obtained as the first few millilitres of urine will wash contaminants away. However, this study has not been validated by NICE and therefore it is important to adhere to the guidelines while remaining up to date with future research.

In Carl's case, it is important to explain what is meant by a midstream urine sample. Many departments have a urine collection kit with a funnel attached to a sterile container.

Advise Carl to wash his hands.
Connect the funnel to the sterile container without contaminating the inside of the pot or funnel.
Explain to Carl that he should first wash the tip of his penis with the cotton wool balls and water provided, and pat dry. As he starts to pass urine he should allow a small amount of urine to pass into the toilet before using the container to collect urine.
The nurse should be close by, wearing gloves, to take the container from Carl, removing the funnel and placing the cap on the bottle.

During urinalysis, the nurse should carefully follow the protocol depending on the urinalysis machine used in his/her department provided s/he is trained to do so. Carl's name and details are entered into the machine and a printout can be obtained. After the urinalysis is completed, local protocols will indicate whether the sample needs to be sent to the laboratory. Results must be documented into Carl's notes.

NB: Carl's parent will be anxious to know the result of the urine test and provided you are competent to do so, or in discussion with a more senior practitioner, it is important to discuss the findings with Carl and his mother.

Medication Alert

Ibuprofen combines anti-inflammatory analgesic and antipyretic properties. It has fewer side effects than other non-steroidal anti-inflammatory drugs (NSAIDs); however, its anti-inflammatory properties are weaker.

Ibuprofen is generally well tolerated and the majority of people do not experience any side effects. The most common side effects are related to stomach irritation and include abdominal pain, indigestion and nausea. These can mainly be avoided by taking ibuprofen with food. Rarely, serious side effects, e.g., ulceration or bleeding of the stomach or intestines, may occur. If the child experiences any sign of bleeding from the stomach or bowels after taking this medicine, e.g., vomiting blood (haematemesis) and/or passing black/tarry/blood-stained stools, consult a doctor immediately.

Testicular torsion

The principal cause of testicular torsion is when the tunica vaginalis fails to encase the testicle and the testis hangs free from the vascular structures leading to a partial or complete venous occlusion. This can lead to ischaemia (tissue death) and could result in a loss of one or both testicles. It is estimated that 1 in 4000 males under 25 years of age will experience testicular torsion, with a peak onset of 13 years (Ta *et al.*, 2016). It can affect babies prenatally and neonates (Fehér & Bajory, 2016). There are a number of predisposing factors relating to testicular torsion. Often it is spontaneous, but it can sometimes follow direct trauma.

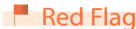

Testicular torsion is a surgical emergency and requires urgent surgical intervention. Most hospital trusts will have a protocol and nurses must ensure that surgeons are informed immediately a child/young person attends with testicular pain. It is important that the parent and child are warned that the surgeons may react very quickly if torsion is suspected. In Carl's case, he was in the emergency department less than 20 minutes before he was rushed to theatre.

Signs and symptoms

- Testicular or lower abdominal pain – in young boys, always consider testicular symptoms (Memik *et al.*, 2012).
- A recent pain in testicles that resolved – there may have been an episode of testicular pain, which may indicate an episode of spontaneously resolving testicular torsion.
- Pain is severe, often associated with vomiting and child can exhibit signs of shock.
- May or may not have been associated with trauma, e.g., kicked in the testicles.

Physical examination

- This should be carried out by surgeon, A & E senior doctor, or A & E or surgical consultant.
- Ultrasound does not provide adequate information and should not be used to diagnose torsion. However, some researchers (Yusuf & Sidhu, 2013) advocate the use of colour Doppler ultrasound (CDUS) or high-resolution ultrasonography (HRUS). As Fehér and Bajory (2016) point out, both these methods may well diagnose torsion or rule it out, but it is important that the technology is used and interpreted by an expert. The authors, following an extensive review of the literature, concluded that history and examination and speed is more important.
- Testicle may or may not appear swollen.
- Testicle may or may not feel hot.
- Testicle may feel hard.
- PEWS may be normal or a tachycardia and hypotension may indicate early shock. Pyrexia may be present.
- Urinalysis should be performed to rule out infection but should not delay surgery, if required.

Treatment options

- Orchiopexy – this is carried out on a viable testicle, i.e., one where the blood supply is intact. The testicle is released and fixed to the inner scrotal wall.
- Orchiectomy – the testicle is removed and a prosthetic implant is inserted at a later date.

The physical care required to treat the patient is essential and any delay in providing surgical intervention can have serious repercussions in the post-operative period. The importance of psychological care associated with an emergency surgical intervention is outlined in the following box.

Psychological Care

- Rapid assessment and move to the operating theatre
- Scar on scrotum
- Possible loss of testicle
- Possible further surgery
- Reduced fertility

The speed of the assessment and the need for rapid surgery can be very traumatic for the child/young person and their families. In Carl's case his time in the emergency room was less than 20 minutes. Because the time from diagnosis is so short there is little opportunity to discuss theatre and pre- and post-operative care with the young person or the parent.

The removal of a testicle can cause both physical and psychological trauma to the young man and his family. Apart from the physical difference in his scrotum, there are also psychological effects. Although a prosthetic can be fitted so the scrotum looks normal, there is the undecided issue of future fertility.

Many sexual health services focus solely on women but there are some local services, and nationally the Brook Centres offer counselling around a range of sexual issues.

Female reproductive health issues

The female reproductive system is more complex than the male reproductive system. Similarities exist between both systems, with the endocrine system producing hormones required for biological development, sexual arousal and puberty. The female reproductive system is predominantly hidden inside the body and the urinary system is collocated but not a part of the sexual organs. The female reproductive system is made up of the ovaries, fallopian tubes, uterus, vagina, and external genitalia (see Figs 14.3 and 14.4). The breasts are also part of the female reproductive system.

The function of the female reproductive system is to produce ova and allow fertilisation of the ova to take place and the fetus to grow inside it. After birth, the reproductive system also prepares the breasts to feed the infant.

As with the male reproductive system, it is expected that the reader has an in-depth knowledge of the anatomy and physiology of the system including the issues of puberty and menstrual cycle.

There are a range of conditions affecting female reproductive health and this chapter will concentrate on some of the most common (see Table 14.2).

Menstrual problems

Menarche, or the first period, has been described in the literature as a major milestone in a girl's life and many cultures celebrate the transition into womanhood (Pitangui et al., 2013; Pateriya & Kanhere, 2014). It should be a normal part of life but the aforementioned authors suggest that problems in menstruation are responsible for loss of education as girls frequently do not seek medical help with significant health problems relating to abnormalities.

Pitangui et al. (2014) describe dysmenorrhoea or pain during menstruation as the most common gynaecological complaint of women. Primary dysmenorrhoea can be described as painful menstruation in women with a normal pelvic anatomy. Secondary dysmenorrhoea refers to pain due to a disorder in the pelvis. The physiology behind dysmenorrhoea is an increased production of the hormone prostaglandins by the endometrium causing uterine contraction and pain. Dysmenorrhoea affects more than 80% of women (Pitangui et al., 2014).

Disorders of the reproductive systems Chapter 14

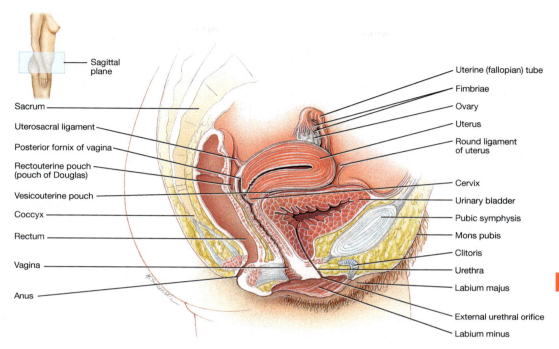

Figure 14.3 The female reproductive system. *Source:* Peate & Gormley-Fleming 2015. Reproduced with permission of Wiley.

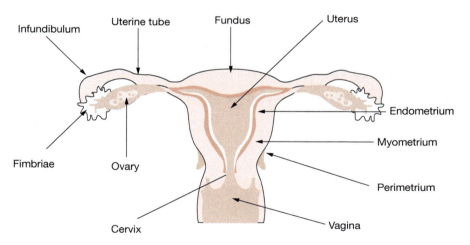

Figure 14.4 The uterus and associated structures. *Source:* Peate & Gormley-Fleming 2015. Reproduced with permission of Wiley.

Table 14.2 Some common female reproductive conditions

- Menstrual problems
- Abdominal pain
- Vulvovaginitis
- Sexually transmitted infections
- Unprotected sexual activity
- Female genital mutilation

Pain begins shortly before menstruation commences and can last 1–3 days. The pain can be associated with cramps, nausea and vomiting, and syncope (fainting). It can be very debilitating for some women and has been associated with missed days in school and a deficit in education (Azurah *et al.*, 2013). The literature also indicates that girls and adult women are unlikely to seek medical help and endure symptoms that may indicate an underlying pathology.

Menstruation is a normal part of everyday life for women. However, it would appear that girls do not always discuss problems with their parents, and nurses need to use opportunities to take a menstrual history from girls whenever an overall health history is taken and allow girls and their parents to discuss any issues relating to dysmenorrhoea.

Abdominal pain in girls

Almost all girls will have abdominal pain at one time or another. The pain can be anywhere between the chest and groin. Most of the time, it is not caused by a serious medical problem; however, sometimes abdominal pain may be a sign of something serious.

Red Flag

Abdominal pain in adolescent girls can be difficult to diagnose as there are a number of causes, some of which are gynaecological, which can lead to severe onset of abdominal pain (see Table 14.3).

Abdominal pain presentations in adolescent girls are outlined in Table 14.3.

The young person with abdominal pain requires a thorough examination and history taking is key. However, the history involves asking personal questions in a manner that is both respectful and non-judgemental. It is important to establish a rapport, and it may be advantageous to have time alone with the young person to allow them to give you information that they may not want shared with their parent (Forcier, 2009). History should include:

- description and location of pain including timing and any repetitive history
- urinary history
- bowel history

Table 14.3 Examples of abdominal pain presentation in adolescent girls

	Acute	Chronic
Gynaecological	Ectopic pregnancy Miscarriage Pelvic inflammatory disease Ovarian cyst rupture	Dysmenorrhoea Endometriosis Pelvic inflammatory disease Adhesions
Gastrointestinal	Gastroenteritis Appendicitis Perforation Bowel obstruction	Constipation Irritable bowel syndrome Lactose intolerance Coeliac disease
Urological	Pyelonephritis Cystitis Urethritis UTI (urinary tract infection)	Chronic cystitis
Other		Abdominal migraine

Source: Bean & Rowell 2014.

- menstrual history
- stress
- sexual activity.

With pre-pubescent and pubescent girls, a urine test for urinalysis and a pregnancy test are required to rule out infection and pregnancy. This can be a difficult subject to broach with both the young person and her parent/carer as some parents feel it is totally unnecessary and insulting. It is particularly difficult in families where sex has never been discussed and sex education in school has been denied. In most cases parents make a joke of it and give consent; however, some parents will try to refuse consent. Generally, medical staff will not be able to proceed with an exploration of the causes of abdominal pain without the pregnancy test and most parents accept this.

Consent

Consent for treatment must be given serious consideration. The nurse and other members of the multidisciplinary team have to understand the key issues associated with consent.

1. Who can give consent?
2. What age is a child considered to be Gillick competent?
3. What is the difference between the Fraser guidelines and Gillick competency?

It is essential that the nurse is able to provide answers to these three questions in order to provide safe and effective, patient-centred care. Informed consent is one aspect of a person's human rights.

Abdominal pain is not only a symptom of gynaecological ill health, but it is important to understand that it will be one of the differential diagnoses to consider. Equally it is important to highlight that it is not the only cause of abdominal pain in adolescent girls.

Vaginal discharge

One of the most common presentations in both primary care and emergency departments, is vaginal discharge in children aged 4–8 years (McGreal & Wood, 2013), although it is also seen in younger and older children. Striegel *et al.* (2006) commented that the anatomy and physiology of the pre-pubertal vagina offers some explanation for the causes of vaginal discharge.

- Vaginal mucosa has a neutral pH
- The vagina lacks antibodies to fight infection
- The vagina is short – 3–4 cm
- The labia minora is small
- Labial fat pads are not present to help combat infection
- The vagina lies in close proximity to the rectum.

Signs and symptoms associated with vaginal discharge

- Discharge, which may be seen by parent on underwear
- Discharge may be foul smelling
- Discharge may look green or have a pus-like appearance
- Pruritus (itch)
- Erythema (redness)/irritation around the labia
- Urinary symptoms, such as dysuria or frequency

Causes of vaginal discharge

There are a wide variety of causes for vaginal discharge in children.

- Idiopathic – following investigation, there is no known cause.
- Vulvovaginitis – irritation around the vulval area, which may be exacerbated by obesity, tight-fitting underwear or irritants such as bubble bath.
- Foreign body – history taking is very important as children may admit that they put something into their vagina or they may not remember. It is not unusual to find Lego, plastic, tissues and other items as the cause for the discharge.
- Infection – often due to poor hygiene. Often occurs when the child starts becoming independent with toileting.
- Sexual abuse – sexual abuse should always be considered when a child presents with a vaginal discharge but it is rare.

There are several factors that predispose young girls to acquire vaginal infections (as discussed by McGreal & Wood, 2013), such as:

- lack of labial fat pads and pubic hair
- neutral vaginal pH (6.5–7.5)
- epithelium is thin and dry in the pre-pubertal vagina.

Making a diagnosis

- History taking from parent and child is important. McGreal and Wood (2013) commented that although obtaining a history from a child may be difficult, it is important to include her in the discussions, particularly if an examination is required.
- History of toileting behaviour is vital, particularly when establishing if the child wipes her own bottom unsupervised.
- Swabs may be taken but high vaginal swabs are rarely indicated.
- Urinalysis is to rule out a urinary tract infection.
- If discharge is bloodstained McGreal and Wood (2013) state that this is an indication for a gynaecology referral.
- Examination should be carried out by a paediatric specialist or a gynaecologist. If the child will cooperate and will put her legs in the 'frog leg' position, that may allow a visual inspection of the perineum and may indicate a pooling of discharge that can be easily swabbed. A play specialist carrying out distraction therapy may mean the child will allow the doctor to separate the labia and visualise the lower vagina. This may reveal a foreign body although this is unlikely to be successfully removed without sedation, such as ketamine or a general anaesthetic.
- Swabs are most likely to grow anaerobic bacteria, followed by group A beta haemolytic streptococcus.

Medication Alert

Ketamine sedation is used very successfully in emergency departments and day units as a means to avoid full anaesthesia.

Route of administration: intramuscular.

Dose: refer to British National Formulary for Children (BNFC) – latest edition.

Disorders of the reproductive systems — Chapter 14

> Caution: ketamine must only be administered by senior medical or anaesthetic staff.
>
> Contra-indications: head trauma, hypertension, cardiac disease.
>
> Side effects: diplopia, hallucinations, nausea, nightmares, tachycardia, transient psychotic effects, vomiting.
>
> Side effects (rare): arrhythmias, bradycardia, respiratory distress.
>
> Caution for administration: nurses should note that ketamine is a controlled drug and should be stored appropriately.
>
> There are different strengths of ketamine and errors have occurred.
>
> Children should be recovered in a dark and quiet area to reduce side effects.
>
> Children may be discharged once they have eaten and passed urine.
>
> Parents should be appraised of the likelihood of nightmares.
>
> Ketamine is an excellent alternative to a general anaesthetic.

Treatment

- Treat cause
- Antibiotics for infection – antibiotic regimes will vary depending on the causative organism
- Removal of foreign body – under sedation or general anaesthetic
- Diagnosis of abuse – suspicion of abuse will result in safeguarding protocols being put into action and will involve police and social services. It is likely to be very upsetting for the child as she may be taken into care pending investigation.

Health promotion advice

For many children vaginal discharge is due to poor hygiene or irritants and can be treated with advice about the contributing factors. This is an important aspect of the nursing care of any child with vaginal irritation regardless of the cause.

- Good toileting hygiene, always wipe from front to back after using the toilet.
- Encourage the child to sit on the toilet with her legs apart when urinating.
- Daily warm baths are very helpful without the addition of scented bubble baths and thorough gentle drying of the area is important.
- Wearing cotton underwear that is not too tight.
- Avoid wearing pants in bed.

Psychological care

There is little written about the effect on parents of being asked if their child may have been abused, but it is a question that may be asked in the course of the investigation of vaginal discharge. Parents may feel very shocked and angry, especially when a cause other than abuse is found. It is important to acknowledge to parents that they are no longer suspected. Children who have had an intimate examination may also feel very vulnerable and upset. However, with treatment for the discharge, it is hoped that this will be short-lived. All nurses must be aware of the effects of hospitalisation on families and they must strive to make a hospital admission as pleasant as it can be.

Health promotion advice in this case is extremely important and it can be time-consuming to explain it to children and their families. There are many advice leaflets available, which are produced either nationally or locally.

Sexual health: both girl and boys

There is a wealth of literature addressing issues regarding sexual health or sexual ill health. It is important to recognise some of the issues:

- Young people are having sex
- Sex education may not always adequately prepare young people for this stage in their life
- Parents do not always want to accept their children as sexual beings
- Nurses are often perceived by young people as being uncomfortable around issues relating to sexual activity
- Discrimination towards lesbian, gay, bisexual and transgender young people is both common and unacceptable for nurses (Nursing & Midwifery Council [NMC], 2015).

Schalet has written comparing the attitude of Dutch parents with that of American parents, and highlights an acceptance by Dutch parents of teenage sexual behaviour, which results in discussions and less risky behaviours. The Dutch have consistently had the lowest rates of teenage pregnancy and sexually transmitted infections in Europe (Schalet, 2011).

There is an overwhelming amount of literature looking at various aspects of young people and sexual behaviour, enough to fill an entire book, but in essence, the rest of this chapter is an attempt to highlight some of the issues and hopefully encourage you to read more widely around the subject. The following issues are discussed in more detail in this chapter: sexually transmitted infections (STIs), emergency contraception in the under-age teenager, and female genital mutilation (FGM).

Sexual activity

Sexual activity in young people is monitored statistically using two measures: the rate of sexually transmitted infections and the teenage pregnancy rate (Schalet, 2011). There is a flaw to this measurement as it is a 'guestimate' based on those two measures.

Teenage pregnancy rates

The UK still has the highest pregnancy rate in Europe even though there has been a fall in rates. Table 14.4 provides the most recent teenage pregnancy figures with a comparison to the 1970 figures.

Sexually transmitted infections continue to rise despite government screening and treatment campaigns aimed at the under 25s. For in-depth information regarding sexually transmitted diseases, please see www.brook.org.uk.

Table 14.4 Teenage conception statistics

Year	Age (yrs)	Rate per 1000	Outcome	% reduction
1970	15–19	82.4	Unknown	
2012	15–19	44.2	40% ended in termination	6.8% reduction
2012	13–15	5.6	60% ended in termination	10% reduction

Source: Adapted from Brook 2014.

Contraception

There are a number of different methods of contraception available. For further details please go to www.fpa.org.uk for an in-depth explanation of what is available.

Emergency contraception

This is a complex issue for children's nurses for many reasons. The philosophy of family-centred care with a partnership between parents and young people is integral to our way of working, but this is challenged when young people seek emergency contraception or if you have to suggest emergency contraception following an assault.

Case Study

Emergency contraception

The following case study highlights many of the issues faced by children's nurses. Mary is a 15-year-old girl who arrives at a children's emergency department on a Sunday morning at 10 a.m. She refuses to say why she is seeking medical help and says it is personal. Mary is seen by a staff nurse and is triaged; she asks for emergency contraception. The department has a nurse-led protocol so the triage nurse carries out the first part of the protocol before she is seen by another nurse. A baseline set of observations is taken:

- Temperature: 36.5 °C
- Pulse: 100 beats per minute
- Respiration: 20 breaths per minute
- Blood pressure 90/60 mmHg
- PEWS score = 0

The nurse asks for a urine sample and asks for consent to carry out a pregnancy test, consent is given. A senior nurse interviews Mary and takes a full medical and sexual history:

Allergies = nil
Medication = nil
Medical history = nil

Sexual history:
Mary has a 15-year-old boyfriend called Tom. They have been seeing each other for 6 months. They had not previously had sexual intercourse. Mary had discussed the idea of starting contraception with her mother who told her father and he was very angry and said as she was not 16, she could not have sex, and if she did have sex, Tom would go to prison.

Mary's parents went away for the weekend and Mary was supposed to have a friend come to stay but she became unwell and Mary asked Tom to stay. They had not intended to have sex on this occasion but 'it just happened' as they had drunk some cider. They tried to use a condom but it fell off and Mary is petrified of getting pregnant. She is adamant that her parents must never find out and she wants emergency contraception. Mary said she wanted to have sex with Tom and they had sex a few times. The nurse clarified if they meant to have sex and what sexual activity took place, it was penetrative sexual intercourse. Mary refuses to discuss this with her mother. Mary is prescribed levonorgestral as sexual intercourse took place less than 12 hours ago and she is advised to attend the genito-urinary medicine clinic in 3 weeks for STI screening and a family planning clinic as soon as possible to acquire contraceptive advice.

Mary is required to take the drug in front of the nurse as per protocol to avoid the risk of a young girl obtaining emergency contraception for another young person.

The side effects were discussed and what to do in the event of her vomiting in the next hour. Mary leaves the department feeling happy.

An example of emergency contraception protocol used in a local hospital Trust

Emergency Contraception Protocol for girls under 16 years (O'Grady 2011)

Introduction
This protocol has been produced in conjunction with A & E consultants, paediatric consultants, GUM consultants, Child Protection Police, Named Nurse for Safeguarding and paediatric senior nurses.

Emergency contraception for girls under the age of 16 may raise issues of both sexual health and child protection. As a result of this a thorough assessment is required to rule out any exploitation.

Confidentiality
Explain to the young person that you may have to refer them to another agency or refer them to another specialist.

A letter will be sent to their GP but GPs are bound by confidentiality and this will not be revealed to her parents/carers.

Ask the age of the young person. If she is under 13 years old, she is deemed to have been raped in the eyes of the law and regardless of the age of the partner is considered to be at risk. Emergency contraception can still be dispensed but safeguarding team/Children Schools and Families and Child Protection Police need to be contacted immediately.

Exploitation – sole interview
Many young people are accompanied by their boyfriend or even an older man who may or may not be their parent/carer. It is important that you are able to interview your young patient alone at least for part of the consultation in case she is being coerced in some way. If the accompanying man does not want this to happen, insist on it and if the young girl leaves the department, seek urgent advice from police/Children's Schools and Family and report the action.

Fraser competent (often referred to as Gillick competent)
Fraser competent:
  You need to be satisfied

1. That your young person, although under the age of 16 years understands your advice;
2. That you cannot persuade her to tell her parents that she is seeking contraceptive advice;
3. That she is likely to continue having sexual intercourse with or without contraceptive treatment;

Disorders of the reproductive systems — Chapter 14

4. That unless she receives contraceptive advice/treatment her physical or mental health or both are likely to suffer;
5. That her best interests require contraceptive advice and treatment to be given without parental consent.

The young person turning up and asking for emergency contraception does not necessarily indicate understanding.

It is not enough to understand the nature of the treatment sought, you must be comfortable that she is mature enough to understand what is involved.

Talking to the young person will help you to assess competence.

Sexual intercourse

Has sexual intercourse actually taken place?

The young person needs to describe her sexual activity, which can be embarrassing for her but you should remain professional and help her to understand that you are not judging her.

No emergency contraception is required for masturbation.

The exact timing of the sexual intercourse is important as it will inform your choice.

If sexual intercourse has taken place in less than 72 hours levonorgestral (Levonelle) needs to be prescribed.

If sexual intercourse has taken place between 72 and 120 hours, ulipristal (ellaOne) needs to be prescribed.

If more than 120 hours has passed it is too late for emergency contraception and the young person should be referred to the gynaecology team.

Age of the sexual partner

This table is a guideline. Two 13-year-old girls might present on the same day but be very different in their emotional maturity. This table is to help you consider the age gap with a view to sexual exploitation. If you do not feel comfortable to proceed, follow your instinct and seek advice from consultant colleagues.

NB: Sexual intercourse with a 12 year old or younger is classified as statutory rape.

Age of young person (yrs)	Age of partner (yrs)	Action
12	Immaterial	Refer CSF/EDT/Police
13	13–15	Proceed if happy
13	16–17	Proceed with caution
13	18+	Refer
14	13–15	Proceed if happy
14	16–18	Proceed with caution
14	19+	Refer
15	14–16	Proceed if happy
15	17–18	Proceed with caution
15	19+	Refer

Consensual sex
The following questions need to be asked:
- Did you intend to have sex?
- Where did you have sex?
- Do you remember having sex?
- Is your partner a boyfriend/known to you?
- Were you under the influence of any other substances, including drugs or alcohol?

Medical assessment
A pregnancy test is required and consent should be obtained.

If it is negative, proceed with the medication but remember to explain to the young person that a negative test does not mean they are not pregnant from a previous encounter or indeed emergency contraception does not always guarantee no pregnancy. Advice should be given with regard to action to take if their period is late.

If positive give the young person time and space and provide information on services to help her, such as Brook Advisory Centre or Family Planning or their GP. Try to persuade her to talk to her parents/carers.

Sexual responsibility
Does the young person intend to continue this sexual relationship?

Have they considered they have put themselves at risk of contracting a sexually transmitted disease?

Refer to local family planning and GUM services to obtain contraceptive advice and undergo sexual health screening. Explain the confidentiality related to both these services.

Medication/treatment
There are two different medications available to young people:

1. Levonorgestral – effective up to 72 hours but may have a lesser effectiveness up to 120 hours. Dose to be repeated if vomited within 2 hours.
2. Ulipristal – effective up to 120 hours. Dose to be repeated if vomited within 3 hours.

The other alternative for emergency contraception is the insertion of an intrauterine device. However, this will not be done in the emergency department but the young person could arrange to go to a local Family Planning Clinic.

Which doctor?
Ideally a doctor should be able to prescribe the medication and a nurse can dispense this. If the doctor wants to see the young person, he/she needs to be accompanied by a nurse to support the young person.

The doctor needs to be staff grade/registrar level or above. At the weekend there may be no staff grade available or willing to help, and in this case the paediatricians may help.

If there is likely to be a significant delay, speak to the consultant on call.

Can a nurse refuse to dispense emergency contraception?
Under the Abortion Act 1967, all nurses and doctors can refuse to dispense emergency contraception if they feel it is morally wrong to do so. This has also been upheld by the NMC Code (2015).

However, remember that this may be a vulnerable young person and there may be safeguarding concerns. As a result, all nurses can assess the young person but are not required to dispense the medication. This can be delegated to another member of staff.

Disorders of the reproductive systems — Chapter 14

Medication Alert

Levonorgestrel
Route: orally

Dose: 1.5 mg taken as soon as possible after sexual intercourse, preferably within 12 hours but no later than 72 hours.

Ulipristal acetate
Route: orally

Dose: 30 mg taken as soon as possible after sexual intercourse, preferably within 12 hours but no later than 120 hours.

Side effects both drugs: nausea, vomiting, abdominal pain, back pain, headaches

Further drug information available, see BNFC 2016 or latest edition.

It is important to note that Gillick competency can be used to discuss a child or young person's competence to give consent whereas Fraser guidelines can only be used in relation to sexual/contraceptive issues. Lord Fraser intended that nurses and doctors would always try to persuade young people to try to discuss this with their parents. The case study regarding emergency contraception highlights some of the issues for nurses faced with this dilemma. Nurses should also be aware that if a young girl has been assaulted or is found drunk and cannot remember if she had sex, it is recommended that emergency contraception is offered.

Female genital mutilation

The World Health Organization (WHO, 2018) defines female genital mutilation (FGM) as follows: 'FGM comprises all procedures that involve partial or total removal of external female genitalia, or other injury to the female genital organs for non-medical reasons'. There is much written about the fact that FGM is a traditional rather than a religious practice. This has made it far more difficult to combat. The reasons given by mothers for allowing this to happen to their daughters include:

- FGM is a social convention and mothers are pressurised by their society and family to conform.
- It can be considered a part of raising a young girl.
- It is believed that it reduces a girl's libido and prevents her from wanting sex before marriage.
- It increases marriageability – in some cultures a man would not marry a girl who is not circumcised.
- FGM is associated with beauty and modesty with the thought that the girl is more hygienic.
- Some religious leaders promote FGM while others oppose it, and others decline to be involved as it is clearly not a religious practice.
- It is a cultural tradition – often an argument for its continuance in some cultures.

Female genital mutilation is classified into four types, see Table 14.5.

Table 14.5 Classification of female genital mutilation

- **Type I:** Also known as clitoridectomy, this type consists of partial or total removal of the clitoris and/or its prepuce.
- **Type II:** Also known as excision, the clitoris and labia minora are partially or totally removed, with or without excision of the labia majora.
- **Type III:** The most severe form, it is also known as infibulation or pharaonic type. The procedure consists of narrowing the vaginal orifice with creation of a covering seal by cutting and appositioning the labia minora and/or labia majora, with or without removal of the clitoris. The appositioning of the wound edges consists of stitching or holding the cut areas together for a certain period of time (e.g., girls' legs are bound together), to create the covering seal. A small opening is left for urine and menstrual blood to escape. An infibulation must be opened either through penetrative sexual intercourse or surgery.
- **Type IV:** This type consists of all other procedures to the genitalia of women for non-medical purposes, such as pricking, piercing, incising, scraping and cauterization.

Source: Royal College of Nursing (RCN) 2015.

Consequences for girls who have undergone FGM

There are both short- and long-term consequences relating to FGM.

Short term:

- severe pain
- haemorrhage
- shock
- septicaemia

Long term:
Physical:

- chronic pain
- chronic pelvic infections
- development of genital abscesses, cysts, and genital ulcers
- excessive scar formation
- urinary tract infections
- problems in child birth

Sexual:

- decreased libido
- painful intercourse
- fertility issues

Psychological:

- post-traumatic stress disorder.

In terms of the pathophysiology of FGM, the difficulties faced by the woman will be related to the type of FGM and the time since it occurred (Ismail, 2009). As Ismail (2009) points out, after the initial risks of shock due to pain and haemorrhage, and infection in the first 10 days, there are other issues facing women in the future.

Dysmenorrhoea – this can be due to the inability of the blood to escape leading to stagnation of blood causing bacteria to spread into the vagina and reproductive tract.

Recurrent urinary infections are due to the flap of skin obstructing the urethra, this obstruction prevents normal micturition leading to a stagnation of urine.

When the woman marries infibulation may prevent sexual penetration occurring, which leads to painful sexual intercourse or further cutting to allow penetration to take place.

Scar tissues in the reproductive tract due to surgery and infection lead to painful sexual intercourse.

Disorders of the reproductive systems Chapter 14

During pregnancy, an opening of the infibulation may be required to prevent complications during labour, for example. midwife will be unable to assess dilatation of the cervix.

Women who have received no antenatal care may require a caesarean section due to the small infibulation opening.

During labour the vaginal canal may have lost its elasticity and pelvic floor muscles are rigid prolonging second stage of labour.

There are many other complications relating to safe delivery of a baby and postnatal complications are common.

It is impossible to imagine the psychological trauma inflicted on a young girl whether she is 5 or 14 years, and it is a very real issue. It is a traumatic event that some girls report causes them to relive the pain for years. Girls often describe the anger felt towards their mothers who have persuaded them that this is a good thing. There may be a requirement for long-term counselling from a therapist who has some understanding of this issue. In addition, there is a requirement to identify and educate women who have undergone FGM to persuade them not to inflict it on the next generation.

FGM: the legal position

- FGM has been illegal in the UK since 1985.
- Legislation was further strengthened with the Female Genital Mutilation Act 2003.
- In 2015, *Female Genital Mutilation Risks and Safeguarding: Guidance for professionals* was published.

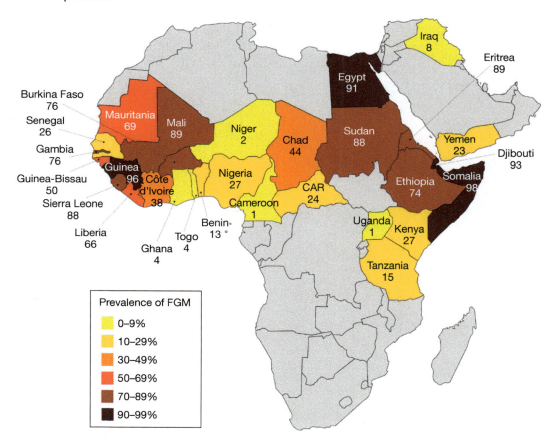

Figure 14.5 Prevalence of FGM (Africa). *Source:* www.data.unicef.org. Courtesy of UNICEF.

- As a result of this and five further reports published that year, the following clarification was enacted:
  - FGM is a form of child abuse
  - Identification of women who have undergone FGM should be reported as there is a risk to other girls within that family
  - Girls under 18 who have undergone FGM are to be referred to the police
  - Women who have undergone FGM are victims of crime
  - Every case of FGM must be reported in the NHS, GP practice and mental health trusts.

The nurse and FGM

It is important that nurses within the UK recognise two things:

1. Three million girls undergo FGM every year in Africa.
2. It is estimated that 60 000 girls aged 0–14 years were born to mothers who have undergone FGM in the UK (Macfarlane & Dorkenoo, 2015).

See Figs 14.5 and 14.6 for prevalence of FGM in Africa and globally.

FGM is a global issue for women, and nurses in the UK should be vigilant for signs of girls who might be about to be abducted to their country of origin to be forced to undergo FGM. With an increase in the migrant population, it is important to consider an intensification of the problem in the UK. FGM is a complex cultural issue that some may feel is beyond

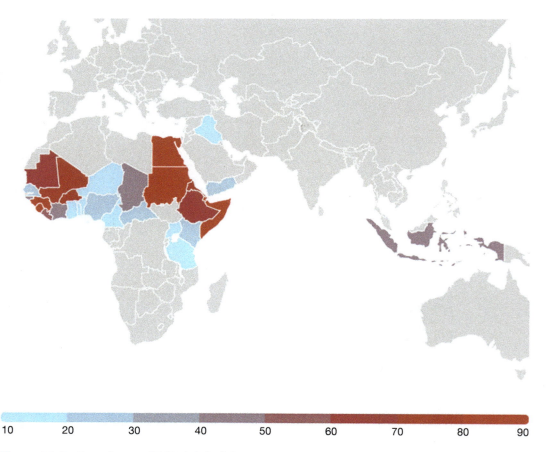

Figure 14.6 Prevalence of FGM (globally). *Source:* www.data.unicef.org. Courtesy of UNICEF.

their comprehension. FGM is so common in some countries that it has the same legitimacy as male circumcision. There is little doubt that nurses have a part to play in the global fight against a practice that has horrific consequences for its victims.

Conclusion

Reproductive health and ill health is a significant part of nursing children and young people; however, it is important to acknowledge that it is often difficult to treat reproductive health in the same way as other systems because of the sensitive nature of the conversations while trying to obtain a better picture of the health of your patient.

The area of reproductive ill health, particularly relating to sexual health, requires all practitioners to keep updated on the latest research and become comfortable in talking to both young patients and their parents and carers.

The challenges faced by children's nurses in dealing with the reproductive health and ill health of the patients and families in their care should be faced head on in order to provide these people with the care and treatment they deserve.

References

Azurah, A.G.N., Sanci, L., Moore, E. & Grover, S. (2013). The quality of life of adolescents with menstrual problems. *Journal of Pediatric and Adolescent Gynecology* 26(2), 102–108.

Bean, J.F. & Rowell, E. (2014). Evaluation of the adolescent female with acute lower abdominal pain. *Clinical Pediatric Emergency Medicine* 15(3), 243–247.

British National Formulary (2016). British Medical Association and Royal Pharmaceutical Society of Great Britain, London.

Brook (2014). Teenage conceptions: Statistics and trends. Available at: https://www.brook.org.uk/images/brook/professionals/documents/page_content/factsheets/factsheet2_2014_Teenage_conceptions.pdf (last accessed April 2018).

Fawzy, F., Hussein, A., Eid, M.M., El Kashash, A.M. & Salem, H.K. (2015). Cryptorchidism and fertility. *Clinical Medicine Insights: Reproductive Health* 2015(9), 39–43.

Fehér, Á.M. & Bajory, Z. (2016). A review of main controversial aspects of acute testicular torsion. *Journal of Acute Disease* 5(1), 1–8.

Forcier, M. (2009). Emergency department evaluation of acute pelvic pain in the adolescent female. *CPEM* 10(1), 20–30.

Glasper, A. & Richardson, J. (2006). *A Textbook of Children's and Young People's Nursing*. Churchill Livingstone, London.

Ismail, E. (2009). Female genital mutilation survey in Somaliland. Edna Adan Maternity Hospital, Hargeisa.

Kolon, T.F., Herndon, C.D.A., Baker, L.A., et al.; American Urological Association (2014). Evaluation and treatment of cryptorchidism: AUA guideline. *Journal of Urology* 192(2), 337–345.

Leser, K.A. & Francis, S.A. (2014). Mother–child communication about sexual health, HPV and cervical cancer among antenatal clinic attendees in Johannesburg, South Africa. *African Journal of Reproductive Health* 18(1), 123–126.

Macfarlane, A. & Dorkenoo, E. (2015). *Prevalence of Female Genital Mutilation in England and Wales: National and local estimates*. City University and Equality Now, London.

Memik, Ö., et al. (2012). Testicular torsion: Case report. *Konuralp Tip Dergisi* 4(1), 35–37.

McGreal, S. & Wood, P. (2013). Recurrent vaginal discharge in children. *Journal of Pediatric and Adolescent Gynecology* 26(4), 205–208.

National Institute for Health and Clinical Excellence (NICE) (2007). Urinary tract infections in under 16s: diagnosis and management. Clinical guideline [CG54]. NICE, London.

Nursing and Midwifery Council (NMC) (2015). *The Code: Professional standards of practice and behaviour for nurses and midwives*. NMC, London.

O'Grady, M. (2011). Renal and reproductive problems. In: Glasper, A., McEwing, G. & Richardson, J. (eds). *Emergencies in Children's and Young People's Nursing*. Oxford University Press, Oxford.

Pateriya, P. & Kanhere, A. (2014). A study of menstrual patterns in adolescent girls. *Journal of Evolution of Medical and Dental Sciences* 3(23), 6345–6351.

Peate, I. & Gormley-Fleming, E. (2015). *Fundamentals of Children's Anatomy and Physiology*, 1st edn. Wiley, Oxford.

Pitangui, A.C.R., Gomes, M.R.A., Lima, A.S., *et al.* (2013). Menstruation disturbances: prevalence, characteristics, and effects on the activities of daily living among adolescent girls from Brazil. *Journal of Pediatric and Adolescent Gynecology* 26(3), 148–152.

Robinson, J., Finlay, J. & Lang, M. (2014). Urinary tract infection in infants and children: diagnosis and management. *Paediatric Child Health* 19(6), 315–319.

Rogers, A.A., Ha, T., Stormshak, E.A. & Dishion, T.J. (2015). Quality of parent-adolescent conversations about sex and adolescent sexual behaviour: An observational study. *Journal of Adolescent Health* 57(2), 174.

Royal College of Nursing (RCN) (2015). *Female Genital Mutilation. An RCN Guidance for Nursing and Midwifery Practice*, 2nd edn. RCN, London.

Schalet, A. (2011). *Not Under My Roof: Parents, Teens, and the Culture of Sex*. University of Chicago Press, Chicago.

Striegel, A.M., Myers, J.B., Sorensen, M.D., Furness, P.D. & Koyle, M.A. (2006). Vaginal discharge and bleeding in girls younger than 6 years. *The Journal of Urology* 176(6), 2632–2635.

Ta, A., D'Arcy, F.T., Hoag, N., D'Arcy, J. P. & Lawrentschuk, N. (2016). Testicular torsion and the acute scrotum: current emergency management. *European Journal of Emergency Medicine* 23(3), 160–165.

Wilson, E.K. & Koo, H.P. (2010). Mothers, fathers, sons, and daughters: gender differences in factors associated with parent–child communication about sexual topics. *Reproductive Health* 7(1), 31.

World Health Organization (WHO) (2018). Female genital mutilation. Fact sheet. WHO, Geneva. Available at: http://www.who.int/mediacentre/factsheets/fs241/en/(last accessed April 2018).

Yusuf, G.T. & Sidhu, P.S. (2013). A review of ultrasound imaging in scrotal emergencies. *Journal of Ultrasound* 16(4), 171–178.

Chapter 15

Disorders of the musculoskeletal system

Liz Gormley-Fleming

Aim

The aim of this chapter is to enable the reader to develop their understanding and knowledge of the musculoskeletal system. This will include understanding the function and malfunction of the system.

Learning outcomes

On completion of this chapter, the reader will be able to:

- Identify the structure of a bone and understand the mechanism of bone healing.
- Describe the key functions of the skeleton.
- Discuss the normal and abnormal pathophysiological changes that occur in the child's musculoskeletal system.
- Be conversant with a number of common disorders of the child's musculoskeletal system.
- Articulate the stages of healing in a bone fracture.
- Care for children with a range of musculoskeletal disorders.

Keywords

- dysplasia
- fracture
- epiphysis
- metaphysis
- diaphysis
- subluxation

Fundamentals of Children's Applied Pathophysiology: An Essential Guide for Nursing and Healthcare Students, First Edition.
Edited by Elizabeth Gormley-Fleming and Ian Peate.
© 2019 John Wiley & Sons Ltd. Published 2019 by John Wiley & Sons Ltd.
Companion website: www.wileyfundamentalseries.com/childpathophysiology

- traction
- cartilage
- abduction
- adduction
- rotation

Test your prior knowledge

1. List the bones of the upper extremity.
2. List the bones of the lower extremities.
3. Describe the developments that occur within the bone from birth to adolescence.
4. Describe the six types of bones that are found in the human skeleton.
5. How many bones are there in a baby's skeletal system?
6. Discuss the function of the various types of joints found in the human body.
7. What is the function of the epiphysis and metaphysis, where are they located?

Introduction

Musculoskeletal disorders of childhood occur as a result of trauma, infection, malignancies or are congenital in nature. Some may occur for no known reason. Bone disorders can range from those that cause extreme pain and restrict mobility to those that have little effect on the child's life. Musculoskeletal injury is common due to the active nature of children and their associated developmental stage.

The skeleton of the child continues to develop post birth and will do so until adulthood is reached. This series of adaptations is essential to facilitate walking and ossification of the bones. Bone growth occurs from the growth plates. This is a vulnerable area of the bone so any interference with this process can have lifelong consequences, hence an understanding of this is important for the healthcare professional when undertaking a physical assessment of the child who presents with a potential musculoskeletal disorder.

The child's skeleton is more pliable and elastic than that of an adult. The bones have a greater tolerance and permit a greater degree of deformity so may simply bend or buckle (torus fracture) making diagnosis challenging.

The periosteal sleeve is greater in diameter that that of an adult so the child's bone has the ability to remodel; the child's skeleton has the innate ability to heal itself. Remodelling of the bones leads to old bone being removed, which is replaced by new bone. During this process other bone disorders may occur which can either improve or remain constant as the child grows. It is these distinguishing features of the child's musculoskeletal system that leads to the distinct musculoskeletal conditions that are unique to childhood.

This chapter provides an outline of a number of musculoskeletal conditions and the associated care is discussed. For detailed revision of the anatomy of the child's skeleton and muscles, please refer to Chapters 16 and 17 in Peate and Gormley-Fleming (2015).

Fractures

A fracture is a break or discontinuity in the bone. In children, the management and diagnosis of fractures is distinct from that of adults due the uniqueness of the anatomy of their bones. In children, bones heal more rapidly than those of adults as bone growth is more rapid. Fractures are very common in children and account for 25% of all childhood injuries,

Disorders of the musculoskeletal system Chapter 15

with a fractured radius and ulna being the most common type of injury. Boys sustain significantly more fractures than girls (Hart, Luther & Grottkau, 2006; Cooper et al., 2004).

Fractures in children usually occur as a result of a traumatic incident and tend to be age-related, for example, toddlers from falls, running into objects or climbing; school-age children – falls from bicycle, skateboard, scooter or motor vehicle accidents, and from climbing; young people – motor vehicle accidents, skateboard, and sport injuries. As the child matures, the incidence of fractures peaks at the 10–16 years age group.

Case Study

Ross is a 9-year-old boy who is normally fit and well. He enjoys school life and has a range of interesting hobbies. He plays ice hockey and is very good at it. During a match he is pushed over by an older player at high speed and crashes to the floor. He cries very loudly and shouts 'my leg, my leg'. The first aider arrives, Ross is unable to move his right leg, it is abducted and there is a swelling mid-thigh. An ambulance is sent for and Ross, following a full assessment, is given Entonox®, with very good effect. He has his leg placed in a splint for transport to the nearest A & E department.

On arrival at the children's A & E department, and following assessment, insertion of a cannula and administration of morphine and intravenous fluids, he is X-rayed. A fractured midshaft of femur is confirmed. He is initially placed in simple traction and transferred to the children's ward while awaiting surgical fixation in theatre the following day.

What support do you think Ross will need over the coming weeks?
What support will his family need at the time of injury and surgery?

Vital signs:

On admission to A & E, Ross's vital signs were recorded. They were:

Vital sign	Observation	Normal value
Temperature	35.7 °C	36.0–37.2 °C
Heart rate	118 beats per minute	80–120 beats per minute
Respiratory rate	28 breaths per minute	20–25 breaths per minute
Blood pressure	96/57 mmHg	90–110 mmHg
Oxygen saturation	97% in air	98–100 % in air
Level of consciousness	Alert on AVPU scale	Alert on AVPU scale
Pain score (1–5)	3	1 (no pain)

Ross's PEWS score is 1 (Fig. 15.1). Why do you think his temperature was 35.7 °C? His heart rate was 118 beats per minute, what explanation can you give for this?

Types of fractures

When a bone fractures it will consist of fragments of bone. These fragments will either lie *distally* (further from the midline) or *proximally* (closer to the midline) to the middle of the bone. If the fragments are separated it will be a *complete* fracture or *incomplete* when the fragments remain partially attached.

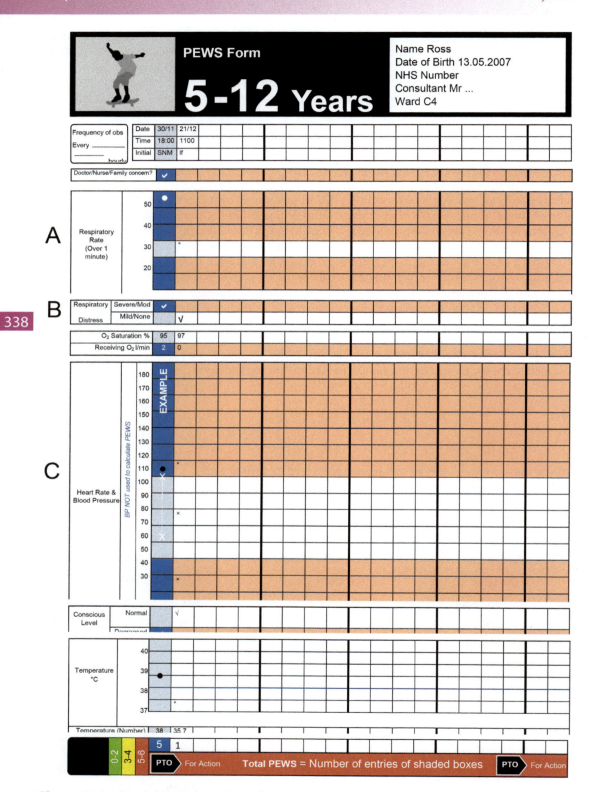

Figure 15.1 Ross's PEWS chart. Reproduced by kind permission of NHS Innovations.

Disorders of the musculoskeletal system   Chapter 15

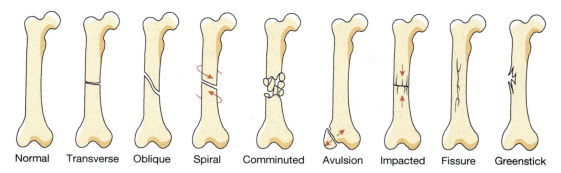

Figure 15.2 Fracture types.

Fractures are either simple or complicated, open, or closed. A complicated fracture will have bone fragments that may damage underlying organs, for example, lungs. An open fracture will have exposed bone visible through a wound in the skin. This is usually as a result of high-impact trauma and will necessitate surgical intervention.

If the fracture is across the bone it is called a *transverse* fracture. An oblique fracture is slanting but straight. A *spiral* fracture is slanting and circular twisting around the shaft of the bone (Fig. 15.2). A spiral fracture may result from physical abuse as a result of twisting a limb and will always warrant further investigation.

🚩 Red Flag

A spiral fracture may result from physical abuse as a result of twisting a limb and will always warrant further investigation.

A *comminuted* fracture occurs when small fragments of bone from the fractured shaft lie in the surrounding tissues.

A *Greenstick* fracture occurs when the bone is angulated beyond its capacity to bend and is an incomplete fracture. This is common in young children due to the pliability of their bones.

Torus or *buckle* fractures occur when one side of the bone buckles on itself without disrupting the other side. They heal more quickly than greenstick fractures.

An *impacted* fracture occurs when a fragment of bone is firmly driven into the other. This is usually as a result of landing feet first from a height.

A *fissure* is a crack on the surface of a bone but not extending through the bone.

An *avulsion* fracture is the separation of a small segment of bone from the cortex at the insertion site of a ligament or tendon.

🚩 Red Flag

Fractures in infancy and early childhood are rare and are usually the result of a fall from a height or from a motor vehicle accident. Bone injury in an infant or young child will always require further investigation. Physical abuse will need to be excluded. Detailed radiological imagining will be required.

Osteogenesis imperfecta should be considered as a possible diagnosis if multiple fractures are identified. Other associated features, e.g., blue sclera and hearing loss may also be present.

Features of fractures in children

Table 15.1 outlines the type, cause and features of fractures in children in relation to their location.

Diagnosis of a fracture

In addition to the history taken and systematic assessment, radiological imaging will be required. This is normally an X-ray in the first instance, and in the case of serious trauma a CT scan will be performed. The signs of a fracture include (Dandy & Edwards, 2003):

- deformity that is visible or palpable
- swelling at the fracture site
- abnormal movement and impaired function in the affected limb
- tenderness over the fracture site
- crepitus or grating between the bone ends
- bruising around the fracture
- pain on any movement, bending or compression.

Certain age groups and fractures may not necessarily display classic signs and can be missed. The young child may not be able to communicate their injury so signs of injury need to considered, for example, refusal to use a limb. In cases of physical abuse the parents or carers may not volunteer information or may give false information in relation to the presenting signs and symptoms. Equally the older child may not identify the exact mechanism of injury if risk-taking behaviour has been involved.

An undisplaced fracture may have no evidence of a deformity; a fracture within a capsule may not have any sign of bruising. Some fractures, such as those of the radial head and scaphoid, are difficult to diagnose (Whiteing, 2008). Non-verbal children will be unable to report pain so changes in behaviour should not be ignore. Untreated fractures can lead to life-changing consequences.

Pathophysiology of a fracture

A bone fractures when a force is applied to it and the bone is unable to absorb the force. Once the fracture has occurred, the muscles immediately contract in an attempt to splint the injured area (Hockenberry, Wilson & Winkelstein, 2005). A result of this is deformity of the bone produced secondary to the muscles pulling the bone out of place. Bleeding occurs at the site of injury resulting in haematoma formation, which is essential to healing.

Healing occurs in three or four distinct but overlapping stages (Fig. 15.3):

1. Early inflammatory stage
2. Repair stage (fibrous)
3. Bony callus formation
4. Remodelling stage.

Early inflammatory stage

In the inflammatory stage a haematoma develops from the fracture site in the immediate aftermath of the fracture. Macrophages, monocytes, lymphocytes, polymorphonuclear cells and fibroblasts infiltrate the bone under prostaglandins mediation (Kalfas, 2001). Granulation tissue forms and mesenchymal cells arrive at the injured site. Nutrients and oxygen supply are provided by the exposed cancellous bone and muscle.

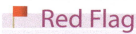

Red Flag

The use of NSAIDs in the early phase may alter the inflammatory response and delay bone healing.

Table 15.1 Location and features of fractures

Location of fracture	Features
Skull and facial bones	Requires significant impact to fracture skull. Types of fractures include: linear: straight line fracture depressed: bone is pushed inwards towards brain (may require surgical involvement) diastatic: a fracture that has spread to more than one bone of the skull as they are not yet fused properly basilar: a fracture in the base of the skull; can lead to spinal cord damage. Facial bone injury is usually as a result of high-energy trauma
Wrist and forearm	Common injury in the over 5 age group Usually resulting from a fall on an outstretched arm Midshaft and distal fractures of radius usually; ulna frequently involved Majority are simple transverse fractures requiring immobilisation in a cast or splint for 4–6 weeks
Epiphyseal injuries	Accounts for up to a quarter of all skeletal injuries Radius and ulna are the most frequent sites of injury 10–15-year age group most affected Usually resulting from a fall on an outstretched arm
Clavicle fracture	Shaft of clavicle usually affected Common injury from falls and sport injury as a result of excessive compression to the shoulder Treatment is supportive in the form of analgesia and application of a sling to immobilise Reduction is required in extreme cases of displacement only Can occur during the birth process if baby is large and mother has small pelvis
Humerus	Supracondylar fractures are the most common usually as result of impact to the elbow from a fall; can lead to significant vascular injury and compromise 10% of humeral fractures occur at the shaft – in the infant and young child this may be as a result of twisting so requires detailed investigation. In the older child it maybe as a result of direct trauma The mechanism of injury in fractures of the humerus is usually a fall onto an outstretched hand Proximal humeral fractures are rare with distal humeral fractures involving the lateral epicondyle more than the medial Treatment will depend on the injury with supracondylar fractures usually requiring open reduction
Rib cage	Rare but could occur as a result of high-energy impact or direct physical trauma (physical abuse)
Spinal fractures	Rare in childhood Resulting from significant trauma: fall from a height, motor vehicle accidents, diving, and sports injury Cervical spine most likely to be injured
Pelvis	Rare but associated with crush injury (horse-riding fall) and motor vehicle accidents Expect damaged to associated organs: bladder, bowel, blood supply
Hip	Rare but may occur as a result of motor vehicle accidents or fall from a height Can lead to avascular necrosis of the femoral head and damage to the growth plates
Femur	Common site of injury in young children. Peaks at 2–3 years of age. Usually femoral shaft involved. Motor vehicle accident or fall from a significant height is the usual cause. Management will depend on the age of the child and the type of injury and fracture
Patella	Rare but may occur as a result of high-energy trauma May be a single crack or multiple cracks, which is called a 'stellar' fracture More common in males than females
Tibia and fibula	Most common lower extremity fracture is midshaft of tibia and fibula Majority are non-displaced and will be managed in a cast and non-weight bearing Tibia fractures in preschool children are commonly as a result of a rotating mechanism injury to the lower limb
Ankle	Young people most likely to fracture ankles Growth plate involved in 1 of every 6 fractures Males more likely to fracture ankles Direct trauma (sport) is most common cause
Foot	Metatarsals account for 50% of fractures of the foot. Most are non-displaced Mechanism of injury is as a result of direct and indirect trauma, falls and jumping from a height and twisting injuries

Adapted from Nettina 2010.

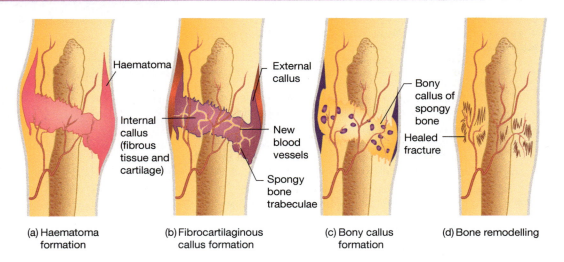

Figure 15.3 Stages in bone healing.

Repair stage (Fig. 15.3)

Vascular ingrowth is supported by the presence of fibroblasts. A collagen matrix is laid down and osteoid is secreted and mineralises with calcium salts, which leads to the formation of very soft callus around the fracture. On X-ray this has a cloud-like appearance. The callus is very weak and needs to be protected during this stage, which usually takes 4–6 weeks by internal fixation, traction or a cast. Failure to protect the newly formed callus could result in unstable fibrous union leading to deformity. The callus then ossifies and a bridge of woven bone is formed between the ends of the fracture fragments.

Remodelling

Remodelling is when the fractured bone has healed to its original shape, structure and strength (Kalfas, 2001; McRae & Esser, 2002; McRae, 2006). This is a slow process and takes place over a period of months to years. The amount of stress placed on the bone during this phase is important in remodelling. Bone is laid down where it is required as the fracture site is exposed to the axil loading force. Adequate strength is normally achieved within 3–6 months.

Traction

The use of traction has somewhat gone into demise as technology has evolved to produce fixation devices that allow partial or full mobility. Surgical interventions are now used more frequently further reducing the length of time and use of traction. However, it is important that the healthcare professional understands the principles of traction to be able to provide appropriate care for children who may still be required to be immobilised by this method.

Traction means to pull and in order to be effective there must be a counter-traction (pull in the opposite direction) (Fig. 15.4).

The general purpose of traction is to provide rest to a limb, treat a dislocation or correct a deformity, immobilise a specific area of the body, promote alignment either pre- or post-operatively.

Traction can be applied to the upper extremities, lower extremities or to the cervical area (Table 15.2). It can be applied manually by hand, directly to the skin surface via

Disorders of the musculoskeletal system Chapter 15

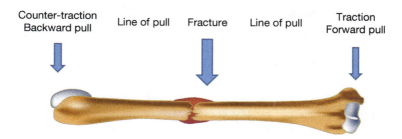

Figure 15.4 Application of traction to maintain bone alignment.

Table 15.2 Types of traction and examples of each

Traction	Type
Upper extremity	Overhead Dunlop traction
Lower extremity	Gallows/Bryant Bucks Russell 90/90 Balanced Skeletal
Cervical	Halo brace Halo vest Crutchfield tongs

adhesive bandages, or to the skeleton by wire, pins or tongs inserted through the diameter of the bone.

The care of a child in traction includes:

- Checking the traction system daily to ensure weights are hanging freely, cords and knots are intact, pulleys are working effectively, that counter-traction is being maintained and end of the bed is elevated.
- Outer bandages should be removed at least daily, limb inspected, washed and dried and outer bandage reapplied.
- Neurovascular status should be assessed and documented.
- Pressure area care administered.
- Passive and active exercises performed along with breathing exercises, e.g., blowing bubbles, balloon to prevent chest infections.
- General physical and personal care needs will be delivered in conjunction with parental/carer involvement.
- Relief of boredom is also an important aspect of care as is maintaining educational needs.

External fixation

If a fracture cannot be reduced and managed by traction or the application of a cast, then external fixation may be used. This is now common when there is associated soft tissue involvement and bone loss. The external fixator holds the bone in alignment as the bone and bone fragments are held in place by metal pins, which are attached to an external metal frame. This frame can be in situ for a number of months thus restricting mobility and activity. An important aspect of caring for a child with an external fixator in place is to ensure their neurovascular status is intact and that the pin sites are inspected and cleaned as per local policy. Early detection of pin-site infection will need prompt treatment. Management of pain is essential as is the provision of psychological care as acceptance of the external frame and the altered body image associated with this may take some time for the child and family.

Distraction

Distraction is the process of separating opposing bone to encourage regeneration of new bone. Distraction osteogenesis is used to treat non-union of fractures, for limb lengthening and malalignment. The bone is surgically 'broken', K wires are inserted proximal and distally to the fracture. Manual distraction is achieved by adjusting the telescopic rods on the rings to increase the distance between the rings. A percutaneous ostomy is performed to create a false growth plate at the same time. Histogenesis of muscle, nerves and skin occurs simultaneously with the development of the new bone (Ilizarov & Rozbruch, 2007). The Ilizarov frame (Fig. 15.5) has been used since the 1960s and its use has been extended to manage acute trauma to the limb where skin integrity has been reduced.

Scrupulous pin care is essential and the child and family will often assume responsibility for this once the child has recovered post-operatively. They will need to be taught to recognise signs of infection and for loosening of the pins. The child and family will also learn how to adjust the frame to achieve distraction. The child will be able to mobilise partially weight-bearing on crutches. As the Ilizarov frame will be in situ for months, the child will need support to return to their normal activities of living. Significant support is often required as the device is obvious, thus body image and self-esteem are challenged. The Ilizarov frame is removed under general anaesthetic and the child will need to carry on using crutches post removal for up to 4–6 weeks.

Care and management

A systematic and holistic assessment is required and initial interventions are directed at assessing and managing airway, breathing, circulation, disability and exposure prior to dealing with the fracture (Frazer, 2007). Once the child is stable the fracture can be assessed.

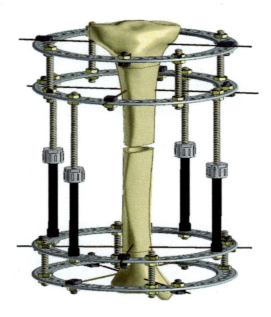

Figure 15.5 Ilizarov frame.

The extent of the injury may be assessed using the 5 Ps to identify vascular compromise. These are:

- **P**ain – administer analgesia
- **P**ulse – palpate pulses distal to the fracture
- **P**allor – the limb
- **P**aresthesia – sensation distal to the fracture site
- **P**aralysis – movement distal to the fracture site.

Neurovascular status should be rechecked on a frequent basis.
The principles of management are the same for all fractures:

- reduction – to restore normal alignment
- immobilisation – to promote healing of the bone
- rehabilitation – to normal function or to assist with impaired mobility.

Open wounds should be covered with a sterile dressing initially. It is likely that open wounds will require surgical intervention. Antibiotics will need to be administered to prevent infection and the development of osteomyelitis.

Avoid moving the affected limb if possible, particularly if it has not been splinted. Soft splints, such as folded towels, may be used until a more definitive splint is applied. The child may require sedation prior to the application of any splinting device and will need continuous cardiovascular monitoring during this procedure.

The child and family are likely to be very anxious and traumatised by the events that have brought them to the hospital and they will need reassurance and an explanation of the plan of care. Once the plan of care is established, it is likely that parental involvement will be significant in relation to personal care, play, and in passive exercises of the limbs. Education in the use of mobility aids will be required as will preparation for discharge.

Limping in childhood

There are a number of conditions that present with a limping child. Limps can be classed as either painful or painless (Lissauer & Clayden, 2007). The cause of the limp will need to be investigated and treated accordingly. Limps can present at any stage in childhood from age 1 year up to adulthood. Table 15.3 outlines some of the causes.

Slipped capital femoral epiphysis

Slipped capital femoral epiphysis (SCFE) is a relatively common disorder of the child or young person's hip, but it is a condition where correct diagnosis and immediate treatment is critical if bone integrity is to be maintained (Katz, 2006). There is displacement of the epiphysis of the femoral head postero-inferiorly (Fig. 15.6) (Lissauer & Clayden, 2007). The metaphysis also slips downwards and backwards.

Occurrence is more common in boys than girls, usually between 10 and 16 years of age. A downward trend in the age of occurrence has been reported, and the suggested rationale for this is the phenomenon of children maturing at a younger age (Azzopardi, Sharma & Bennet, 2010). The risk of SCFE is increased in children who are obese. Children with Down syndrome, adiposogenital syndrome, hypothyroidism, pituitary tumours and decreased growth hormone levels are also more predisposed to developing SCFE.

One hip or both may be involved, with 20% of children having bilateral involvement. Of the children who present with one-sided SCFE initially, 20–30% will develop a contralateral SCFE within 12–18 months (Nettina, 2010).

Table 15.3 Some causes of limp in childhood

Age	Painful limp	Painless limp
1–3 years of age	Trauma both accidental and non-accidental Osteomyelitis Septic arthritis Transient synovitis	Developmental dysplasia of the hip Neuromuscular defects, e.g., cerebral palsy Juvenile idiopathic arthritis
3–10 years	Trauma both accidental and non-accidental Osteomyelitis Septic arthritis Transient synovitis Perthes disease Malignant disease Juvenile idiopathic arthritis	Juvenile idiopathic arthritis Developmental dysplasia of the hip Neuromuscular defects – Duchenne's muscular dystrophy
11–18 years	Slipped capital femoral epiphysis Trauma Juvenile idiopathic arthritis Osteomyelitis Septic arthritis Bone tumours	Juvenile idiopathic arthritis Slipped capital femoral epiphysis Dysplastic hip Neuromuscular defects, e.g., cerebral palsy

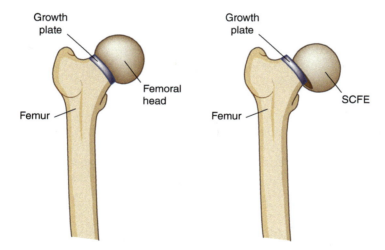

Figure 15.6 Normal femur and femur with slipped capital femoral epiphysis.

The child may present with hip pain, mid-thigh pain, knee pain, sudden, insidious onset of a limp and a decreased range of motion in the hip.

🚩 Red Flag

The goal of treatment is to prevent complications such as avascular necrosis and necrosis of cartilage. Accurate diagnosis is paramount and prompt treatment is essential. Delay in diagnosis and treatment can have life-changing effects.

Disorders of the musculoskeletal system   Chapter 15

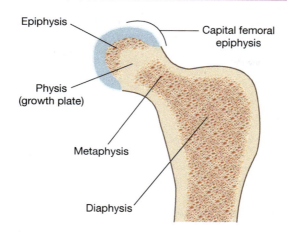

Figure 15.7 Growth plates of the femur.

Pathophysiology

The exact aetiology is unknown but it is thought that there are predisposing risk factors such as inactivity, periods of rapid growth spurts, overweight.

The epiphyseal growth plate widens unusually and there is a zone of hypertrophy. In addition to this there is abnormal cartilage maturation, endochondral ossification and instability of the perichondral ring. This leads to inadequate organisation of the cartilage columns. Slippage then occurs through this weakened area. During adolescence the proximal physis changes from horizontal to oblique. This redirects the forces felt through the hip from compression to shear (Zupanc, Krizanic & Daniel, 2008). In children who present with SCFE, a disorganisation of collagen fibrils and an accumulation of glycoproteins with the growth plates have been identified, but the exact role of this is unknown.

The femoral neck slips off the proximal femoral epiphysis and it remains contained within the acetabulum. This is one of the few joints in the body where the epiphysis is within the joint capsule (Fig. 15.7). This is referred to as a Salter–Harris type physeal fracture.

Classification

SCFE is classified by the duration of the symptoms. There are three elements to this:

1. Acute is defined as sudden onset and symptoms have been present for less than 3 weeks.
2. Chronic is the presence of symptoms lasting 3 weeks or more with changes.
3. Finally, an acute exacerbation of symptoms.

It is essential to determine if the child can weight bear with stable hip, or will be non-weight bearing with unstable hip.

Classification will identify the percentage of displacement of the hip in relation to the neck of femur and radiological interpretation (Georgiadis & Zaltz, 2014), see Table 15.4.

Diagnosis

The definitive diagnosis is confirmed by radiological evaluation, X-ray, CT scan, MRI and bone scan if avascular necrosis is suspected. A full physical examination of the child is required, including examination of the hip joint.

Table 15.4 Radiological classification of SCFE

Classification	% displacement
Type I	Less than 33% displacement
Type II	33–50% displacement
Type III	>50% displacement

Care and management

A detailed nursing assessment should be carried out including the onset of symptoms along with the characteristics and location of pain. Hip movement and associated restrictions should be noted.

Control of pain is an essential aspect of nursing care. An age-appropriate pain assessment tool should be used and analgesia administered as prescribed with effectiveness monitored. This is a requirement in the pre- and post-operative period.

Immobilisation through bed rest will be required and activity restricted as directed. This may include the application of skin traction. The provision of mobility aids, for example, crutches or a wheel chair should be considered.

The child and family should be prepared for surgery in accordance with local policy. Post-operative care will be determined by the procedure carried out.

Support for the child and family in following any pre- and post-operative restrictions is required in order to prevent lasting damage to the femur and hip joint (Nettina, 2010). Assistance with mobilisation will be needed so early introduction to the physiotherapy team is recommended.

The management options for SCFE will be dependent on the severity of the slip. Surgical intervention will be required. Fixation permits early stabilisation of the slippage, preventing further slippage and amelioration of potential risks (Georgiadis & Zaltz, 2014). For mild to moderate slips, percutaneous fixation is required and there may be prophylactic pinning of the contralateral hip using either Kirschner wires or cannulated screws (NICE, 2015).

In severe cases, open fixation of the growth plate with a bone graft is required. The aim of this procedure is to relocate the capital femoral epiphysis to its central position in the acetabulum and preserve the blood supply to the epiphysis thus reducing the risk of avascular necrosis. This may involve surgical dislocation of the hip, removal of bone from the metaphysis of the femoral neck, adduction and rotation of the limb, or realignment of the epiphysis to its normal position within the acetabulum, which is kept in situ with cannulated screws or Kirschner wires.

Perthes disease

This is a self-limiting condition of the proximal femur characterised by interruption of the blood supply to the capital femoral epiphysis. This results in avascular necrosis. This loss of blood supply is temporary and revascularisation and re-ossification occurs over a period of 24–48 months (Joseph, 2015; Lissauer & Clayden, 2007).

Boys are five times more likely to be affected than girls and it is more common in the 5–10-year age group. Ten to 20% of cases are bilateral. The exact aetiology of Perthes disease remains unknown but early recognition and treatment is essential in preserving the femoral head deformation.

Pathophysiology

While the aetiology is unknown, it is known that there is interruption to the vascular supply to the femoral head leading to necrosis. Perthes disease has four identified stages:

Disorders of the musculoskeletal system Chapter 15

- Stage 1 Avascularity
- Stage 2 Revascularisation
- Stage 3 Reossification
- Stage 4 Healing

Stage 1: Avascularity

Vascular occlusion is triggered spontaneously and the capital femoral epiphysis is deprived of blood. This results in the osteoblasts in the epiphysis dying and a cessation in bone growth. As a result of this, there is widening in the joint space. Synovitis, hypertrophy of the articular cartilage and hypertrophy of the ligamentum teres occurs (Joseph, 2015). The soft tissue changes and muscle spasm results in the femoral head extruding from the acetabulum laterally. Weight bearing causes stress and further muscle contractions within the hip joint and onto the extruded part of the avascular femoral head. This results in the trabeculae collapsing, leading to an irreversible deformity of the femoral head (Joseph et al., 2003) (Fig. 15.8). The greater the degree of extrusion of the femoral head, the greater the propensity for deformation. This stage may last for weeks to several months. The child may show signs of the disease at this stage by walking with a limp or altered gait.

Stage 2: Revascularisation

This stage may also be referred to as fragmentation. X-ray appearance of the femoral head will show a flattened femoral head. Necrotic bone is reabsorbed and replaced with woven bone initially. The head of the femur is particularly vulnerable during this stage as it is

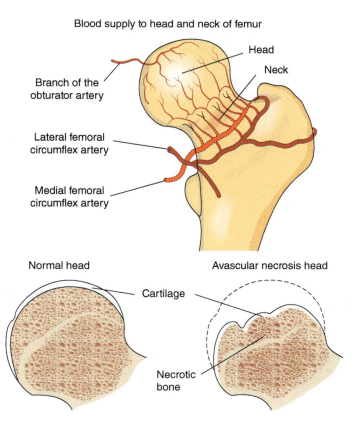

Figure 15.8 Avascularity of the femoral head.

lacking in strength so is prone to pathological fractures. Any abnormal force to the weakened epiphysis can lead to progressive deformities (Nettina, 2010). If more than 20% of the width of the epiphysis extrudes outside the acetabulum, damage is likely to be irreversible (Joseph *et al.*, 2003). This stage may last for 1–2 years.

Stage 3: Reossification
The head of the femur gradually begins to reshape as new stronger bone develops. The nucleus of the epiphysis breaks up into tiny fragments. New bone develops at the medial and lateral aspects of the epiphysis. All of the necrotic bone is now replaced and this stage, the longest, lasts 2–4 years.

Stage 4: Healing
Bone regrowth is complete and the femoral head will have reached its final shape. The reshaped femoral head may or may not resemble the desired spherical shape. This is dependent on a number of factors:

- extent of damage that occurred during the fragmentation stage;
- age of the child at the onset of the disease;
- instigation of treatment.

Treatment that is instigated after fragmentation or in the latter stages of fragmentation is likely to prevent further damage to the femoral head and is said to be remedial in nature (Joseph, 2015).

Diagnosis
The child is likely to present with a history of limp or pain in their hip. This may have been present for a period of time and may worsen with activity. There may be referred pain in their knee, thigh or groin. On examination the child will have limited abduction (Fig. 15.9) in the affected hip and it will be internally rotated.

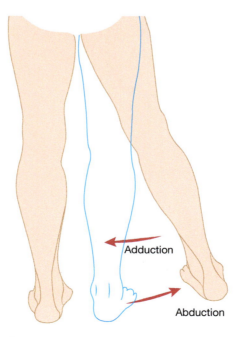

Figure 15.9   Abduction of lower limb.

Disorders of the musculoskeletal system   Chapter 15

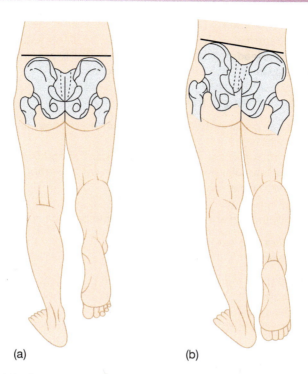

(a)   (b)

Figure 15.10 Trendelenburg gait. (a) Normal hip joints. (b) There is a dip on the opposite of the pelvis when weight bearing on the affected side.

On examination of the hip joint, the child is likely to develop muscle spasm on internal rotation. Trendelenburg gait will be evident; when the child is weight bearing on the affected limb, there will be a dip on the opposite side of the pelvis (Fig. 15.10).

Investigations

X-ray will be required following a full physical examination. The child with Perthes disease will need several X-rays during the course of treatment, which can last 2 years or longer. The X-ray required of the hip joint will be anteroposterior view and a frog-leg lateral. The X-ray will identify the extent of epiphyseal involvement, its condition, and will enable the doctor to identify the stage of the disease. It is important to note that as the condition progresses, the X-rays of the hip joint may look worse before any improvement is seen. Early X-ray may not show any abnormality. The young child with Perthes disease who is being managed through observation will require an X-ray every 3–4 months to monitor progress of the disease.

Magnetic resonance imaging has limited use in the detection of infraction of the bone, and is less beneficial in identifying the stages of healing.

Bone scanning may be required to confirm diagnosis if X-ray is questionable. Ultrasound may be useful if joint effusion is suspected in the early stages.

Care and treatment

The goal of treatment with Perthes disease is to relieve pain, protect the shape of the femoral head by containment and restore normal hip movement. Containment of the femoral epiphysis well into the acetabulum in order to protect the epiphysis is the desired outcome of any intervention (Joseph, 2015). Treatment early in the disease process is key to a positive outcome. If left untreated the femoral head will be deformed, inadequately positioned with the acetabulum, leading to the likelihood of the early onset of arthritis. The child and family need to be aware that the treatment is long term.

There are many treatment options for Perthes disease and the plan of treatment will be dependent on the following factors:

- age of child at the onset of the disease – younger children have greater potential for developing new bone;
- the degree of damage to the femoral head. If more than 50% of the femoral head has been affected by avascular necrosis the prospect for bone regrowth and special shaping of the femoral head is diminished;
- the range of motion of the hip joint;
- the stage the disease is diagnosed. Ideally this needs to be achieved early in stage 1.

Treatment is either non-surgical or surgical.
Non-surgical treatment will involve:

- Observation entailing regular monitoring on an outpatient basis with X-ray of the hip. This will continue while the condition is stable and until the head of the femur has completely healed.
- Reduction of activity such as running, jumping or any activity that has high impact on the hip joint. This may include periods of bed rest and skin traction if the femoral head is not in a satisfactory position or if there is loss of function of the joint and muscle spasm. Braces and cast may also be used to restrict movement. Parental involvement in the care of the child will be required as one of the challenges with caring for the child with Perthes disease is that they are well and active but need to have their activity restricted.
- Analgesia, non-steroidal anti-inflammatory medication to reduce inflammation of the hip joint.
- Physical therapy to restore range of movement in the hip joint. This may include hip abduction and exercises to promote internal rotation of the hip joint and hydrotherapy.

Surgical treatment will be required to re-establish the alignment of the femoral head in the acetabulum and thus the function of the hip joint. It may be required if non-surgical interventions have been unsuccessful or the child meets the criteria set out earlier. It includes:

- Soft tissue release – this will improve movement within the hip joint as the tight muscles within the groin are released.
- Shelf acetabuloplasty – e.g., a bone graph is used to enlarge the acetabulum so the femoral head will have more covering to protect it and it fits more securely into the newly formed acetabulum.
- Pelvic osteotomy – the acetabulum is reoriented so it covers the anterolateral aspect of the femoral epiphysis.
- Femoral osteotomy – the head of the femur is repositioned into the acetabulum by cutting through the femur and the alignment is held by plate and screws until after the healing stage of the disease has occurred.

Post-surgery (osteotomy), the child is usually placed in a cast to protect the alignment for 6–8 weeks. In the initial post-operative period, opioid analgesia will be required so close monitoring of the child's condition is necessary. Blood transfusion may be required (Hockenberry et al., 2005).

Disorders of the musculoskeletal system   Chapter 15

 Red Flag

Healthcare professionals need to be aware that some children may not be able to take non-steroidal anti-inflammatory medication (NSAIDs). Examples of these are: ibuprofen, naproxen, indomethacin and diclofenac acid. As an effective analgesia in musculoskeletal disorders, the lowest dose of NSAID should be used (BNFC, 2016). NSAIDs have both an analgesic and anti-inflammatory effect. The relief of pain is usually within a short time frame once the NSAID has been consumed, but the anti-inflammatory effect may not be achieved for up to 3 weeks. This can be longer in some conditions, e.g., juvenile idiopathic arthritis.

NSAIDs reduce the production of prostaglandins, which inhibit the enzyme cyclo-oxygenase. There are different types of cyclo-oxygenase and inhibition of cyclo-oxygenase 2 will reduce gastrointestinal intolerance. Gastrointestinal symptoms are unusual with short-term use of NSAIDs (BNFC, 2016).

NSAIDs should be used with caution in children with asthma, angioedema, urticaria, rhinitis and allergic disorders. For children with renal, cardiac or hepatic impairment caution is required when prescribing NSAIDs.

NSAIDs are contraindicated in children with severe heart failure and gastric ulceration. However, children do appear to tolerate NSAIDs better than adults and gastrointestinal side effects are less commonly reported.

While there is no consensus on treatment for Perthes disease, treatment should aim to prevent the deformation of the femoral head in order to minimise the risk of secondary arthritis, which might necessitate hip replacement at a later stage.

Developmental dysplasia of the hip

Developmental dysplasia of the hip (DDH) is a spectrum of disorders relating to abnormal development of the hip. These can range from dysplasia, to subluxation, to complete dislocation of the hip (Table 15.5). A common congenital malformation, it is an important cause of disability in childhood and contributes to 9% of all primary hip replacements (Dezateaux & Rosendahl, 2007). DDH is more common in girls and in the left hip (Paton, 2005). Bilateral involvement is evident in 50% of cases and it is more common in Caucasians (Nettina, 2010).

Neonatal screening identifies the majority of babies with DDH, but not all as it may not be possible to detect if the acetabulum is only mildly shallow. The rapid development of ultrasound has led to speedy and accurate diagnosis in the neonatal period. Not all dysplastic or instable hips will require treatment.

A number of risk factors are known and these include:

- breech birth
- first born
- large baby

Table 15.5 Key terms associated with DDH

Instability: a diagnosis made on examination where passive manipulation caused the hip to subluxate or dislocate.
Subluxation: partial dislocation of the femoral head from the acetabulum. There is incomplete contact between articular surfaces of the femoral head and acetabulum. Usually diagnosed by ultrasound.
Dysplasia: an abnormality of the development of the acetabulum. This usually results in a shallow and dysmorphic acetabulum.
Dislocation: complete loss of contact between the articular surfaces of the femoral head and acetabulum.

- oligohydramnios
- positive family history of DDH
- intrauterine malposition that leads to other musculoskeletal disorders, e.g., tortocolis, metatarsus adductus
- cultural swaddling of babies where legs are adducted.
- underlying neuromuscular disorders.

Diagnosis

Neonatal screening for DDH will detect the majority of cases, but not all. Diagnosis in the older infant and child can be challenging as the disorder can be advanced by the time the condition is suspected (McCarthy, Scoles & MacEwen, 2005). Unilateral DDH is more likely to be detected early as asymmetry of the lower limb will be more obvious and likely to concern the parents/carers. Other signs that may be apparent in the older infant and child are:

- limited abduction
- limb length discrepancy
- asymmetries of the thigh skin folds
- asymmetry of buttocks
- crawls with difficulty
- delayed walking
- difficulty sitting astride adult's legs or bicycle
- stands or walks with external rotation
- limp evident if able to walk, or waddling gait.

Care and treatment

The primary aim of treatment is to achieve reduction of the hip, which will increase the chances of having a functioning hip joint and therefore a normal range of movement. Early diagnosis is likely to, but may not necessarily avoid the need for surgical intervention.

Splinting is usually the initial treatment modality and the infant will be placed in a Craig splint or Pavlik harness (Fig. 15.11). If hip reduction can be maintained, the acetabulum appears to be able to develop around the head of the femur. This results in improved sta-

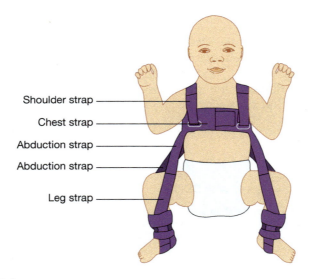

Figure 15.11 Pavlik harness.

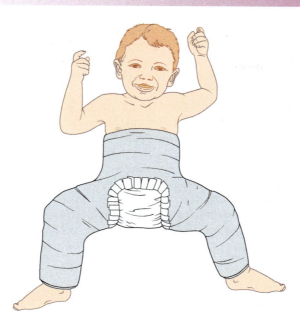

Figure 15.12 Hip spica.

bility of the hip and associated dysplasia (Paton, 2005). The splint may be in situ for a number of months. The position of the infant in the splint is important as the blood supply to the femoral head is easily compromised and could lead to avascular necrosis or deformity of the femoral head. The straps of the harness prevent the hips abducting beyond the midline and flexion is maintained between 90° and 100°. Close monitoring will be required and the infant will need to have ultrasound to monitor their progress and for development of complications. For hips that are severely subluxed and not reducible the infant will require weekly ultrasound scanning while the splint is in situ. The infant with a dysplasia of their hips will normally have an ultrasound every 3 weeks.

However, if the child's hip is not responding to this treatment, it should be discontinued because of the risk of developing avascular necrosis (Clarke & Sakthivel, 2008).

If diagnosis is delayed and the hip is unstable, a hip spica (Fig. 15.12) following closed reduction may be used (Lissauer & Clayden, 2007). The child may have a period of traction prior to this. Hoop traction and serial abduction traction is now outdated (Clarke & Sakthivel, 2008). The hip spica places the hip in a secure position, promoting good blood flow thus avoiding the risk of avascular necrosis. An arthrogram and/or abductor tenotomy will often be performed at this stage giving a more detailed picture of the hip. The hip spica will be in situ for 3 months but it will be changed under general anaesthetic at 6-weekly intervals to examine the hip because the child will be growing, and the hip spica is likely to be soiled. Parental education and support will be needed to enable them to meet their child's care needs while h/she is in the hip spica.

If correction is not achieved by the aforementioned methods, the child will need an open reduction at a later stage. Diagnosis after 24 months of age will require surgical treatment, and surgery is effective up to the age of 8 years.

In addition to the care the child requires pre- and post-surgery, nursing care interventions for a child with DDH should focus on skin integrity, mobility and family care. The parents/carers will need explanation about the conditions and treatments. The parents/carers will need to be comfortable with applying the Pavlik harness. Competency in handling their child in a hip spica will be required before the child can be discharged. This will include transporting the child and attending to their personal hygiene needs. The mother may need assistance with breastfeeding as positioning can be more difficult due to the weight of the cast.

Neurovascular status will need to be monitored and this should be explained to the parents prior to discharge.

Skin integrity is important and normal hygiene habits should be maintained. Pressure points should be checked while the child is in the Pavlik harness. The condition of the skin in the perineal area, abdomen and lower limbs should be checked for developing pressure ulcers. The condition of the hip spica around the perineal area should be checked as it can get soggy from urine if the correct size nappy is not used. Additional padding may be required overnight to avoid urine leaking into the cast.

The child in a hip spica will need assistance to turn as they will be unable to do this themselves initially. Tummy time is also important for those under 6 months to assist with developing their head control. They will be unable to crawl while in their hip spica so activities that encourage foot action and upper body engagement will be beneficial.

Investigations

Barlow test: The hip is adducted and gentle pressure is applied to the hips. A 'clunk' will be felt as the hip subluxes out of the acetabulum (Fig. 15.13). This is a positive test.

Ortolani test: The thumb is placed over the inner thigh and the index is placed on the greater trochanter. The hip is then abducted and gentle pressure is placed on the greater trochanter. A 'clunk' will be felt when the hip is reduced (Fig. 15.14). This is a positive test.

Both tests are only suitable on infants younger than 6 weeks of age. The fingers should not leave any marks on the infant's skin and the test should be performed gently. One hip at a time should be tested. The Barlow test should be performed first and then the Ortolani test.

If either test is positive, then the baby must be referred for ultrasound to confirm diagnosis.

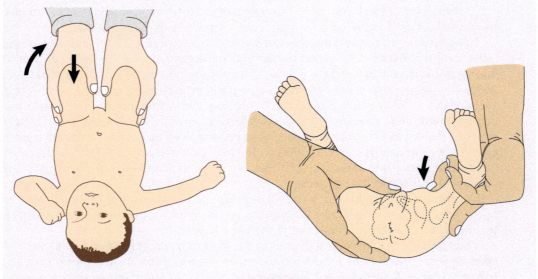

Figure 15.13 Barlow test.

Figure 15.14 Ortolani's test.

Disorders of the musculoskeletal system   Chapter 15

Conclusion

This chapter has provided insight into the anatomy and pathophysiology of a number of musculoskeletal conditions that are common in childhood. The focus has been on providing information that is pertinent for the delivery of effective care by enhancing the reader's understanding of the pathophysiological changes that occur either as a result of injury or those due to abnormal development, and the impact that this has on the child and family or carers.

References

Azzopardi, T., Sharma, S. & Bennet, G.C. (2010). Slipped capital femoral epiphysis in children aged less than 10 years. *Journal of Pediatric Orthopaedics* 19(1), 13–18.

British National Formulary for Children (BNFC) (2016). [online] Available at: https://bnf.nice.org.uk/ (last accessed April 2018).

Clarke, N.M.P. & Sakthivel, K. (2008). The diagnosis and management of congenital dislocation of the hip. *Paediatrics and Child Health* 18(6), 268–270.

Cooper, C., Dennison, E.M., Leufkens, H.G., Bishop, N. & Van Staa, T.P. (2004). Epidemiology of childhood fractures in Britain: a study using the general practice research database. *Journal of Bone and Mineral Research* 19(12).

Dandy, D.J. & Edwards, D.J. (2003). *Essential Orthopaedics and Trauma*, 4th edn. Churchill Livingstone, Edinburgh.

Dezateux, C. & Rosendahl, K. (2007). Developmental dysplasia of the hip. *Lancet* 369, 1541–1552.

Frazer, A. (2007). Major trauma: assessment prioritization and initial treatment. In: Evans, C. & Tippins, E. (eds). *The Foundation of Emergency Care*. Open University Press, Maidenhead.

Georgiadis A.G. & Zaltz, I. (2014). Slipped capital femoral epiphysis: how to evaluate with a review and update of treatment. *Pediatric Clinics of North America* 61(6), 1119–1135.

Hart, E.S., Luther, B. & Grottkau B.E. (2006). Broken bones: common pediatric lower extremity fractures – Part III. *Orthopaedic Nursing* 25(6), 390–407.

Hockenberry M.J., Wilson, D. & Winkelstein, M.L. (2005). *Wong's Essentials of Pediatric Nursing*, 7th edn. Elsevier Mosby, St. Louis.

Ilizarov, S. & Rozbruch, S.R. (2007). *Limb Lengthening and Reconstruction Surgery*. Informa Healthcare, New York.

Joseph, B. (2015). Management of Perthes disease. *Indian Journal of Orthopaedics* 49(1), 10–16.

Joseph, B., Varghese, G., Mulpuri, K., Narasimha Rao, K. & Nair, N.S. (2003). Natural evolution of Perthes disease: a study of 610 children under 12 years of age at disease onset. *Journal of Paediatric Orthopedics* 23, 590–600.

Kalfas, I.H. (2001). Principles of bone healing. *Neurosurgical Focus* 10(4), E1.

Katz, D.A. (2006). Slipped capital femoral epiphysis: the importance of early diagnosis. *Pediatric Annals* 35(2), 102–111.

Lissauer, T. & Clayden, G. (2007). *Illustrated Textbook of Paediatrics*, 3rd edn. Mosby/Elsevier, London.

McCarthy, J.J., Scoles, P.V. & MacEwen, G.D. (2005). Development dysplasia of the hip (DDH). *Current Orthopaedics* 19, 223–230.

McRae, R. (2006). *Pocketbook of Orthopaedics and Fractures*, 2nd edn. Churchill Livingstone, Edinburgh.

McRae, R. & Esser, M. (2002). *Practical Fracture Treatments*, 4th edn. Churchill Livingstone, Edinburgh.

National Institute for Health and Clinical Excellence (NICE) (2015). Open reduction of slipped capital femoral epiphysis. Interventional procedures guidance [IPG511] Available at: https://www.nice.org.uk/guidance/ipg511 (accessed 1 December 2016).

Nettina, S. (2010). *Lippincott Manual of Nursing Practice*. Wolters Kluwer/Lippincott Williams & Wilkins, Philadelphia.

Paton, R.W. (2005). Management of neonatal hip instability and dysplasia. *Early Human Development* 81, 807–813.

Peate, I. & Gormley-Fleming, E. (eds) (2015). *Fundamentals of Children's Anatomy and Physiology*, 1st edn. Wiley, Oxford.

Whiteing, N.L. (2008). Fractures: pathophysiology, treatment and nursing care. *Nursing Standard* 23(2), 49–57.

Zupanc, O., Krizanic, M. & Daniel, M. (2008). Shear stress in epiphyseal growth plate is a risk factor for slipped capital femoral epiphysis. *Journal of Pediatric Orthopedics* 28(40), 444–451.

Chapter 16

Disorders of the skin

Liz Gormley-Fleming

Aim

This chapter provides an overview of the anatomy and physiology of the skin. The chapter introduces the reader to altered pathophysiology and the impact this may have on the child, young person and family. The condition of the skin can often be the first sign of an underlying health issue.

Learning outcomes

On completion of this chapter, the reader will be able to:

- Describe the anatomy of the skin.
- Articulate an accurate description of a skin condition/rash.
- Outline the care of children with a wound.
- Articulate the difference between healing by primary intention and secondary intention.
- Understand the physiological changes that occur during wound healing.
- Explain the physiological change that occurs when a child has eczema.
- Understand the body's response to a burn injury, identify the classification of a burn injury and know how to calculate.

Keywords

- integument
- epidermis
- dermis
- epithelialisation
- inflammatory
- proliferation
- maturation
- keloid
- hypertrophic scar

Fundamentals of Children's Applied Pathophysiology: An Essential Guide for Nursing and Healthcare Students, First Edition.
Edited by Elizabeth Gormley-Fleming and Ian Peate.
© 2019 John Wiley & Sons Ltd. Published 2019 by John Wiley & Sons Ltd.
Companion website: www.wileyfundamentalseries.com/childpathophysiology

Chapter 16 — Disorders of the skin

Test your prior knowledge

1. Describe the functions of the skin.
2. List the layers of the epidermis.
3. Identify the different types of glands and their location.
4. List the accessory organs of the skin.
5. Identify the cells in the epidermis and their function.
6. Discuss how wounds heal.
7. Discuss the mechanism of injury in relation to burns.
8. Highlight the impact burns can have on a child physically and psychologically.
9. Discuss the life cycle of head lice.
10. Describe the role of the healthcare professional when providing care to a child with a disorder of their skin.

Introduction

The skin is the largest organ in the human body. It has several vital functions that are essential to sustain life. The skin, also known as the integumentary system, is a complex organ that is essential for human survival due to it physiological functions. It undergoes significant changes from birth to adulthood, such as thickening of the dermis and increased activity of the sebaceous glands. The most dynamic changes occur within the first 3 months of life (Hoeger & Enzmann, 2002). At birth the skin of a term baby is developed to cope with extra-uterine life.

As a system, the skin has contributions from basic germ layers: the ectoderm and the mesoderm. The ectoderm forms the surface epidermis and the associated glands while the mesoderm forms the underlying connective tissue of the dermis and subcutaneous layer (Chamley *et al.*, 2005). It is also populated with melanocytes and sensory nerve endings. These different tissues perform many specific functions: thermoregulation, synthesis of vitamin D, excretion, and immunity.

Frequently referred to as the largest organ in the body, the skin covers all of the body's external surfaces and is approximately 10% of the body mass. By adulthood the skin will be almost 2 square meters. The ratio of skin surface to body weight is highest at birth and this will decline progressively during infancy. At birth, the surface area is nearly three times greater than that of an older child, whereas at 37 weeks' gestation or less, it is proportionally five times greater than that of a term baby (Wong, 1999).

The skin is the first line of defence against the environment. Skin disorders of childhood vary greatly in both symptoms and severity. They can be permanent or temporary, painful or painless, minor to life-limiting. They are frequently associated with viral or bacterial infections, for example, slapped cheek syndrome, meningococcal septicaemia. Some of the more common conditions are identified in Table 16.1. Empirical evidence has demonstrated that loss of skin integrity in infants and children is most commonly attributed to wounds secondary to congenital conditions, thermal injury, extravasation injury, epidermal stripping and pressure ulcerations (McCullough & Kloth, 2010).

Disorders of the skin are normally described by the type of lesions that appear on the skin, the shape of the lesion, the colour and the configuration. Noting the type, shape, location and colour of the lesion is an essential component of obtaining a history of the rash or skin condition. Therefore it is important to be able to describe accurately the details of any rash an infant or child presents with, for example, a generalised, macular erythematous rash, hot to touch.

Disorders of the skin   Chapter 16

Table 16.1 Skin conditions of childhood

Congenital/present at birth	Infections	Acquired/trauma
Epidermolysis bullosa	Cellulitis	Surgery
Haemangioma	Herpes simplex	Burns
Eczema	Rubeola (measles)	Epidermal stripping
Café au lait spots	Verrucas	Pressure ulcerations
Port wine stains	Necrotising fasciitis	Blunt force trauma
Mongolia blue spots	Impetigo	Nappy rash
Lymphatic malformations e.g., cystic hygroma	Molluscum contagiosum	Melanoma
Albinism	Pilonidal sinus	Acne
Vitiligo	Shingles	Urticaria
	Ringworm	Friction
	Chicken pox	Sunburn

Type of lesion

Lesions may be described as either primary or secondary.

Primary lesions

- Macule – flat distinct discoloured area usually <1 cm diameter.
- Papule – a solid raised lesion, distinct border <1 cm diameter.
- Pustule – small raised area of skin containing cloudy purulent fluid.
- Wheal – a raised (itchy) area of the skin.
- Nodule – a solid raised area under the skin that is filled with fluid or tissue.
- Vesicle – small fluid-filled sacs.
- Petechiae – non-raised red-brown non-blanchable lesions.
- Bulla – vesicle or blister >1 cm in diameter.
- Plaque – solid and elevated lesion on the skin >1 cm in diameter.
- Cyst – soft, firm mass in the skin that will be filled with fluid or semi-solid material in a sac.

Secondary lesions

- Crusts – covering formed by drying serum, blood or pus.
- Scales – excessive dead cells that are produced due to an abnormality or inflammatory change.
- Lichenification – thickening of the skin.
- Fissures – cracks in the skin as a result of prolonged drying of the skin.
- Ulcer – destruction of the epidermis and part of the dermis.

Colour

- White – leukoderma, hypomelanosis
- Red – erythema
- Pink – hypermelanosis
- Brown
- Blue
- Grey
- Black

Shape
- Round
- Oval
- Annular – ring-shaped
- Irregular
- Guttate – drop-like

Arrangement
- Grouped – clustering of lesions
- Disseminated
- Generalised – widespread
- Discrete – lesions remain separate
- Linear – in lines
- Multiformed – more than one type of lesion
- Telangiectasia – dilated cutaneous vessels that are thread-like or lines

Epidermolysis bullosa

Epidermolysis bullosa (EB) is an inherited disorder that occurs in 1 : 17 000 children in the UK. It is a group of skin-blistering conditions and it is characterised by blisters, skin breakdown, pain, deformity, infection that can lead to secondary complications and an increased risk of squamous cell carcinoma (Watson, 2016). The epithelial lining of other organs may also be affected and blister as a result of minimal trauma. A lifelong condition, the child with EB will require lifetime healthcare input.

Epidermolysis bullosa is generally an inherited autosomal dominant disorder in that it relies on only having one affected parent for transmission. If a parent is a carrier, there is a 50% chance of having a child from each pregnancy who will inherit EB. Males and females are affected equally.

It may also be autosomal recessive so each parent would carry the affected gene and the risk of having a child born with EB would be 25% for each pregnancy.

It may also occur as a new disorder with no parent carrying an affected gene by genetic mutation.

Diagnosis

Diagnosis is by immunohistochemistry (Tenedini *et al.*, 2015). A definitive diagnosis will require a skin biopsy, possibly imaging and endoscopy if there is thought to be involvement of the gastrointestinal tract (Bruckner-Tuderman *et al.*, 2014). This is essential even in the presence of a complete history and assessment in order to prescribe the correct plan of treatment. Blood sampling for genetics may be obtained. Amniocentesis may be performed for prenatal diagnosis as early as the 10th week of gestation (National Institute of Arthritis and Musculoskeletal and Skin Diseases [NIAMS], 2013).

Types of epidermolysis bullosa

There are various types of epidermolysis bullosa ranging in severity from mild to life-limiting. Currently there are more than 30 types of EB so categorisation is ongoing as research develops in this area. International consensus was agreed in 2008 on the currently used names. Classification is dependent on the layer of skin at which blistering occurs (Fig. 16.1), as follows:

- Epidermolysis bullosa simplex (EBS)
- Junctional epidermolysis bullosa (JEB)

Disorders of the skin   Chapter 16

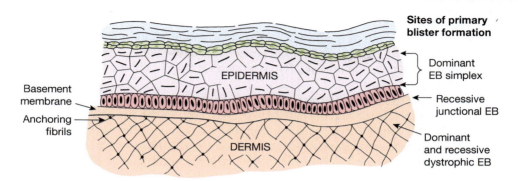

Figure 16.1   Cross-section of the skin and primary sites of blister formation.

- Dystrophic epidermolysis bullosa (DJB)
- Multiple levels of blistering – Kindler syndrome.

Epidermolysis bullosa simplex

Epidermolysis bullosa simplex (EBS) is a generalised form and is usually present at birth with blisters occurring primarily on the hands and feet. Blistering may be more widespread in sub-types of EBS. The cells of the epidermis are normally supported by keratins, which give the cells their shape and support. The keratin, usually type 5, type 14, or rarely plectin, is absent or present in insufficient amounts. In the presence of friction the cells rupture causing fluid to leak, which forms a blister. Finger and toenails may be absent. Blisters may occur inside the mouth. There may be thickening of the skin on the palms of the hands and soles of the feet. Anaemia may be present. In general the blisters are small but plentiful and approximately 2 cm in size. EBS accounts for 70% of cases (British Association of Dermatologists [BAD], 2015).

Junctional epidermolysis bullosa

Junctional epidermolysis bullosa (JEB) is usually severe and the child will have large blisters on its face, trunk and legs. It can be life-threatening because of the risk of infection and fluid loss. Blisters may also be present in the upper airway, oesophagus, lower intestinal system and urogenital system. This may lead to life-threatening episodes.

Absent finger and toenails may be in evidence and the skin may have a very thin appearance (atrophic scarring). Alopecia may occur following blistering of the scalp. The child will have delayed growth secondary to malnutrition. Anaemia is common. Involvement of soft tissues of the nose and mouth will be identified. JEB accounts for 5% of all cases, (BAD, 2015).

Dystrophic epidermolysis bullosa

Dystrophic epidermolysis bullosa (DEB) occurs in approximately 25% of cases (BAD, 2015). This may be either the autosomal dominant or recessive forms of DEB. In the dominant and mild recessive forms, blisters will be present on the hands, feet, elbows, and knees. There will be milia present on the trunk and limbs. The oesophagus is usually affected. Nails will be present but misshapen.

In severe DEB there will be blisters over large areas of the body surface. In addition, there will be loss of nails, pruritus, scarring, anaemia and delayed growth. There may be inflammation of the eyes and corneal erosion. The gastrointestinal tract and the oral cavity are likely to be affected. Early loss of permanent teeth occurs. Pseudosyndactyly – fusion of the fingers and toes – will affect most suffers of this type of DEB. Squamous cell carcinoma has been reported in young people with recessive DEB (NIAMS, 2013).

Kindler syndrome

Kindler syndrome is a rare type of EB. In addition to blistering, there are changes to the appearance of the skin – poikiloderma (breakdown of the skin) – and involvement of the gastrointestinal tract and the eyes. Hyperkeratosis of the soles of the feet and the palms of the hands will occur.

Kindler syndrome is usually diagnosed by the age of 1 year, with the presence of blisters on the hands and feet being the initial cause of concern. By the age of 5 years, the skin will be considerably thinner and more wrinkled than that of an unaffected child. It occurs as a result of a defect in the gene *KIND1* (also called the *FERMT1* gene) and is an autosomal recessive disorder (Genetic Reference, 2016). Children with Kindler syndrome are more susceptible to skin damage from sunlight so treatment plans and education on safety in the sun need to be provided.

Pathophysiology

Cytolysis, which is the destruction of cells by either rupture or disintegration, occurs. This causes blisters to form in the epidermis or basement membrane. It is the result of a genetic mutation, which affects the protein at the epidermal–dermal junction.

In EBS, cytolysis leads to blister formation in the basal or spinous layers of the epidermis. The keratinocytes have abnormal keratin filaments and they may also be structured inadequately. In JEB, there is separation of the epidermis from the basal lamina. The protein structures, hemidesmosomes, which are thread-like fibres, are absent or reduced; thus the epidermis is not firmly anchored to the base membrane. As a result of this, the tissues separate and blistering occurs in the upper area of the base membrane, the lamina lucida. In cases of DEB, the basal lamina and the epidermis are attached but a blister cavity forms below the lamina densa of the dermo–epidermal junction (Nettina, 2010). The hemidesmosomes (anchoring fibrils) are abnormal, reduced in number, or completely absent.

Case Study 1

Harry is 8 years old and has epidermolysis bullosa simplex, which was diagnosed when he was an infant. He has a severe form of epidermolysis bullosa simplex. As a baby and toddler he had frequent admissions to hospital. He attends his local lower school and tries his best to get involved in a range of activities as he dislikes not being able to participate. His mum has requested that he does not play football during the lunch break but Harry does not want to feel left out. He borrows some trainers and develops even more blisters on his feet. Harry has multiple blisters at the moment as the weather has become warmer. These are located on his hands, feet, trunk, legs, arm, face, and in his mouth. He does not want to tell his mum about these new blisters. His mum normally bursts new blisters to reduce the risk of infection.

After a few days, he is complaining of a lot of pain in his feet and when his mum takes his socks off to look at his feet she notices that the skin is red, hot and there is yellow/greenish fluid draining from the lateral malleolus on his left foot and from the dorsum of his right foot. He is not eating or drinking very much at the moment either, and is generally not himself. His mum knows that he needs to be seen by a doctor and takes him to the local hospital. He is also a patient at a specialist centre for EB and has regular appointments there with a dermatologist and an EB nurse specialist.

A full history is taken and his vital signs are recorded (see Table 16.2).

Disorders of the skin Chapter 16

Table 16.2   Harry's vital signs

Vital sign	Harry's observations	Normal range
Temperature	38.5 °C	36.0–37.2 °C
Pulse	130 beats per minute	80–120 beats per minute
Respiration	20 breaths per minute	20–25 breaths per minute
Blood pressure	100/60 mmHg	90–110 mmHg
Oxygen saturation	97%	98–100%
Pain score (1–5)	3	0

Table 16.3   Harry's blood test results

Test	Harry's results	Normal range
White blood cells (WBC)	16.4	4.5–13.5 WBC $\times 10^9$/L
Neutrophils	9×10^9/L	1.5–8 $\times 10^9$/L
Lymphocytes	8.4×10^9/L	1.5–7.0 $\times 10^9$/L
Red blood cells (RBC)	4.8×10^{12}/L	4.0–5.2 $\times 10^{12}$/L
Haemoglobin (Hb)	11.1 g/100 mL	11.5–15.0 g/100 mL
Platelets	240×10^9/L	150–450 $\times 10^9$/L
C-reactive protein	25 mg/L	<5 mg/L

As he is pyrexial the paediatrician arranges for Harry to have blood drawn for a full blood count and C-reactive protein level; the results are shown in Table 16.3.

Care and management

A holistic, systematic assessment is required based on the individual's needs. Care will be planned and implemented in accordance with findings. In addition to treating any infections, the aim of care should be to prevent any further trauma and blistering to the skin by any of the care interventions.

Pain

The pain score will indicate the type of analgesia required. This will need to be reassessed on a regular basis and the appropriate analgesia administered as required. Opiates are frequently used to control pain and prior to change of dressings. Appropriate monitoring will need to be considered to ensure the safety of the child.

Infection

There is a very high probability that a secondary infection is present so antibiotics will need to be prescribed. These may be oral, usually a penicillin-based antibiotic or clarithromycin if there is a known allergy to penicillin (BNFC, n.d.), or topical antibiotics may be prescribed. The choice of oral or topical antibiotics will be determined by the clinical assessment. A swab of the infected area is required for culture and sensitivity. This will identify the organism and indicate if the antibiotics prescribed are suitable.

Hydration and nutrition

Hydration is important when there is a loss of skin integrity and fluid loss from blisters. Oral fluids should be encouraged. A petroleum-based product should be used to protect the lips. If oral hydration is not possible, intravenous fluids will be required. Utmost care is required when inserting a cannula; use of a tourniquet is not recommended. Adhesive dressing must not be used to secure the cannula once in situ.

Because of the presence of blisters in the mouth and oesophagus, oral intake may be insufficient. A naso-gastric tube should not be used. The presence of a naso-gastric tube will cause additional blistering both on insertion and while in situ. The dietician is an integral member of the care team, and will usually suggest high calorific and protein-fortified drinks and food. These will replace the protein lost from the fluid that drains from the blisters. Nutritional supplements may also be prescribed, such as minerals and vitamins. The dietician can also advise on foods and fluids that will prevent and assist with constipation.

Blisters and skin care

The objective of care is to reduce pain and prevent discomfort, excessive loss of body fluid, and infection, and to promote healing.

If not lanced, blisters will continue to enlarge (Abercrombie et al., 2008). Apply very gentle pressure with soft gauze to the blister. A sterile hypodermic needle 14 or 16 gauge is inserted at the lowest point of the blister, and passed through it to create an exit point. Fluid will then drain from the blister. Heavy drainage from the blisters can irritate the skin further so it is important that this is absorbed and removed. If the roof of the blister is intact then leave it exposed. The needle should not be resheathed prior to disposal. Parents/carers are generally educated to pierce their child's blisters in the home environment.

Daily cleaning of the skin is important. The skin should be patted, not rubbed. Using antiseptic washes is thought to help reduce the risk of contracting skin infections (BAD, 2015). Adding salt to bath water is also beneficial in reducing pain, infection and odour (Thomas, 2010). The amount of salt in the water has not been determined and is not of significance.

Clothing should be soft, loose and made of natural fibres. Overheating should be avoided. Shoes should be well fitting and made of natural material.

Dressings must be non-adherent (silicone-based) and cut to size. Hydrogel dressing will assist with cooling blistered areas. Dressings should be secured using a tubular bandage or silicone-based tape. Dressings must be changed when strike-through occurs. If silicone tape is in situ it should be rolled back. An appropriate dressing removal spray should be used or the dressing should be soaked off in a bath. Fingers and toes should be dressed individually (Denyer & Murrell, 2010).

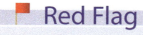
Red Flag

Opiates are frequently required to control pain and prior to change of dressings. Appropriate monitoring will need to be considered to ensure the safety of the child.

Medicines management

- Topical medications maybe antibiotics, anti-fungal, analgesia, steroids or anaesthetic. These are applied directly to the affected area. They include creams, ointments, sprays, lotions and patches.
- Care must always be taken when applying topical medication to protect both the child and the nurse/parent. The manufacturer's instruction should be followed. The dose to administer must be checked carefully.
- The wearing of gloves is normally advised so adherence to local policy is essential. Gloves can potentially drag the skin of a child with EB so sprays are preferable as they will reduce the risk of further trauma to the child's skin.
- Most topical medication is provided in tubes. These do not have child-proof caps so safe storage in the home needs to be discussed with parent/carers.

Atopic eczema

Atopic eczema usually develops in early childhood and often has a genetic predisposition. It is a chronic inflammatory pruritic condition, which follows a pattern of acute episodes and periods of remission. It is often erratic and varies in severity. The skin's natural barrier is broken down, which makes it susceptible to trigger factors, such as allergens, chemicals and irritants. While rarely serious, it does have a significant impact on the child's and parents'/carers' quality of life.

Pathophysiology

There is a genetic predisposition to developing atopic eczema. If both parents have the condition there is an 80% chance that one of their children will be affected. However, the aetiology is multifactorial with the environment, immunological and physical factors all possibilities in its development.

Immunoglobulin IgE will be elevated. An increased amount of histamine is released from the basophils, and hyper-reactive T cells secrete proinflammatory cytokines.

Various dendritic cells, such as Langerhans cells, inflammatory epithelial cells, or plasmocytoid cells, all play a role in determining the impact of the underlying mechanism (Allam & Novak, 2006). Corneocytes separate in the epidermis and reduces the epidermal lipids. It is thought that this disruption to the epidermal barrier is a result of a mutation in the *FLG* gene (filaggrin). Filaggrin is found in the upper layers of the stratum corneum (Darsow, Eyerich & Ring, 2013).

The epidermis already has an inability to retain water so fluid leaks from the cells. This makes the skin dry and the skin barrier is now less effective. Bacteria can penetrate, which results in an inflammatory response. As a result of the inflammatory response, erythema and oedema occur in the epidermis. There is increased blood flow, which in turn causes the white blood cells to leak into the dermis. This causes vesicles and blistering of the epidermis. When this is scratched and the skin breaks, weeping occurs.

Itching is an important factor in diagnosing eczema (Rudolf, Lee & Levene, 2007), it is referred to as the 'itch that becomes a rash'.

Diagnosis

There is no single marker that will definitely diagnose atopic eczema. It is a clinical diagnosis based on the evaluation of signs, symptoms and history. It is diagnosed when the child presents with an itchy skin condition and three of the following (NICE, 2007):

- Visible flexural dermatitis in the skin creases, or in the case of a child <18 months of age, dermatitis on the cheeks and/or extensor surfaces.
- History of flexural dermatitis or dermatitis on the cheeks and/or extensor surfaces in a child <18 months of age.
- Personal history of asthma, allergic rhinitis or positive family history of atopic eczema in children <4 years of age; family in this case refers to parents and/or siblings.
- Onset of symptoms before 2 years of age.

Assessment

A holistic approach must be taken when assessing a child with atopic eczema. This includes noting the severity of the eczema and the impact of this on the child's quality of life. The impact on the parents/carers should also be assessed. A range of quality of life scoring tools for infants and children with eczema is available and an age-appropriate tool should be utilised.

Trigger factors

A range of triggers has the potential to irritate the skin and lead to an exacerbation of eczema. With atopic eczema likely triggers are:

- food allergens (eggs, milk, fish)
- contact allergens (wool, synthetic fabrics, house dust mite, animal dander, heat/cold)
- inhalant allergens (dust, trees)
- irritants (soaps)
- skin infections.

Treatment

The goals of treatment are to improve skin integrity, identify and eliminate trigger factors, control pruritus, and prevent infection (Kiken & Silverberg, 2006). A stepped care plan is recommended so treatment is adjusted up or down according to the severity of the eczema (NICE, 2007). Emollients, followed by topical steroids are the predominant treatment agents. Topical calcineurin inhibitors are recommended if topical steroids do not control the atopic eczema. Occlusive dressing-bandages are recommended for short-term use. These are applied over an emollient or topical steroid cream.

Phototherapy may be recommended in severe cases when quality of life is severely impacted. Antihistamines are not recommended for routine use. They may have a role to play when sleep disturbance is significant or when itching is severe. Bacterial infections will require systemic antibiotics and herpes infections will require systemic acyclovir.

Wounds

A wound is a breach in the surface of the skin necessitating the healing process to commence. The majority of wounds in children are relatively minor and healing occurs without significant impact on the child. Today, the increasing complexity of medical and surgical care provided to infants and children has resulted in an increase in the risk of complications from wounds that may be non-healing, and also from pressure ulcers, intravenous extravasation injury and moisture-associated skin damage. The extremely low-birth-weight neonate is at significant risk of skin breakdown because of the fragility of their skin. Life-threatening sepsis secondary to wound infection is a further potential risk. Wounds may be caused by trauma, surgery, friction, pressure, chemical injury, biological injury and infection.

Revisit Chapter 19 in Peate and Gormley-Fleming (2015) to revise the anatomy and physiology of the skin.

Age-dependent factors need to be considered in wound care as the physiology of the skin (Table 16.4) alters significantly over the period from newborn to young person.

Table 16.4 Age-related factors to consider in skin care

Age	Factors to be considered
Premature infant	• Impaired epidermal barrier so trans-epidermal water loss and electrolytes imbalance • Thermoregulation • Immature immune system • Potential to absorb topical agents as body surface area to weight ratio is greater • Enhanced susceptibility to irritants
Term infant	• Fragile skin • Thermoregulation • Immature immune system • Potential to absorb topical agents as body surface area to weight ratio is greater
Toddler	• Potential to absorb topical agents as body surface area to weight ratio is greater • Possible removal of dressings • Contamination of wound and dressings through normal activities and exploring environment • May not co-operate at dressing changes making assessment and care planning more difficult due to fear and anxiety
Child	• Possible removal of dressings • Contamination of wound and dressings through normal activities and exploring environment • Developmental delay may compound wound healing • May not co-operate at dressing changes making assessment and care planning more difficult due to fear and anxiety

Source: Adapted from King et al. 2014.

Case Study 2

Kate, aged 10 years, was climbing over a fence and sustains a laceration to her right thigh (6 cm) from some wire that was not visible to her. This happened at school and following first aid she is brought to her local minor injuries unit. In triage a complete assessment is undertaken and her vital signs are normal. Her wound is exposed and it is noted that she has an 'L'-shaped laceration on the medial aspect of her thigh and it is deep. Following analgesia, the wound is irrigated with sterile water to remove the dressing that was applied at school. It is decided that this wound should be sutured because of its location and depth. Kate is part of a cheerleader team and needs to get back to training soon. She is anxious about having a scar. Consent is obtained from Kate and her mum who has arrived by this time. Following the instillation of local anaesthetic, 12 absorbable sutures are inserted using a septic non-touch technique. Entonox® is administered during the procedure. Kate's immunisations are up to date so no tetanus is required.

Wound healing

Wound healing is a complex and dynamic process and occurs by either primary intention (healing) or secondary intention. In children, wound healing tends to occur more rapidly than in young people and adults because of the numbers of neutrophils, lymphocytes and monocytes present in the inflammatory phase (Pajulo *et al.*, 2000).

Wound healing involves four stages:

1. coagulation and haemostasis
2. inflammation
3. proliferation
4. maturation/regeneration.

A series of overlapping stages and complex processes will occur during healing and its duration is variable. There are a number of factors that will determine this: general health, nutritional status, ischemia, and infection.

Primary healing (intention)

Primary healing occurs when the wound repairs following minimal destruction of the tissues, the edges of the wound are in close apposition, for example, a surgical incision (Waugh & Grant, 2014), and the healing process is generally unremarkable. The wound edges are normally sterile, there is minimal tissue damage and the wound edges are routinely sutured (Fig. 16.2). Scar formation is typically minimal but keloid may develop.

Secondary healing (intention)

The wound is left opened so healing can occur spontaneously or the wound may be sutured at a later date. A burn injury, trauma injury, pilonidal sinus, ulcer or infected wounds (Fig. 16.3) are examples of wounds that would be allowed to heal by secondary

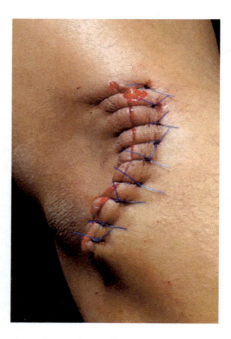

Figure 16.2 Wound healing by primary intention.

Disorders of the skin   Chapter 16

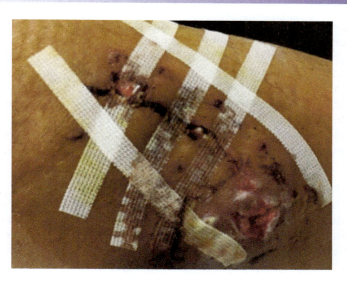

Figure 16.3 Healing by secondary intention-infected wound.

intention. The cavity fills with granulation tissue and eventually closure will be achieved by the formation of a scar. Scars tend to be wider in wounds that heal by secondary intention.

Inflammatory stage

This is a non-specific local reaction to tissue damage as a result of trauma or infection. As an essential part of wound healing, the body's defence mechanism is activated at the time of injury. Vascular and cellular activity is immediately initiated. Vasoconstriction occurs and this is transient, lasting for 5–10 minutes. This reduces the blood flow and is followed by a release of von Willibrand factor from the platelets and endothelia cells. After this a fibrin platelet clot is formed. This assists with control of bleeding, and is part of the clotting cascade (Deely, 2012). The complement and the kinin systems are triggered by the release of the Hageman factor during the clotting cascade (Marieb & Hoehn, 2010).

Growth factors are involved in the healing process and they are released from the platelets. The role of growth factor is to stimulate cell proliferation (Deely, 2012).

The kinin system is activated and kininogen is activated to bradykinin. Dilatation of the microcirculation follows with red blood cells, leukocytes (neutrophils), plasma proteins and plasma fluids leaving the microcirculation. They permeate the injured area to cause redness, warmth, oedema and pain (Nettina, 2010). Following this, neutrophils and monocytes enter the wound and begin to destroy the wound debris. They are attracted to the wound by kinins. Neutrophils squeeze through the capillary walls into the tissues and can be found at the wound site within half an hour of sustaining the injury. Once they have destroyed any bacteria present by phagocytosis, the neutrophils decay, as they are unable to regenerate.

Macrophages will be evident at the injured site and they will also be involved in digesting the debris and decaying neutrophils as they have a longer life span than phagocytosis. Oxygen is required for both macrophages and neutrophils to function at their optimum (Cherry, Harding & Ryan, 2000). T lymphocytes migrate to the wound and their role is to influence the activity of the macrophages. They produce colony-stimulating factor, which encourages the macrophages to produce cytokinins and enzymes.

The activation of the plasma protein leads to the release of histamine, prostaglandins and serotonin from the mast cells. This results in vasodilation and an increase in capillary permeability. Fluid then flows into the injured area and this is referred to as exudate.

Inflammation will continue for 4–5 days. It requires energy and nutrition. The sensation of pain in the wound is often absent at the time of injury but once the kinin system becomes activated pain will be experienced. The presence of prostaglandins, which causes chemical irritation, will also enable the sensation of pain to be felt (Deely, 2012). If the inflammatory stage is prolonged, the risk of hypertrophic scarring is increased. This stage may continue into the proliferation stage.

Proliferation stage

This stage is characterised by the development of granulation tissue. Fibroblasts multiply and migrate across the fibrin strands. This serves as a matrix. Angiogenesis is an essential component of wound healing and is controlled by the action of the chemical mediators, physical factors, the extracellular matrix, and metabolic factors (Arnold & West, 1991). Endothelial buddying occurs on the blood vessels, which are in close proximity, and angiogenesis occurs. These then penetrate and supply nourishment to the injured tissue.

Collagen is synthesised by the fibroblasts on day 2–7 post injury. Macrophages produce various growth factors including fibroblast growth factor. These then stimulate fibroblasts production, which later divide and collagen fibres are produced (Deely, 2012). Type III collagen can be found in the wound in the early stages of wound healing; this will later change to be Type I.

Fibroblasts are essential to the proliferation stage of wound healing. They also produce cellular matrix, which is visible in the wound bed as granulation tissue (Harding, Morris & Patel, 2000). The fibroblasts are responsive to the localised oxygen levels. Poor vascularisation will delay wound healing. The surface of the wound will have a low oxygen tension that encourages the macrophages to produce growth factors and this will initiate the angiogenesis process. Capillary loops are formed from the undamaged capillaries beneath the wound, which forms buds that project towards the surface of the wound. Collagen is required for the formation of these capillary loops (Cherry *et al.*, 2000; Nettina, 2010). The wound gains tensile strength and by week 3 post injury it will have recovered 30% of its pre-injury tensile strength.

The process of contraction is enabled by the role of the fibroblasts and occurs at day 5 post injury. This involves the rearrangement of the extracellular matrix. The exact mechanism is unknown. The surface area of the wound is reduced by the contraction and this accounts for closure of a large amount of the cavity wounds. The risk of the contraction process is that it may lead to contracture development from shallow wounds. This process is more apparent in wounds that heal by secondary intention.

The number of macrophages and fibroblasts decreases as the capillary network is formed and the wound fills with granulation tissue.

Maturation/remodelling stage

This is the final stage. The wound's vascularity is reduced, as there is no longer a need to transport cells to the wound site. Collagen fibres undergo a process of lysis and regeneration. They become more organised, align more closely to each other and thus increase tensile strength. This process peaks at 14–21 days (Cherry *et al.*, 2000). Collagen production slows down and the wound site matures. Its appearance will change from red, raised and hard to a flat, soft and pale scar. The scar will only ever have a tensile strength of 70–80% of normal tissue.

Disorders of the skin   Chapter 16

Complications of wound healing

The majority of wounds heal effectively and within normal time frames. However, healing may be impaired. This can result in:

- Hypertropic scars – excessive fibrous tissue response leading to excessive collagen being deposited and to a larger scar forming.
- Keloid – excessive fibrous response, may take time to form, more common in children and dark skin. They do not flatten out and need further treatment.
- Contractures – wound contraction that continues after re-epithelialisation has occurred leading to loss of function, appearance and mobility. Will require additional treatment.
- Acute to chronic wound – delayed healing due to underlying aetiology.

Epidermal stripping

Epidermal stripping is a common form of iatrogenic skin injury in neonates and children. This can be as a result of their fragile skin or because of an impaired epidermal barrier. The neonate has attenuated rete ridges so adhesive products adhere more forcefully to the epidermis (McCullough & Kloth, 2010). Not only can this lead to an increase in discomfort but it can also lead to an increase in morbidity. The correct dressing choice must be made, for example, soft silicone (King *et al.*, 2014) to avoid epidermal stripping in the first instance. Once it has occurred, it is necessary to consider how epithelialisation can be promoted so careful choice of dressing is essential.

Burns

Burns are a common cause of damage to the skin and underlying tissues and can have devastating life-changing consequences for a child and their family. A burn is an injury caused by energy transfer from a heat source to the body (Burns *et al.*, 2004). That heat source may be from a thermal, radiation, chemical or electrical source. A scald is a burn that occurs as a result of steam or liquid coming into contact with the skin.

The severity of the burn injury correlates to the rate of heat transferred to the skin. This is also dependant on the mechanism of transfer, duration of transfer of heat and the conductivity of heat through the tissues. When the skin is burnt or scalded continuity is lost, damage to the stratum corneum will permit entry of micro-organisms, and damage to the Langerhans cells will diminish the immune response making the child susceptible to serious infection. Thus any burn of size has the ability to make the child seriously ill.

Incidences

The incidence of burns and scalds to children in the UK remains high. Approximately 250 000 people will sustain a burn injury per annum in the UK. A significant amount of these will be as a result of thermal injury and scalds. Children aged 1–4 years will account for 20% of this total and 70% of these will be due to scalds. It is estimated that 110 children per day will be seen in A & E in the UK following a burn injury (Children's Burns Trust, 2016). Each year, 500 children are admitted to hospital following scalds (Royal Society for the Prevention of Accidents, 2016). Most burns occur in the kitchen in early evening. Boys are more at risk than girls (Hettiaratchy & Dziewulski, 2004a).

Flame-retardant bed wear and bed clothing has seen a reduction in the number of burn injuries due to flames. The 5–12-year age group account for 10% of the total population of burn injury patients; this is most likely to be a flame injury often as a result of using an accelerating agent (e.g., lighter fluid, aerosols).

Mechanism of injury

The mechanism of injury will be:

- Thermal: scalds, flames or contact heat, e.g., iron or cooker ring
- Electrical: domestic electricity, high-tension injury or flash injury
- Chemical injury
- Non-accidental injury. Three to 10% of burn injury in infants and children are due to non-accidental injury. These are more common in the under 3 age group. The suspicion of non-accidental burn injury should lead to immediate safeguarding procedures being implemented.

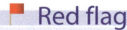

Red flag

Non-accidental injury should be suspected if the following injury pattern is present:
- Obvious patterns of burn injury from irons, cigarettes, cooker rings
- Burns to genitals, perineum, soles of feet, buttocks
- Uniformity of depth and symmetry
- No splash marks in a scald injury
- Absence of burn injury to flexion creases as child may be defending themselves by curling into fetal position
- 'Doughnut' marks – absence of scald injury to an area that has been in contact with a surface as a result of the child being held down, e.g., in a bath of hot water. There may be an area of unaffected skin as it was in direct contact with the bath.

The mechanism of injury will determine the treatment required. This may be resuscitation (if necessary), analgesia, burn treatment and ongoing supportive treatment as indicated by the child's condition.

Classification of burns

The child's survival and outcome is dependent on the following factors: size and depth of burn, age, presence of inhalation injury and comorbidities. Burn injury is classified according to the depth of injury to the skin (Fig. 16.4) and the severity of injury (Table 16.5). The depth of the burn injury is classified as degrees (Table 16.5).

Burn depth is related to the temperature of the source of the heat and the duration of contact with that source. The child's thin skin makes it more difficult to assess the depth of burn injury (Sharma & Parashar, 2010). A burn injury that may appear to be partial thickness may in fact be a full thickness burn. A temperature below 44.4 °C will cause no local damage unless exposure is prolonged whereas exposure to a temperature of 70.6 °C for less than one second will lead to a third-degree burn in a child. Burns may also be classified as minor, moderate or major. The percentage of injured and lost skin is reported as total body surface area (TBSA). Burns severity classification is outlined in Table 16.6.

Calculation of the burn injury area

The TBSA is based on the age of the child as this identifies the changes in body surface area, which alters as the child grows. In the young child, the head constitutes a greater proportion of the surface area compared to the lower limbs. As a rough estimate the palm of a child's hand with the fingers extended can be considered equal to 1%. The 'rule of 9s' is not appropriate for use in young children but may be acceptable for use with the child <10 years of age. The Lund and Browder chart (1944) is a more accurate assessment tool to use for calculating the percentage of burn injury in children (Fig. 16.5).

Disorders of the skin   Chapter 16

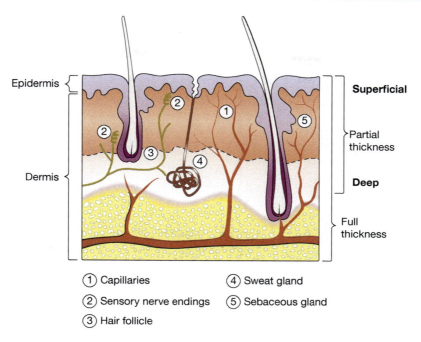

Figure 16.4 Degree of burn injury.

Table 16.5 Classification of burns and presentation of injury.

Classification	Presentation
First degree Superficial	The burn injury only affects the epidermis, the skin will be red and there are no blisters. An example of a first-degree burn is mild sunburn. Healing will occur in 7–10 days. There will be no scarring.
Second degree Partial thickness	The epidermis and some of the dermal layer will be injured. There will be blistering. Swelling and pain will be present. The appearance will range from pink to red to shiny to pale to mottled. Some of the dermal appendages will remain and spontaneous epithelialisation will occur (Nettina, 2010).
Third degree Full thickness	The dermis and epidermis are destroyed; underlying structures may also be destroyed, such as the subcutaneous layer. The injured area will appear white or charred. This is the core of the burn-zone of coagulation. Scarring will be significant and skin grafting required.
Fourth degree	This will involve injury to ligaments, muscles and bones. As nerves will have been destroyed sensation may be reduced or absent. Scarring will be significant as will loss of function. Skin grafting required.

Table 16.6 Burn severity classification

Classification	Percentage of TBSA	Description
Minor	10%	First- and second-degree burn
Moderate	10–20% 2–5%	Second-degree burn Third-degree burn not involving ears, eyes, face, hands, feet or genitals Excludes circumferential burns
Major	20% 5–10%	Second-degree burns Third-degree burns All burns involving face, eyes, hands, ears, feet and genitals All electrical burns Burns with other associated injuries, e.g., fractures, head injuries High-risk groups, e.g., diabetes

Area	Birth–1 year	1–4 year	5–9 year	10–14 year	15 year	Adult	2"	3"	Total	Donor Area
Head	19	17	13	11	9	7				
Neck	2	2	2	2	2	2				
Art. Trunk	13	13	13	13	13	13				
Post. Trunk	13	13	13	13	13	13				
R. Buttock	2½	2½	2½	2½	2½	2½				
L. Buttock	2½	2½	2½	2½	2½	2½				
Genitalia	1	1	1	1	1	1				
R.U.Arm	4	4	4	4	4	4				
L.U.Arm	4	4	4	4	4	4				
R.L.Arm	3	3	3	3	3	3				
L.L.Arm	3	3	3	3	3	3				
R.Hand	2½	2½	2½	2½	2½	2½				
L.Hand	2½	2½	2½	2½	2½	2½				
R.Thigh	5½	6½	8	8½	9	9½				
L.Thigh	5½	6½	8	8½	9	9½				
R.Leg	5	5	5½	6	6½	7				
L.Leg	5	5	5½	6	6½	7				
R.Foot	3½	3½	3½	3½	3½	3½				
L.Foot	3½	3½	3½	3½	3½	3½				
						TOTAL				

AGE vs. AREA — Initial Evaluation — UMC.519a, Rev 3.99

Cause of Burn _____
Date of Burn _____
Time of Burn _____
Age _____
Sex _____
Weight _____
Height _____
Date of Admission _____
Signature _____

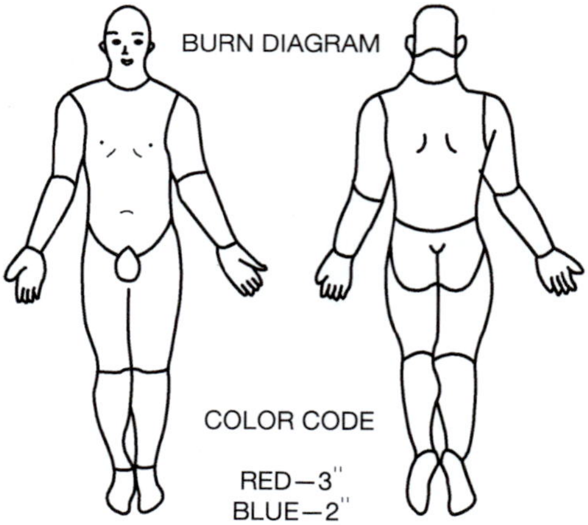

BURN DIAGRAM

COLOR CODE
RED—3"
BLUE—2"

Figure 16.5 Chart to determine extent of burn injury.

Pathophysiology of burns

It is important to know the mechanism of burn injury in order to provide the correct treatment and to anticipate the physiological response that may occur.

All burn injuries will result in both a local and systemic response. The physiological reaction to a burn injury is very similar to the inflammatory process.

The intact blood vessels adjacent to the site of the injury dilate; this leads to redness, which will blanch, on the application of direct pressure. Leukocytes and platelets adhere to the endothelium. There is an increase in the permeability of the capillaries, which results in oedema. Monocytes and polymorphonuclear leukocytes flood the site of injury. Immature fibroblasts, new capillaries and new collagen fibrils appear within the wound to form granulating tissue (Nettina, 2010). Once granulating tissue has begun to form, skin graft can be placed on the wound.

Local response

There are three zones of burns (Fig. 16.6) and these are evident on the first day after the burn injury. These were first described by Jackson in 1947 (as cited by Hettiaratchy & Dziewulski, 2004a) as:

- zone of coagulation
- zone of stasis
- zone of hyperaemia.

Zone of coagulation

The zone of coagulation is the central zone and has the most contact with the heat source and therefore the point of maximum damage. The centre consists of dead cells and damaged tissue. Tissue loss is irreversible as a result of coagulation of the constituent protein so blood flow is absent. It usually appears white or charred.

Zone of stasis

The zone of stasis is usually red and there will be decreased tissue perfusion. Balancing may be evident on the application of pressure initially but this may not persist. Circulation through the superficial blood vessels may cease after a couple of days leading to further loss of tissue if perfusion is not maintained. One of the aims of burns resuscitation is to increase tissue perfusion to prevent further tissue loss, so any challenge to this has the potential to result in more tissue loss (Hettiaratchy & Dziewulski, 2004a). Prolonged hypotension, oedema and infection will impact on the zone of stasis and may lead to extensive tissue loss if not treated. Coagulation occurs leading to vascular occlusion. Prostaglandins, histamine and bradykinins are the chemical mediators in this progressive vascular occlusion. Oedema occurs as the endothelial cells are altered, as is the basement membrane function so permeability is increased. If ischaemia persists the burn will become a full-thickness burn injury.

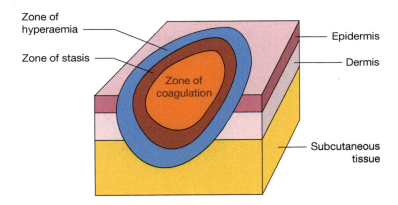

Figure 16.6 Jackson's burns zones.

Zone of hyperaemia

This is the outermost zone and there is increased perfusion to the tissue. As long as this tissue remains free from infection and perfused the likelihood of recovery is high.

Systemic response

If the burn injury is >10% of the TBSA, there will be a systemic impact. This will involve the majority of body systems Fig. 16.7.

Cardiovascular system

Children have almost three times the body surface area to body mass ratio of adults. This has significant implications as fluid loss will be greater in children than in adults, which is a major consideration in the resuscitation process (Sharma & Parashar, 2010).

A function of the epidermis is to act as a water-vapour barrier. If this is damaged, fluid may be lost from the non-functioning epidermis. The fluid volume deficit will be directly proportional to the depth and extent of the burn injury. Capillary permeability is increased, which will result in a loss of intravascular protein and fluid into the interstitial compartments. This occurs in the first 24–36 hours. This protein-rich fluid will ooze from the injured site in the presence of second- and third-degree burns. Recognition and treatment of this fluid loss is essential as the intravascular volume is reduced. Hypovolemic shock will result if it is left untreated.

The protein that is lost to the interstitial space will remain there for a number of weeks before it returns to the intravascular space. When this happens, it will either result in a diuresis in children who have good cardiac and renal functions, or for those who have less than optimal cardiac and renal functions, there is a risk of pulmonary oedema and fluid overload.

Haemoviscosity occurs as a result of the red blood cell (RBC) mass reducing. This is due to destruction of the RBC from the burn injury, which results in the blood becoming concentrated and fluid leakage from the capillary walls. The haematocrit rises and the impact of this is a sluggish blood flow. This can result in capillary stasis, leading to tissue necrosis.

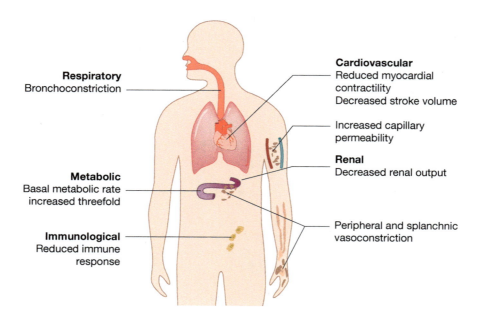

Figure 16.7 Systemic impact of burn injury.

Decreased cardiac output occurs as a result of the reduced circulating blood volume. The child will have an increased heart rate. Stroke volume is decreased due to vasoconstriction in the peripheries, leading to a significant increase in peripheral resistance. There is a decrease in the contractility of the myocardium as a result of the release of tumour necrosis factor α. This together with fluid loss will lead to systemic hypotension and may result in end-organ hypoperfusion, i.e., renal failure (Hettiaratchy & Dziewulski, 2004a). The body will attempt to compensate for the loss of circulating volume by further constricting vessels and withdrawing fluid from undamaged tissues. This will present as thirst in the patient.

Electrolyte imbalance is probable and hyponatremia will be present due to fluid shift from the intravascular to the interstitial space. Hyperkalaemia is likely because of initial cell destruction, but this may change to hypokalaemia as a result of fluid shifting and not being replaced (Pham, Cancio & Gibran, 2008). Anaemia is likely due to the destruction of RBCs at the time of injury.

Thermoregulation
Hypothermia is likely because of the large BSA to body mass ratio in children. Children <2 years of age lose heat more rapidly as they have thinner layers of skin and subcutaneous tissue than an older child. In the very young child, thermoregulation is based on non-shivering thermogenesis. As a result of this the metabolic rate will be increased, which makes additional demands on oxygen consumption leading to the production of lactate.

Respiratory system changes
As this chapter is concerned with the skin, inhalation injuries will not be considered. However, the impact of major burn injury will lead to hyperventilation and therefore an increase in oxygen consumption. The outcome of this is respiratory alkalosis, which can change to respiratory acidosis due to pulmonary insufficiency. Bronchoconstriction may occur due to the release of inflammatory mediators.

Renal system changes
If blood flow to the renal system is compromised, the impact may be either diuresis or oliguria. Oliguria will result in decreased creatinine clearance. Glomerular filtration may also be decreased. The presence of haemoglobin and possibly myoglobin (deep muscle damage) as a result of an electrical burn injury may lead to tubular necrosis. Monitoring of urine output is therefore an essential aspect of nursing care.

Metabolic changes
The release of catecholamine is the primary mediator of the metabolic response in a child with a burn injury. Initially, the greater demand on the metabolic system is due to increased oxygen consumption (Hettiaratchy & Dziewulski, 2004b). Pyrexia is common in the days following a burn injury (moderate and major burns). The healing process also requires energy so there will be an accelerated demand on glucose. However, total body stores of glucose are limited and glucose stored in the liver and muscles as glycogenesis is quickly exhausted thus increasing gluconeogenesis in the liver.

Insulin levels decrease and hyperglycaemia ensues shortly after the burn injury. As a result of gluconeogenesis, hyperglycaemia will persist even after insulin levels increase. Protein is mobilised from visceral and skeletal sources. This will attempt to meet the increased demand for nutrition.

Initially the child's weight may increase post burn due to the adequate fluid resuscitation; however, once the fluid begins to mobilise, weight will reduce and nutritional support will be required to ensure metabolic demands are met to facilitate the healing process.

Gastrointestinal tract

The sympathetic nervous system response to the burn injury may result in a decrease in peristalsis leading to vomiting and gastric distension. Gastric ulceration may also occur due to ischaemia of the gastric mucosa (Nettina, 2010; Hettiaratchy & Dziewulski, 2004b).

Immunological system

Sepsis following a burn injury is a major threat to the long-term outcome and survival of the child. Burnt skin is sterile for approximately 24 hours (Marieb & Hoehn, 2010). Cell mediation and humoral pathways are affected by alterations in the immune response (Hettiaratchy & Dziewulski, 2004b). The effectiveness of the immune system is reduced after 1–2 days post burn injury. The removal of the skin as a barrier facilitates bacterial and fungal growth. The abnormal inflammatory responses following a burn injury lead to a reduction in the delivery of oxygen and white blood cells to the injured area. Hypoxia, thrombosis and acidosis in the injured area further reduce resistance to pathogenic bacteria. Serum albumin, complement and other immunoglobulins are reduced after the burn injury as are the number of lymphocytes, which may lead to lymphocytopenia. Susceptibility to fungi, viruses and gram-negative organisms is increased. This can lead to systemic septicaemia, which would require aggressive treatment to prevent loss of life.

Pediculosis (lice)

Three types of lice affect human beings: head, body, and pubic lice. Children are most commonly infected with head lice, body lice are rare, and pubic lice may be found in sexually active young people. Lice generally remain confined to their designated area. They are transmitted by close personal contact or by contact with infected bed clothing or clothes. Head and pubic lice are not a sign of poor hygiene or poor health. Body lice are capable of transmitting disease. Head lice are most common in the 3–10-year age group.

Diagnosis is by identification of the presence of head lice or their eggs. These can be seen with the naked eye. The child may be seen to be scratching their head or report the presence of lice. Nits and eggs can be found on the hair shaft when there is an active infection with head or pubic lice. This is usually 1 cm from the skin and the lice are firmly adhered to the hair shaft.

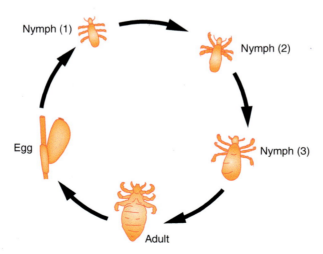

Figure 16.8   The life-cycle of head lice.

The head louse has a 30-day life span (Mumcuoglu, Miller & Gofin, 1990). The egg will produce one single nymph that will develop into a louse (Fig. 16.8). The louse feeds on blood by inserting tiny, fine needle-like structures from their mouths into the scalp of the infected child (Leung & Robson, 2008). Saliva is excreted during this feeding process, which irritates the skin and is the cause of the itchy scalp. Infection is unlikely unless a broken area of scalp becomes contaminated with bacteria transmitted via itching.

Early detection and treatment is essential to ensure infestations are contained. Treatment is either chemical with over-the-counter agents or with 'wet combing'. Compliance with the chosen treatment is essential to ensure complete eradication.

Conclusion

Skin conditions in childhood can be listed as congenital, acquired through injury, surgery or infection, or as a result of non-accidental injury. Many of the congenital skin conditions will range in severity from life-limiting to minor birthmarks. Burn injury is common in the younger age group and injury from trauma can also result in significant loss of skin integrity. Whatever the cause, recognition of the systemic impact of loss of skin integrity is of paramount importance when assessing the child. Understanding the physiological changes that occur is essential in enabling the healthcare professional to perform a holistic assessment and in planning appropriate treatment. Supportive care for the child and family is required as is ongoing education to enable self-care or care by family where possible.

References

Abercrombie, E., Mather, C., Hon, J., Graham-King, P. & Pillay, L. (2008). Recessive dystrophic epidermolysis bullosa. Part 2: care of the adult patient. *British Journal of Nursing* 17(6 Suppl 3), S6–20.

Allam, J.P. & Novak, N. (2006). The pathophysiology of atopic eczema. *Clinical Experimental Dermatology* 31(1), 89–93.

Arnold, F. & West, D.C. (1991). Angiogenesis in wound healing. *Pharmacology & Therapeutics* 52(3), 407–422.

British Association of Dermatologists (BAD) (2015). Epidermolysis bullosa simplex. Patient Information Leaflet. Last updated August 2015. Available at: http://www.bad.org.uk/for-the-public/patient-information-leaflets/epidermolysis-bullosa-simplex (last accessed April 2018).

British National Formulary for Children (BNFC) (n.d.). [online] Available at: https://bnfc.nice.org.uk/ (last accessed 25 April 2018).

Bruckner-Tuderman, L., Eady, R.A., Bauger, E.A., et al. (2014). Inherited epidermolysis bullosa: updated recommendations on diagnosis and classification. *Journal of the American Academy of Dermatology* 70(6), 1103–1126.

Burns, T., Breathnach, S., Cox, N. & Griffiths, C. (eds) (2004). *Rook's Textbook of Dermatology, Volume 1*, 7th edn. Blackwell Science, Oxford.

Chamley C., Carson, P., Randall, D. & Sandwell, W. (2005). *Developmental Anatomy and Physiology of Children*. Churchill Livingstone, London.

Cherry, G., Harding, K. & Ryan, T. (2000). *Wound Bed Preparation* (International Congress and Symposium Series 250). Royal Society of Medicine Press, London.

Children's Burns Trust (2016). Burns database. Available at: http://www.cbtrust.org.uk/burns-database/ (accessed 12 October 2016).

Darsow, U., Eyerich, K. & Ring, J. (2013). Eczema Pathophysiology. World Allergy Organization. Available at: http://www.worldallergy.org/education-and-programs/education/allergic-disease-resource-center/professionals/eczema-pathophysiology (last accessed April 2018).

Deely, C. (2012). *The Care of Wounds: A Guide for Nurses*, 4th edn. Wiley, Oxford.

Denyer, J. & Murrell, D.F. (2010). Wound management for children with epidermolysis bullosa: epidermolysis bullosa: part II – diagnosis and management. *Dermatology Clinic* 28, 257–264.

Genetics Home Reference (2016). Kindler syndrome. [online] Available at: https://ghr.nlm.nih.gov/condition/kindler-syndrome (accessed June 2016).

Harding, K.G., Morris, H.L. & Patel, G.K. (2002). Healing chronic wounds. *British Medical Journal* 324(19), 160–163.

Hettiaratchy, S. & Dziewulski, P. (2004a). ABC of burns: introduction. *British Medical Journal* 328(7453), 1366–1368.

Hettiaratchy, S. & Dziewulski, P. (2004b). ABC of burns: pathophysiology and types of burns. *British Medical Journal* 328(7453), 1427–1429.

Hoeger P.H. & Enzmann C.C. (2002). Skin physiology of the neonate and young infant: a prospective study of functional skin parameters during early infancy. *Pediatric Dermatology* 19(3), 256–262.

Kiken, D.A. & Silverberg, N.B. (2006). Atopic dermatitis in children, part 2. Treatment options. *Pediatric Dermatology* 78(6), 401–406.

King, A., Stellar, J.J., Blevins, A. & Shah, K.N. (2014). Dressing and products in pediatric wound care. *Advances in Wound Care* 3(4), 324–334.

Leung, A.K.C. & Robson, W.L.M. (2008). Pruritus in children. Pediatrics/Consultants Live; http://www.pediatricsconsultantlive.com/pediatric-skin-diseases/pruritus-children (last accessed March 2018).

Lund C.C. & Browder N.C. (1944). The estimation of areas of burns. *Surgery, Gynaecology, Obstetrics* 79, 352–358.

Marieb, E. & Hoehn, K. (2010). *Human Anatomy & Physiology*, 8th edn. Pearson Benjamin Cummings, San Francisco.

McCullough, J.M. & Kloth, L.C. (2010). *Wound Healing: Evidence-Based Management*, 4th edn. F.A. Davis, Philadelphia.

Mumcuoglu, K.Y., Miller, J. & Gofin, R. (1990). Epidemiological studies on head lice infestation in Israel. Parasitological examination of children. *International Journal of Dermatology* 29(7), 502–505.

National Institute of Arthritis & Musculoskeletal & Skin Diseases (NIAMS) (2013). Epidermolyosis bullosa. [online] Available at: https://www.niams.nih.gov/health-topics/epidermolysis-bullosa (accessed 25 April 2018).

National Institute for Health and Care Excellence (NICE) (2007). Atopic eczema in children. Clinical guideline [CG57]. NICE, London.

Nettina, N. (ed.) (2010). *Lippincott Manual of Nursing Practice*, 9th edn. Wolter Kluwer/Lippincott Williams & Wilkins, Philadelphia.

Pajulo, O.T., Puikki, K., Alanen, M.S., et al. (2000). Duration of surgery and patient age effect wound healing in children. *Wound Repair and Regeneration* 8(3), 174–178.

Peate, I. & Gormley-Fleming, E.A. (2015). *Fundamentals of Children's Anatomy and Physiology*, 1st edn. Wiley, Oxford.

Pham, T.N., Cancio, L.C. & Gibran, N.S.; American Burn Association (2008). American Burn Association practice guidelines burn shock resuscitation. *Journal of Burn Care and Research* 29(1), 257–266.

Royal Society for the Prevention of Accidents (2016). Accidents to children. [online]. Available at: http://www.rospa.com/home-safety/advice/child-safety/accidents-to-children/#fires (accessed 14 August 2016).

Rudolf, M., Lee, T. & Levene, M. (2007). *Paediatrics and Child Health*, 3rd edn. Wiley Blackwell, Oxford.

Sharma R.K. & Parashar, A. (2010). Special considerations in paediatric burn patients. *Indian Journal of Plastic Surgery* 43(Suppl), S43–S50.

Tenedini, E., Artuso, L., Bernardis, I., et al. (2015). Amplicon-based next generation sequencing: an effective approach for the molecular diagnosis of epidermolysis bullosa. *British Journal of Dermatology* 173(3), 731–738.

Thomas, S. (2010). *Surgical Dressings and Wound Management*. Medetec Publications, Cardiff.

Watson, J. (2016). Diagnosis, treatment and management of epidermolysis bullosa. *British Journal of Nursing* 25(8), 428–431.

Waugh, A. & Grant, A. (2014). *Ross and Wilson Anatomy & Physiology in Health and Illness*, 12th edn. Churchill Livingstone Elsevier, Edinburgh.

Wong, D. (1999). *Whaley & Wong's Nursing Care of Infants and Children*, 6th edn. Mosby, London.

Index

Note: page numbers in *italics* refer to figures; those in **bold** to tables.

abdominal pain
  case studies 155, 277
  in girls **320**, 320–321
  haemolytic uraemic syndrome 293, 305
abduction, lower limb 350, *350*
A-beta fibres **138**, 140, *140*
ABO blood groups 106
abscesses 94, *94*
accessory muscles, breathing 215
acetylcholine 161
acetylsalicylic acid 204
acquired immunity 97–99, *100*
acquired immunodeficiency syndrome (AIDS) 109–110
acromegaly 237
actin 14
active immunity 99, *100*
active transport 7–8
acute kidney injury (AKI) 290–292, **291**, 293
acute lymphoblastic leukaemia (ALL) **56**, 61, 62–64
acute pain 141–142, 148
acute tubular necrosis 291
adaptive immunity 84, 86, **86**, 97–99
Addison's disease 245–246
adduction, lower limb *350*
A-delta fibres **138**, 138–139, 140, *140*
adenine (A) *29*, 30, 35
adenosine deaminase (ADA) deficiency 49
adenosine triphosphate (ATP) 7–8, 12, 13
adhesive dressings, epidermal stripping 373

adipose tissue 22
adolescents
  causes of limp **346**
  pain assessment **146**
  pain management 154
  pain perception 144
adrenal crisis 246
adrenal disorders 245–247
adrenal gland *236*
adrenaline *see* epinephrine
adrenal insufficiency 59, 245–246
afterload 125, **125**, *126*, 182
airway assessment 130
aldosterone 69, *69*
aldosterone antagonists **184**
alleles 32–33
allergens 101
allergic march 101, *101*
allergy 101–103, **102**, *102*
  penicillin 206
Alport syndrome 285, 287
ambiguous genitalia 246, 249–250
Anadin® **150**
anaerobic metabolism 127
analgesia 149, 150–154
  case studies 155
  non-opioid **150**, **150**
  nurse controlled 152
  opioid 150–152, **151**
  patient-controlled (PCA) 152, **153**
  procedural pain 154
  regional 152–153, **153**
  WHO 3 steps 149
anaphase *40*, 41, 42
anaphylactic shock 121
anaphylaxis 103–105, *104*, 111–112

angiotensin-converting enzyme (ACE) 69, *69*
angiotensin-converting enzyme (ACE) inhibitors **184**
ankle fractures **341**
antenatal screening 74, 281, **281**
antibodies 98, **98**
  deficiencies 108–109
  response to infection 98–99, *99*
anticoagulation **184**
anti-diarrhoeal medications 260
anti-diuretic hormone (ADH; vasopressin) 122, 237–238
anti-emetics 260, 261
antigen-presenting cells (APC) 97
antigens 97
antihistamines 103
aorta, coarctation of *194*, 194–195
aortic atresia 193
aortic stenosis 123, *192*, 192–193
aortic valve *192*, *192*
apnoea 215
appendicitis 263–265
  case studies 110–111, 275–276, 277
  location of pain 264
arachnoid mater *168*
areolar tissue 21
arginine vasopressin (anti-diuretic hormone; ADH) 122, 237–238
arrhythmias, cardiac 182, 208–210
arteries 180

Index

ascending pain pathways 137–139, *138*
ascites 74, 121–122
aspirin 204
asthma 227–230
   acute/severe or life-threatening 230, **230**
   allergic 101, *101*, **102**
   anaphylaxis 103, 105
   assessment 228–229
   care and treatment 229
   difficult 230
   medication 103, 228
   pathophysiology 227, *228*
astrocytoma 56, 171
atenolol **184**
atopic 101
atopic eczema **102**, 367–368
   allergic march 101, *101*
atrial fibrillation 210
atrial kick 129
atrial septal defect (ASD) 187–188, *188*
autoimmune disease 105–106
autosomal dominant diseases 44, 45–46
autosomal recessive diseases 44–46
autosomes 32, 43
AVPU response scale 166, **166**
avulsion fractures 339, *339*
axonal brain injury 168

bacteria 87
balanitis 299, 301
balloon angioplasty 194
balloon septostomy 197, 198, 202
balloon valvuloplasty 192
Barlow test 356, *356*
basement membrane 16, *17*
bases, nitrogenous 30
Battle's sign **165**
BCG (bacille Calmette–Guérin) vaccine 224
Beckwith–Wiedemann syndrome **54**
beclomethasone 228
becotide 228
bed wetting 298–299
behavioural cues, pain assessment 146, **146**
benzylpenicillin 206
beta-blockers **184**, 243
bisphosphonates 59

bleeding *see* haemorrhage
blinatumomab 61–62
blisters 363, 364, 366
blood 23
blood loss 71, 122–123
blood pressure
   post-operative changes **274**
   regulation 69, *69*
   septic shock 117–118
   see also hypertension; hypotension
blood transfusion 123, *124*
blood vessels 180
B lymphocytes 86, **86**, 97, 98
boil 94
bone 21
   growth 336
   healing 340–342, *342*
   remodelling 336, 342, *342*
bone marrow 63, 98
bradycardia
   respiratory distress 217
   shock 119, 120, 121, 129
bradykinin 91, 371, 377
brain injury, traumatic *167*, 167–168
brain tumours 171, **172**
   see also central nervous system tumours
breathing
   assessment 130, 215–216
   paroxysmal 215
   prolonged increased effort 227
bronchiolitis 218–219
bronchopneumonia 220
bronchospasm 227
Brudzinski's sign **174**
Brufen® *see* ibuprofen
buckle fractures 339
bulla 361
burns 373–380
   calculation of area 374, *376*
   classification 374
   depth (degrees) 374, **375**, *375*
   incidence 373
   Jackson's zones **377**, 377–378
   mechanism of injury 374
   pathophysiology 376–380
   severity classification **375**
   systemic response *378*, 378–380

callus 342, *342*
Calpol® **150**

cancer 51–65
   aetiology 53–54, **54**
   biology 52–54
   examples 62–64
   familial 53–54
   incidence 52, *52*
   investigations **58**
   late effects (LE) 64
   outcome and survivorship 64
   pathogenesis 53
   prevention 62
   signs and symptoms 55, *55*
   staging 55–56
   treatment 57–62
capillaries 180
capillary refill time 117, 122, 175
captopril **184**
carbimazole 243
carbon dioxide (CO_2) 72, *73*
carbonic acid 72
cardiac arrhythmias 182, 208–210
cardiac catheterisation 186–187
cardiac failure (CF) 181–184
   cardiogenic shock 125, **125, 126**
   causes 181–183, **182**
   management 184, **184**
   signs and symptoms 183
cardiac index 123
cardiac muscle 24
cardiac output (CO) *128*, 128–129, 379
cardiac tamponade 123
cardiogenic shock **117**, 123–125
   causes 123, **125**
   goals of treatment **127**
   left ventricular failure 125, **126**
   right ventricular failure 125, **125**
   signs and symptoms **126**
cardiomyopathy 206–208
   dilated 207
   hypertrophic 207
   restrictive 207–208
cardiovascular system 180
   burn injury 378–379
carotid sinus massage 210
cartilage 21, *22*
cauda equina syndrome 169
cell cycle *39*

Index

cell division 40, 41
cell-mediated immunity 75, 97
cell membrane (plasma membrane) 3–8
   active transport 7–8
   bilayer structure 4, 5
   functions 5
   movement of substances across 5–8
   passive transport 6–7
   permeability 6
cells 2–14
   characteristics 2–3
   different types 3
   migration 15
   organelles 8–14
   reproduction 9–10, 38–41
   structure 3–14, 4
central blocks 152–153
central nervous system (CNS) 135, 160, **160**, *161*
central nervous system tumours 171–172
   radiation therapy 60
   signs and symptoms 55, **172**
   staging and grading 56, **57**
central venous catheter (CVC) 61
central venous pressure (CVP) **70**
centrioles 14
centromere 31, *31*
centrosomes 39–40
cerebral blood flow 163
cerebral contusions 167
cerebral dysfunction 163–165
cerebral lacerations 167
cerebral palsy 169–170
cerebral trauma 165–168
cerebrospinal fluid (CSF) 163
   shunts 165
C fibres **138**, 138–139, 140
Charcot–Marie–Tooth disease type 1 37
chemoreceptors 72, *73*
chemotaxis 15, 91
chemotherapy 58–59, 63–64
chest movement 215
chest wall recession 215
chest X-ray 226–227
child abuse
   burns and scalds 374
   false accusations 19
   fractures 339, 340
   see also sexual abuse

child mortality 68
Children's Cancer and Leukaemia Group (CCLG) 57
chlorphenamine 104
choking 220, *220*
chromatids 31, *31*, 39–41, *40*
chromatin 30–31, *31*
chromosome disorders 162
chromosomes 29, 30–33
   cell reproduction 9–10
   human complement 31–32, *32*
   interphase 39
   meiosis 41, 42, 43
   mitosis 39–41, *40*
   structure 30–31, *31*
chronic granulomatous disease 90
chronic kidney disease (CKD) 74, 287–289
   causes in children 287, **287**
   clinical consequences **288**
   stages **288**
   treatment 288–289, *289, 290*
chronic pain 141–142, 148
cilia 14
circadian rhythm disturbances 241
circulation, assessment 130
circumcision 301–302
cisternae 10
clavicle fractures **341**
cleft lip and palate 270–271, *271*, **273**
clotting, blood 92
clubbing 196
coarctation of aorta *194*, 194–195
codeine 151, 152
CODE RED protocol 123, *124*
coeliac disease 268–269, **269**
cognitive impairment 144, **146**
collagen 20, 21, 372
columnar epithelium
   simple 17, *17*
   stratified 18
commensal micro-organisms 87–88
comminuted fractures 339, *339*
compensated shock 117–118, *120*, 123, 125
compensatory mechanisms
   dehydration 69, 71
   renal impairment 74

complement system 76, 91
computed tomography (CT) 239, 282
concentration gradient 6
concordance, medication 230
concussion 168
confidentiality 326
congenital adrenal hyperplasia (CAH) 246–247
congenital heart defects (CHD) 181–202
   acyanotic 185, *185*, 187–195
   cardiac failure 181–184
   causes **182**
   classification 184, *184*
   cyanotic 185, *185*, 195–202
   decreased pulmonary flow 195–197
   increased pulmonary blood flow 187–191
   investigations 184–187
   mixed blood flow 197–202
   ventricular outflow obstruction 191–195
conjunctivitis, allergic **102**
connective tissue 20–23
   blood supply 21
   dense 21
   function 15, *17*, 20
   loose 21–23
   types 21–25
conscious level, assessing **166**
consent 321
constipation 260, 298
contraception 325–329
contractures, wound 373
convulsions, febrile 77, 177
coronary artery aneurysms 203, 204
corticosteroids
   adrenal **236**
   allergy 103
   asthma 228
   cancer therapy 59
   Kawasaki disease 204
   nephrotic syndrome 284
cortisol 59
counselling *see* psychological care
craniopharyngioma 239, 240
C-reactive protein (CRP) 106
Crohn's disease 37, **265**, 265–266
croup 219
crusts 361

Index

cryptorchidism 314–315
CT *see* computed tomography
cuboidal epithelium
  simple 16–17, *17*
  stratified 18
cultural aspects, pain 144–145
Cushing disease/syndrome 240
Cushing's triad 164, 165
cyanosis
  congenital heart defects 196, 197, 198
  respiratory distress 216
cyst 361
cystic fibrosis
  genetics 36, 38, 45
  oxygen administration 72–74
  recurrent infections 88
cytokines 90, 95, 96
cytoplasm 4, 8–9
cytosine (C) 29, 30, 35
cytoskeleton 13, 13–14
cytotoxic chemotherapy 58, 63
cytotoxic T cells **98**

daytime wetting 298
dehydration 68–71, *69*
  blood loss 71
  diagnosis **70**, 70–71
  gastrointestinal fluid loss 68–71
  hypovolaemic shock 122
  infections 77
  pre-operative fasting 71
  respiratory infections 222
deletions 36–37
deoxyribonucleic acid *see* DNA
deoxyribonucleotides 29–30
descending pain pathways 139–140, *140*
desmopressin (DDAVP) 238
developmental dysplasia of the hip (DDH) **353**, 353–356
  care and treatment 354, 354–356, *355*
  diagnosis 354, 356, *356*
dexamethasone 59
diabetes insipidus 121, 237–238, 251–252
diabetes mellitus 71, 77–79, 248–249
diabetic ketoacidosis (DKA) 78–79, 122, 248–249
dialysis 288–289, *289*, *290*, 291
diamorphine, intranasal 151
diaphoresis 183

diaphragmatic breathing 215
diaphysis *347*
diarrhoea 259–260
  case study 80
  causes **259**
  dehydration 68–69, 71
  hypovolaemic shock 121
dietary restrictions 294–295
dietary supplements 282, 294–295
diethylstilboestrol (DES) 54
diffusion 6, *7*
DiGeorge syndrome 245
digestive disorders 257–277
digoxin **184**
dilated cardiomyopathy 207
diploid cell 41
disability, assessment 130
dislocation, hip **353**
disorders of sex development (DSD) 249–250
disseminated intravascular coagulation (DIC) 118
distraction, psychological 137, 154
distraction osteogenesis 344, *344*
distributive shock 116–121, **117**
diuretics **184**
DMSA (dimercaptosuccinic acid) scan 282
DNA 29
  cell nucleus 9, *28*
  chromosomal 30–31
  double helix *29*, 29–30
  mutations 36–38
  processing genes 53
  protein synthesis 33–35, *35*
  replication *34*, 39
  structure 29–31, *30*
  transcription 33–35
dominant genes 33, 44
dopamine 161
dorsal horn 137, *140*
double helix, DNA *29*, 29–30
Down syndrome 53, **54**, 162, 195
dressings 366, 373
Duchenne muscular dystrophy 46
ductus arteriosus 123, 190
  maintaining patency 193, 197
  patent (PDA) **190**, *190*, 190–191

duplications, genetic 37
dura mater *168*
dysmenorrhoea 318–320, 330
dysplasia, hip **353**, 355
dystrophic epidermolysis bullosa (DEB) 363, *363*, 364

ECG *see* electrocardiogram
elastic fibres 20
electrocardiogram (ECG) **70**, 129, 202, *203*
electroencephalogram (EEG) 176
electromagnetic radiation 60
embryonal central nervous system tumours 56, 171
emergency contraception 325–329
emotional effects *see* psychological/emotional effects
emotional support *see* psychological care
empyema 222
encephalitis 175
endocarditis, infective 204–205
endocrine disorders 235–253, **236**
  childhood obesity 247
  emotional and psychological effects 250
  hormone therapy 238, 241, 247
  investigations 238–239
  multi-system effects 240–241
endocrine glands 20, 234, *235*, **236**
endocrine system 234, *235*, **236**
endocytosis 5
endoplasmic reticulum (ER) 10, *11*
end-organ perfusion, monitoring 129–130
end-stage renal disease (ESRD) 287, **288**
enuresis 298
enzymes 13
ependymoma 56
epidermal stripping, iatrogenic 373
epidermolysis bullosa (EB) 362–367
  care and management 365–367
  case studies 18–19, 364–365, **365**

Index

diagnosis 362
pathophysiology *363*, 364
types 362–364
epidermolysis bullosa simplex
(EBS) 363, *363*, 364
epididymitis 299–300
epidural analgesia 152–153,
153
epiglottitis 219
epilepsy 176
epinephrine (adrenaline)
adrenal gland **236**
anaphylaxis 103–104, *104*,
111
autoinjector 105
pathophysiology 79, 95
epiphyseal growth plate *347*
epiphyseal injuries **341**
epithelial tissue 15–20, *17*
classification 16–18
glandular 20
simple *16*, 16–17, *17*
stratified 16, *16*, 17–18
Epstein–Barr virus (EBV) 54
erythema marginatum **205**
erythrocyte sedimentation rate
(ESR) 106
Escherichia coli O157:H7 292,
293
eukaryotes 9
exocrine glands 20
exocytosis 11
exploitation, sexual 326
exposure 130
external fixation 343–344
extracellular matrix 20

facial bone injuries **341**
facilitated diffusion 6–7, *7*
Fallot's tetralogy (TOF) *195*,
195–196
Fanconi anaemia **54**
fasting, pre-operative 71
fat tissue 22
febrile convulsions 77, 177
febrile neutropenia 63
feedback control *73, 78*
female genital mutilation
(FGM) 329–333
classification **330**
consequences 330–331
legal position 331–332
prevalence *331, 332*
female reproductive health
issues 318–324, **319**

female reproductive
system 318, *319*
femoral fractures 337, **341**
femoral osteotomy 352
femur, growth plates *347*
fentanyl **153**
fetal alcohol syndrome 162
fever (pyrexia) 77, 95–96
fibrin 91, 92
fibroblasts 21, 92, 372
fibular fractures **341**
filaggrin 367
filgrastim *see* granulocyte
colony-stimulating factor
filtration 7
fission, simple 2
fissures
bone 339, *339*
skin 361
fistula 94
flagella 14
fluid losses 68–71, 121–122,
378
fluid overload 127, **286**, 294
fluid resuscitation 127
fontanelles 70
food allergy 101, *101*, **102**, 103
foot fractures **341**
foramen ovale 187
forearm fractures **341**
foreign body
aspiration 220
vaginal 322, 323
fractures 336–345
case study 337, *338*
diagnosis 340
infancy and early
childhood 339
location and features 340,
341
management 342–345
pathophysiology 340–342,
342
types 337–339, *339*
fragile X syndrome 37
frameshift mutations 37
Fraser guidelines 326–327, 329
free radicals 12
fungi 87
furosemide **184**

gallop rhythm 183
gametes 41
gametogenesis 44
gastric acid 88

gastroenteritis 259–260
gastrointestinal (GI)
disorders 257–277
burn injury 380
case studies *275–276*, 277
hernias 271–274
inflammatory 263–266
malabsorption 268–269
motility 259–263
obstructive 266–268
structural defects
269–271
gastrointestinal fluid
loss 68–71, 121
gastrointestinal
infections 68–69
gastro-oesophageal reflux
(GOR) 261–262, **262**
gate control theory 139–140,
140
gender aspects, pain
assessment 144–145
gender dysphoria 250
genes 29
cancer 53
crossover 42, *42*
dominant 33, 44
loci 32–33
recessive 33, 44
transference 38–43
gene therapy 49
genetic disorders
inheritance 44–47
neurological disorders 162
spontaneous mutations 47
support and
counselling 37–38
genetic mutations *see*
mutations
genetics 27–49
cancer 53–54, **54**
role in inheritance 43–44
genotype 33, 43
gestational diabetes 248
gigantism 237
Gillick competence 321,
326–327, 329
glandular epithelium 20
Glasgow Coma Scale (GCS) 166,
166
glial tumours 171
gliomas 171
glomerular filtration rate
(GFR) 288, **288**
estimated (eGFR) 285, **291**

Index

glomerulonephritis 74, 285–286, **286**
glucagon 77, *78*, **236**, 249
glucocorticoids (GCs) 59
glucose
   blood **70**, 77, *78*, 248
   transport 6–7
gluten 268
glycaemic control 77–78, 79
glycosuria 78
goblet cells 17, 88
goitre 242
Golgi complex *4*, 10–11
gonadotrophin-releasing hormone (GnRH) analogues 250, 251
gonads, disorders of 249–251
graft-versus-host disease 107
granulation tissue 372
granulocyte colony-stimulating factor (GCSF) 61, 89
granulomas 90, 91
Graves' disease 243
gray (Gy) 60
greenstick fractures 339, *339*
ground substance 20
Group B streptococcus 173
growth disorders 237
growth factors 371, 372
growth hormone, human 237
growth plates, femoral *347*
grunting, respiratory 216
guanine (G) *29*, 30, 35

haematoma, fracture site 340, *342*
haematopoietic stem cell transplantation (HSCT) 61
haematuria 287
haemodialysis 289, *290*
haemoglobin (Hb) **70**, 71
haemoglobin A$_{1c}$ (HbA$_{1c}$) 77
haemolysis 7, *8*
haemolytic disease of newborn 106
haemolytic uraemic syndrome (HUS) 292–293, 305, *306–307*
haemophilia 46
Haemophilus influenzae 92, 219
haemorrhage 71, 122–123, *124*
haemorrhagic shock 122–123
hair colour 32, 44
haploid cell 41
hay fever **102**, 103

head bobbing 215
head injury 167–168
head lice *380*, 380–381
Health Play Specialist (HPS) 60
heart
   anatomy 180–181, *181*
   oxygen saturation levels *186*
   pressures within *186*
heart disease 181–211
   acquired 203–211
   congenital 181–203
heart failure *see* cardiac failure
heart rate (HR) 118, 128–129
   post-operative changes **274**
   respiratory distress 216–217
   see also tachycardia
heatstroke 47, *48*
helper T cells **98**, 110
hemidesmosomes 364
Henoch–Schönlein purpura 285, 286
heparin **184**
hepatomegaly 183
herbal remedies 282
hernias 271–274
heterozygous 33
Hickman line 61
hip
   developmental dysplasia **353**, 353–356
   fractures **341**
hip spica *355*, 355–356
Hirschsprung disease 262–263, *263*
histamine 91, 101, 121, 367
histones 30–31, *31*
hives **102**
homeostasis 67–80
homozygous 33
hormones 234
   laboratory tests 238–239
   long-term effects of deficiency 244
   replacement therapy 238, 247
   routes of administration 241
   therapy to suppress or counteract 250
human immunodeficiency virus (HIV) 109–110
human papillomavirus (HPV) vaccine 62
humeral fractures **341**
humoral immunity *75*
Huntington's disease 46

hydration 70, 366
hydrocele *273*, 300
hydrocephalus 164–165
hydrocortisone 59, *104*
hydronephrosis **281**, 295
21-hydroxylase deficiency 246
hypercalcaemia 244
hypercalciuria 287
hypercapnia 72
hypercyanotic spells 196
hyperglycaemia 77, 78, 248, 379
hyperinsulinaemia, congenital (CHI) 249
hypernatraemic dehydration 71, 122
hyperparathyroidism 244
hypersensitivity reactions 99–105, **100**
hypertension 294
hyperthyroidism 242–244, 250
hypertrophic cardiomyopathy 207
hypertrophic scars 373
hypoalbuminaemia 74
hypoglycaemia 79, 249
hyponatraemic dehydration 71, 122
hypoparathyroidism 244–245
hypoperfusion 116, 127
hypopituitarism 237
hypoplastic left heart syndrome 197–202
hypospadias 300–301, *301*, 308
hypotension 69, 74
   cardiogenic shock 123, 125
   neurogenic shock 120
   septic shock 117
hypothalamic disorders 235
hypothalamus 69, 77, 95, **236**
hypothermia 379
hypothyroidism 242
   case study 253
   congenital (CH) 242, 244
hypovolaemia 74
   burn injury 378, 379
   neurogenic shock 120
   third-spacing 121–122
hypovolaemic shock **117**, 121–123
hypoxia 72, 216, 217
hypoxic brain injury 168

ibuprofen (Brufen®) **150**, 286, 316
Ilizarov frame 344, *344*

Index

immune deficiency 107–110
　primary (PID) 107–109, *108*
　secondary 107, *109*, 109–110
immune system 84–112
　adaptive 84, 97–99
　alterations 99–112
　blood cells 85–86, **86**
　burn injury 380
　innate *see* innate immune system
　response to infection *75*, 75–77
immunisation 99
immunoglobulin A (IgA) **98**, 99
immunoglobulin D (IgD) **98**
immunoglobulin E (IgE) **98**, 101, 367
immunoglobulin G (IgG) **98**, *99*
immunoglobulin M (IgM) **98**, *99*
immunoglobulin therapy 108–109, 204
immunosuppressive therapy 107
impacted fractures 339, *339*
infants
　cardiac failure **182**, 183
　dehydration 68–69, 70
　immunity 75–76
　pain 141, 143, **146**, 154
　positioning 262
　respiratory disorders 214, 215
　urinary tract infections **297**
infection control precautions 218
infections 75–77
　autoimmune disease and 105
　defence against 87
　epidermolysis bullosa 365
　immune deficiencies 107, 108
　inflammatory response *76*, 76–77, 92
　intracranial 173–175
　prenatal 162
　primary and secondary response 98–99, *99*
　respiratory 218–219, 220–225
　systemic effects 94–97, *95*
　transplant recipients 107
　see also sepsis; septic shock
infective endocarditis 204–205
infibulation 330, **330**, 331

inflammation 90–97
　acute 90, 91–92
　airway 227, *228*
　alterations 99–112
　atopic eczema 367
　causes 90–91
　chronic 90–91
　fracture site 340
　in infection *76*, 76–77, 92
　process 91, *92*, *93*
　systemic effects 94–97, *95*
　wound healing 91–92, 371–372
inflammatory bowel disease (IBD) **265**, 265–266
inflammatory mediators 91, 117
influenza vaccine 64
infoKID 283
inguinal hernia 272–274, *273*
inhalers 228
inheritance *43*, 43–47
innate immune system 84, *87*, 87–97
　cells 85, **86**
　see also inflammation
inotropic drugs, positive **184**
insect sting hypersensitivity **102**
insertion mutations 37
instability, hip **353**, 355
insulin 77, *78*, *79*, **236**, 248–249
integumentary system 360
interatrial septum 187
interleukin 1 (IL-1) 95
interleukin 6 (IL-6) 95
intermediate filaments 14
International Classification of Diseases for Oncology (ICD-O) 56
interphase 39, *39*, *40*
interventricular septum 189
intracerebral haemorrhage 167
intracranial haemorrhage 167
intracranial infection 173–175
intracranial pressure (ICP), raised *163*, 163–165, 166
intramuscular (IM) injections 151
intrathecal (IT) chemotherapy 58–59, 63
intravenous urogram 282
intussusception *267*, 267–268
ionising radiation (IR) 54, 60
ion transport 6

ischaemic heart disease 183, 204
isonatraemic dehydration 71, 122
itching 367

junctional epidermolysis bullosa (JEB) 363, *363*, 364

Kawasaki disease 183, 203–204
keloid 373
Kernig's sign **174**
ketamine sedation 322–323
kidney
　biopsy 283
　congenital anomalies 74, 281, **281**, 287
　duplex **281**, *282*
　ectopic **281**
　horseshoe **281**
　solitary **281**
Kindler syndrome 364
kinins 91, 371

lactic acid/lactate 127
late effects (LE), cancer 64
left ventricular failure 125, **126**
leukaemia 54, 55
　case study 62–64
　risk stratification 55–56, **56**
　treatment 59, 61–62
levobupivacaine **153**
levonorgestrel 325, 327, 328, 329
lice *380*, 380–381
lichenification 361
lifestyles, healthy 62
Li–Fraumeni syndrome 53, **54**
ligaments 21
limbic system 137
limps, childhood 345–353, **346**
lipid bilayer 4, *5*
lipopolysaccharides (LPS) 117
live vaccines 64
locus, gene 32–33
lower urinary tract *280*
lower urinary tract disorders 280, 297–304
　medical 297–300
　surgical 300–304
Lund and Browder chart 374, *376*
lymphatic system 85, 97
lymph nodes 85
lymphocytes 86, **86**, 97–98

Index

lymphoma 54, 55, 59, 61–62
lysosomes *4*, 11–12
lysozyme 88

macrophages 76, 77, **86**, 88, 90
  inflammation 91, 92
  wound healing 371, 372
macule 361
MAG3 scan 283
magnetic resonance imaging (MRI) 239, 351
major histocompatibility complex (MHC) 107
malabsorption syndromes 268–269
male reproductive system *300*, 312–313, *313*
  development *314*
  disorders **313**, 313–318
mast cells **86**, 91, 101
maturity-onset diabetes of young (MODY) 248
McBurney's point 264, *264*
Medicines and Healthcare products Regulatory Agency (MHRA) 204
medulloblastoma 56, 64, 171
meiosis 9–10, 41–43
melatonin **236**, 241
memory B cells **86**, 98
memory T cells **98**
menarche 318
Mendelian genetics 43–44
meninges *168*, 173
meningitis 173–174, **174**
meningocele 170
meningococcal disease **174**, 174–175
meningoencephalitis 175
menstrual problems 318–320
mental status, assessment 217
metabolic acidosis 77, 78
metabolic disorders 162
metabolic rate, increased 77, 379
metaphase 40, *40*
metaphysis *347*
microfilaments 14
micro-organisms 87–88
microtubules 14
micturating cystourethrogram (MCUG) 283
midstream urine sample 316
mineralocorticoids 59, **236**
missense mutations 36

mitochondria *4*, 12–13
mitosis 9, 15, 38–41, *40*
mitotic spindle 40, *40*
monoclonal antibody (mAb) drugs 61–62
monocytes 88, 90
morphine **151**, 152
motor dysfunction 169–170
MRI *see* magnetic resonance imaging
mRNA (messenger RNA) 29, 34–35
mucosal surfaces 88
mucous membranes 17
mucus 88
multicystic dysplastic kidneys (MCDK) **281**
muscle tissue 15, 23–24
musculoskeletal disorders 335–357
mutations 36–38
  causing cancer 53
  spontaneous 47
  types 36–37
Mycobacterium tuberculosis 91, 224–225
myelinated nerve fibres 138–139, *139*
myelomeningocele 170
myocardial contractility 182, 379
myocardial ischaemia 129, 183, 204
myosin 14
myxoedema 242

nasal flaring 216
nasal secretions, clearing 217–218
National Cancer Research Institute (NCRI) 57
National Institute for Health and Care Excellence (NICE) 95–96, 97
National Patient Safety Alerts (NPSA) 59
natural killer (NK) cells 85, **86**
nausea 261
Neisseria meningitidis 173, 174
neonates
  cardiac failure **182**
  ductus arteriosus-dependent 193
  pain 143, **146**
  skin care **369**, 373

nephrectomy 294, 295–296
nephroblastoma *see* Wilms' tumour
nephron *285*
nephrotic syndrome 284
nerve impulse transmission 161
nervous system 135, 160–161
  development 161–162
  structure **160**, 160–161, *161*
  see also neurological disorders
nervous tissue 15, 24–25
nesidioblastosis 249
neural tube defects 170
neuraxial analgesia 152–153
neuroblastoma 172
neurofibromatosis type 1 (NF1) **54**, 172–173
neurogenic shock 119–121
neuroglia 25
neurological disorders 161–177
  causes 161–162
  endocrine disorders 240
neurological tumours 171–173
neurones (nerve cells) 24–25, *25*, 160
neuropathic pain 141
neurotransmitters 161
neutropenia 63, 89
neutrophils 76, **86**, 88–89, 91, 371
nociceptive pain *136*, 136–139
nociceptors 137
nocturnal enuresis 298–299
nodule 361
non-accidental injury *see* child abuse
nonsense mutations 36
non-steroidal anti-inflammatory drugs (NSAIDs) 286, 316, 340, 353
Noonan syndrome **182**
norepinephrine (noradrenaline) 95, 161, **236**
nucleosomes 30, *31*
nucleus, cell *4*, 9, *28*
nurse controlled analgesia (NCA) 152
nutrition 366

obesity 247
oedema
  burn injuries 377
  cardiac failure 183

390

Index

inflammatory response 91
renal disorders 74, 284
oesophageal atresia *269*, 269–270
oestrogen **236**
oncogenes 53
opioid analgesics (opiates) 150–152, **151**
  epidermolysis bullosa 365, 366
  patient-controlled analgesia (PCA) 152, **153**
  routes of administration 151–152
opioid receptors 150
opioids, endogenous 137
oral secretions, clearing 217–218
Oramorph® **151**
orchiectomy 317
orchiopexy 317
organelles, cellular 8–14
orthopnoea 183
Ortolani test 356, *356*
osmolality, plasma **70**, 71
osmoreceptors 237–238
osmosis 7
osmotic pressure 7
osteogenesis imperfecta 339
osteonecrosis 59
ovaries **236**
overactive bladder 298
ovum (egg) 2, 10, 41
oxidative burst 90
oxygen delivery (DO$_2$) 128, *129*
oxygen saturation (SaO2)
  cardiac failure 184
  effects of clubbing 196
  haemorrhagic shock 123
  within the heart *186*
  respiratory disorders 74, 216
oxygen therapy
  bronchiolitis 218–219
  cardiac failure 184
  chronic respiratory disease 72–74
  respiratory distress 217
  shock 123, 130

p53 gene 53
packed cell volume (PCV) **70**, 71
paediatric early warning system *see* PEWS
Paediatric Glasgow Coma Scale (PGCS) **166**

pain 133–155
  acute 141–142, 148
  anatomy and physiology 135–142
  ascending pathways 137–139, *138*
  chronic 141–142, 148
  definition 134
  descending pathways 139–140, *140*
  effects of unrelieved 147
  effects on vital signs 141
  factors affecting 134–135, **135**, 143
  gate control theory 139–140, *140*
  modulation 137
  myths 141
  neuropathic 141
  nociceptive *136*, 136–139
  perception 137
  procedural 148, 154
  recurrent 142
  transduction 137
  transmission 137
  wound healing 372
pain assessment 142–147
  behavioural cues 146, **146**
  cognitive development and 143–144
  context of pain experience 142
  gender and cultural aspects 144–145
  methods 145–147, **146**
  myths 147
  parents and family 147
  QUESTT approach 145
  self-report 145
pain management 147–154
  epidermolysis bullosa 365, 366
  methods 149
  multimodal approach 150
  myth 149
  non-pharmacological 154
  pharmacological 149, 150–154
  WHO analgesic ladder 149
palate, development 270, *272*
pamidronate 59
Panadol® **150**
pancreas
  disorders 247–248
  endocrine **236**

pancytopenia 58, 63
panda eyes **165**
papule 361
parasympathetic nervous system *161*
parathyroid disorders 244–245
parathyroid gland **236**
parathyroid hormone (PTH) **236**, 244
passive immunity 99, *100*
passive transport 6–7
patellar fractures **341**
patent ductus arteriosus (PDA) **190**, *190*, 190–191
patent foramen ovale 188
pathogens 87
patient-controlled analgesia (PCA) 152, **153**
Pavlik harness 354, *354*, 356
pCO$_2$ 73
peak flow readings 229
pediculosis 380–381
pelvic fractures **341**
pelvic osteotomy 352
penicillin 206
Perfalgan® **150**
perfusion pressure 129
peripheral blocks 153
peripheral blood stem cells (PBSC) 61
peripheral nervous system (PNS) 135, 160, **160**, *161*
peristalsis 24, *24*
peritoneal dialysis 288, *289*
peroxisomes 4, 12
Perthes disease 348–353
  care and treatment 351–353
  diagnosis *350*, 350–351, *351*
  investigations 351
  stages 349, 349–350
pertussis 223
petechiae 361
PEWS (paediatric early warning system) 79, 130
  appendicitis 275–276, 277
  femoral shaft fracture 337, *338*
  haemolytic uraemic syndrome 305, *306–307*
  hypoplastic left heart syndrome *200–201*
  severe sunburn 47, *48*
pH, blood 72, *73*
phagocytosis 5, 88–90, *89*, 91
phenotype 33, 43

Index

phenoxymethylpenicillin 206
phenylketonuria 162
phimosis 301
phospholipids 4, *5*
pia mater *168*
pilonidal abscess 94
pineal gland **236**, 241
pinocytosis 5
pituitary adenoma 239, 240
pituitary disorders 237–240, 251–252
pituitary gland **236**
pituitary tumours 239–240
plaque 361
plasma cells 86, 98
plasma membrane *see* cell membrane
plasma membrane proteins (PMPs) 4, *5*
play, as coping strategy 147
pleural effusions 74
pneumonia 220–222
   bacterial 221
   interstitial 220
   lobar 220
   viral 221
pO_2 73
polyarteritis nodosa 285
porins 13
positioning, infant 262
posterior urethral valves **281**, 303–304, *305*
post-operative vital signs **274**
post-streptococcal glomerulonephritis (PSGN) 285, 286
Potter syndrome **281**
precocious puberty 250
prednisone 59
pregnancy
   female genital mutilation and 331
   teenage 324, *324*
pregnancy test 328
preload 127–128, 181
premature infants **190, 369**
pre-school children
   cardiac failure **182**, 183
   limps **346**
   pain 143–144, **146**, 154
   skin care **369**
primary treatment centres (PTCs) 57, 62–63
procedural pain 148, 154
processus vaginalis 272, *273*

prokaryotes 9
prolactinoma 239, 240
prophase 39–40, *40*, 42
proptosis 243
prostaglandins 77, 95, 193, 197, 372
protein synthesis 33–35, *35*
proteinuria 283, **284**
protozoa 87
pseudopodia 14
pseudosyndactyly 363
psychological care
   cryptorchidism 315
   genetic disorders 37–38
   inflammatory bowel disease 266
   suspected sexual abuse 323
   testicular torsion 318
psychological/emotional effects
   endocrine disorders 250
   female genital mutilation 331
   pain 143–144, 147
puberty
   delayed 251
   precocious 250, 251
pulmonary oedema 127
pulmonary stenosis *191*, 191–192
pulse pressure 118, 123
pus 76, 92, 94
pustule 361
pyeloplasty 295
pyloric stenosis *266*, 266–267, 277
pyogenic bacteria 88, 90, 91, 92
pyrexia (fever) 77, 95–96
pyrogens, endogenous 95

QUESTT approach, pain assessment 145

raccoon eyes **165**
radiation, ionising (IR) 54, 60
radiation therapy 60, 64, 294
radioimmunoassay 238–239
rape, statutory 327
rashes 96, 174
receptor-mediated endocytosis 5
recessive genes 33, 44
red blood cells 9
   antigens 106
   solute concentration effects 7, *8*
reflex arc 139

regional analgesia 152–153, **153**
regulatory T cells **98**
renal agenesis **281**
renal ectopia **281**
renal impairment 74
renal pelvic dilatation (RPD) 281
Renal Registry, UK 287
renal system 280, *280*
   assessment 282–283, **283**
   congenital anomalies 74, 281, **281**, 287
renal system disorders 279–308
   antenatal screening 74, 281, **281**
   burn injury 379
   case studies 305–308
   herbs and supplements causing 282
   lower urinary tract 297–304
   upper urinary tract 283–297
renal transplantation 289, *290*
renin-angiotensin-aldosterone system 69, *69*, 74
reproduction, cell 9–10, 38–41
reproductive health/ill health 311–333
respiration, internal 12
respiratory acidosis 72
respiratory arrest 227
respiratory assessment 215–216
respiratory centre 72
respiratory disorders 213–230
   burn injury 379
   case studies 80, 217–218, 226
   clearance of secretions 217–218
   endocrine disorders 240–241
   infection control precautions 218
   investigations 226–227, 229
   pathophysiology 72–74
   upper airway 219–220
respiratory distress 215–217, 225
respiratory distress syndrome, neonatal **190**
respiratory infections 218–219, 220–225
respiratory noises 216
respiratory rate 215, **274**
respiratory syncytial virus 218

Index

restrictive cardiomyopathy 207–208
reticular connective tissue 22
reticular fibres 20
retinoblastoma, familial 53, **54**
rhesus (Rh) incompatibility 106
rheumatic fever **205**, 205–206
rhinitis, allergic 101, *101*, **102**, 103
rib fractures **341**
ribonucleic acid *see* RNA
ribosomes 10, *11*
right ventricular failure 125, **125**
RNA 10, 29
   DNA transcription to 33–35
   types 34
rough endoplasmic reticulum 10, *11*
rRNA (ribosomal RNA) 34, 35
rule of 9s 374

salbutamol 228
saltatory conduction 161
Sandifer syndrome 262
SBAR (Situation, Background, Assessment, Recommendations) 79
scalds 373
scales 361
school-age children
   cardiac failure **182**, 183
   limps **346**
   pain 144, **146**, 154
   skin care **369**
secretions, nasal and oral 217–218
seizure disorders 175–177
seizures 175–176
self–non-self differentiation 84, 97
sensory nerve fibres **138**, 138–139
sepsis 96–97, 117–119, **119**, 380
septic shock 96–97, 117–119, **119**
   compensated 117–118
   decompensated 117, 119
   life-threatening complications *120*
serotonin 91
Sevredol® **151**
sex chromosomes 31–32, *32*, 43

sex hormones **236**
sexual abuse 312, 322, 323
sexual activity 324
sexual exploitation 326
sexual health 324–329
sexual history 325, 327–328
sexually transmitted infections 324
sexual partner, age of 327
shelf acetabuloplasty 352
shock 115–131
   ABCDE approach 130
   anaphylactic 121
   cardiogenic **117**, 123–125
   classification **117**
   cold 117, 118, 119, *120*
   compensated 117–118, *120*, 123, 125
   decompensated 117, 119, 125
   definition 116
   dehydration 69
   distributive 116–121, **117**
   haemorrhagic 122–123
   hypovolaemic **117**, 121–123
   monitoring end-organ perfusion 129–130
   neurogenic 119–121
   obstructive **117**
   pathophysiology 127–129
   refractory 117
   septic *see* septic shock
   signs and symptoms 70, **70**
   spinal 169
   strategies for managing 129
   warm 117, *120*
short stature 237
sickle cell anaemia 36
simple epithelium *16*, 16–17, *17*
sinus bradycardia 208
sinus tachycardia 208
Situation, Background, Assessment, Recommendations (SBAR) 79
skeletal muscle 23, 24
skeleton 336
skin 18, 360
   barrier to infection 87–88
   biopsy 19
   colour 216
skin care
   age-related factors **369**
   epidermolysis bullosa 366

skin disorders 359–381, **361**
   endocrine disorders 240
   lesion types 361–362
   renal system disorders **283**, 295
skull fractures **165**, 165–166, **341**
sleep problems 241
slipped capital femoral epiphysis (SCFE) 345–348, *346*
   care and management 348
   classification 347, **348**
   pathophysiology 347, *347*
slough 92
smooth endoplasmic reticulum 10, *11*
smooth muscle 23, 24
sodium, plasma **70**, 70–71, 122
sodium cromoglycate 103
sodium retention 74
somatosensory cortex 137, *138*
sperm (spermatozoa) 2, 10, 41
spina bifida 162, 170
spinal cord 137–138, 168
   injury (SCI) 119–121, 168–169
   tumours 171
spinal shock 169
spinal trauma 168–169, **341**
spiral fractures 339, *339*
spironolactone **184**
splinting 345, 354–355
spontaneous mutation 47
squamous epithelium 16, 18
Staphylococcus aureus 91, 92
status epilepticus 176
stratified epithelium 16, *16*, 17–18
strawberry tongue 203
streptococcal throat infection 205–206, 285, 286
Streptococcus pneumoniae 92, 173, 220
Streptococcus pyogenes 91, 92
stridor 121, 216, 219
stroke volume 128, *128*
subarachnoid haemorrhage 167
subarachnoid space *168*
subcutaneous nodules **205**
subdural haemorrhage 167
subluxation, hip **353**, 355

Index

sunburn, severe 47, *48*
support, emotional *see* psychological care
supraventricular tachycardia (SVT) 210
surgery 61, 71
Sydenham chorea **205**
sympathetic nervous system 95, 118, *161*
tumours 171–173
synacthen test 59
synapses 25
systemic inflammatory response syndrome (SIRS) 117, **119**
systemic lupus erythematosus (SLE) 285
systemic vascular resistance (SVR) 117

tachycardia
  extreme or prolonged 128–129
  haemorrhagic shock 122, 123
  septic shock 118, 119
tachypnoea 183
targeted cancer therapies 61–62
Tay–Sachs disease 37
teenage pregnancy 324, **324**
telangiectasia 361
telophase *40*, 41, *42*
temperature, body
  increased 77, 95
  post-operative changes **274**
  recording 95–96
tendons 21
testes **236**
  ascending 314
  ectopic 314
  undescended 314–315
testicular torsion 315, 316–318
testosterone **236**
tetralogy of Fallot (TOF) *195*, 195–196
thalamus 137, 138, *138*
thermoregulation 379
third-spacing 121–122
thirst 69, 238
13q syndrome **54**
thymine (T) *29*, 30, 35
thymosin **236**
thymus gland 97, **236**, 245

thyroid disorders 241–244
thyroid gland **236**
thyroid-stimulating hormone (TSH) 241, 242, 243
thyrotoxicosis 242–244
thyroxine (T4) 12, **236**, 242, 243–244
tibial fractures **341**
tissues 2, 15–25
  repair 25
  types 15–25
T lymphocytes 86, **86**
  functions 97, **98**
  transplant rejection 107
  wound healing 371
topical medications 367
torus fractures 339
total body irradiation (TBI) 64
total body surface area (TBSA) 374
tracheal tug 216
tracheooesophageal fistula (TOF) *269*, 269–270
traction 342–343, **343**, *343*
tramadol **151**
transcription 33–35, *34*
transfusion reactions 106
transitional epithelium 18
translation 33
transplantation 61, 106–107, 289, *290*
transposition of great arteries (TGA) 197–198, *198*
transverse fractures 339, *339*
traumatic brain injury (TBI) *167*, 167–168
Trendelenburg gait 351, *351*
tricuspid atresia 196–197, *197*
tripoding 227
tRNA (transfer RNA) 34, 35
tuberculosis (TB) 91, 224–225
tubulin 14
tumour necrosis factor (TNF) 95, 379
tumour suppressor genes 53
Turner syndrome 162, **182**
22q11.2 deletion syndrome 37

ulcer 361
ulcerative colitis **265**, 265–266
ulipristal acetate 327, 328, 329
ultrasound 239, 282, 317

umbilical hernia 271
unlicensed medicines 204
unmyelinated nerve fibres *139*
upper airway disorders 219–220
upper urinary tract *280*
upper urinary tract disorders 280, 283–297
  medical 283–295
  surgical 295–297
uracil (U) 34–35
urea, plasma **70**
ureteropelvic junction obstruction 295, *296*
ureterostomy, temporary cutaneous 302
ureterovesical junction obstruction 302, *302*
urge incontinence 298
urinalysis **283**, 285, 316
urinary catheters 291
urinary retention 297
urinary tract *see* renal system
urinary tract infections (UTI) 297–298
  signs and symptoms **297**
  surgical urinary tract disorders 296, 303
urine output 119, **283**
urine samples
  collection 297, 298, 315–316
  midstream 316
urticaria **102**

vaccination 64, 99, 224
vaginal discharge 321–324
vaginal examination 322
vaginal infections 322, 323
Valsalva manoeuvre 210
vanillylmandelic acid (VMA) 172
vasopressin (anti-diuretic hormone; ADH) 122, 237–238
veins 180
ventricular septal defect (VSD) *189*, 189–190
vesicle 361
vesicostomy 303–304

vesicoureteric reflux (VUR) 283, 295, 303, *304*
vincristine 58
viral meningitis 173
viruses 54, 87
Voltarol® **150**
vomiting 260–261
   case studies 80, 277
   causes **261**
   dehydration 68–69, 71
vulvovaginitis 322

water retention 74
Wegener vasculitis 285
weight measurement 70

wheal 361
wheeze 121, 216, 228
white blood cells 85–86, **86**
WHO 3-step management of pain 149
whooping cough 223
Wilms' tumour 293–294, **294**
Wolff-Parkinson-White (WPW) syndrome 209–210
wound healing 370–373
   complications 373
   inflammation 91–92, 371–372
   primary (first intention) 92, 370, *370*
   secondary intention 92, 370–371, *371*
   stages *93*, 370, 371–372
wounds 94, 368–373
wrist fractures **341**

X chromosome 31–32, *32*, 43
X-linked recessive disorders *46*, 46–47
X-rays 351

Y chromosome 31–32, *32*, 43

Zika virus 162
Zydol® **151**